T0304691

# CHILDREN'S PALLIATIVE NURSING CARE

Nursing is an essential component of children's palliative care and palliative care is an essential aspect of nursing. Yet the complex inter-disciplinary nature of palliative care brings into sharp focus the work nurses undertake with others in delivering palliative care. This is, however, a book by nurses for nurses.

This comprehensive text presents the essential knowledge and skills required by nurses providing this invaluable care to a growing number of children. The chapters are mapped to the Children's Palliative Care Education and Training standards. These are endorsed by the International Children's Palliative Care Network, a major partner with the World Health Organization in the push to make children's palliative care a universal health right. In its three Parts, *Children's Palliative Nursing Care* covers public and universal care, core nursing and specialist care. The chapters can be read individually or cumulatively to move from engagement in public health and public understanding of palliative care through to delivering nursing care. Topics range from managing symptoms and end-of-life care, to education, research and issues of quality and leadership.

Uniquely each chapter has been written by a team of authors who come from both high-income and low-/middle-income countries. This makes this not just a book by nurses for nurses but a global book for global nursing practice.

**Duncan Randall** has over 20 years' experience in delivering, researching and teaching children's palliative nursing. He has worked on projects such as the Spectrum of Children's Palliative Care, the Involve to Evolve database project, founding the first data group on children's palliative care in the UK. He has also worked extensively with the Children's Palliative Care Education and Training Action Group (CPCET) on the Standards for Education and the Standards for Advanced Care Planning. Duncan has an extensive publication history, including his theoretical work using Pragmatics to set out a theory of children's nursing for children and their childhoods.

**Susan Neilson** has over 30 years' experience in children's palliative nursing care, research and teaching. She is a qualitative methodologist and supervises research students. Sue teaches across undergraduate and post-graduate programmes and also leads interprofessional palliative care workshops. She is Chair of the Royal College of Nursing Children's Palliative Care Community. Her work focuses on education, recently coordinating the Children's Palliative Care Education and Training Action Group and Young Person's Advance Care Plan Collaborative's work on the Education Standard Framework and Standard Framework for Advanced Care Planning.

**Julia Downing** has over 30 years' experience in palliative care, with more than 20 of those working in children's palliative care and internationally in Uganda, Africa, Eastern Europe and globally. She is an experienced palliative care nurse, advocate, educationalist and researcher. She is the Chief Executive of the International Children's Palliative Care Network (ICPCN) and has various visiting and honorary contracts at universities in Uganda, Serbia and the UK. She was part of the Children's Palliative Care Education and Training Action Group (CPCET), supporting the development of the Standards for Education and the Standards for Advanced Care Planning, as well as the Global Paediatric Standards. She has extensive experience in global palliative care, research and education, and is on the editorial boards of *eCancer*, *APM* and the *IJPN*. She serves on the boards of several international organisations, is regularly invited to speak at conferences and has an extensive publication history on global palliative care and nursing.

# Children's Palliative Nursing Care

Edited by
Duncan Randall, Susan Neilson
and Julia Downing

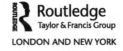

Routledge
Taylor & Francis Group

LONDON AND NEW YORK

Designed cover image: "Self so" by Lynne Davidson, 2024

First published 2025
by Routledge
4 Park Square, Milton Park, Abingdon, Oxon OX14 4RN

and by Routledge
605 Third Avenue, New York, NY 10158

*Routledge is an imprint of the Taylor & Francis Group, an informa business*

© 2025 selection and editorial matter, Duncan Randall, Susan Neilson and Julia Downing; individual chapters, the contributors

*British Library Cataloguing-in-Publication Data*
A catalogue record for this book is available from the British Library

ISBN: 978-1-032-47164-8 (hbk)
ISBN: 978-1-032-47071-9 (pbk)
ISBN: 978-1-003-38486-1 (ebk)

DOI: 10.4324/9781003384861

Typeset in Sabon LT Pro
by KnowledgeWorks Global Ltd.

# Contents

# Contributors

## EDITORS

**Professor Julia Downing** has over 30 years' experience in palliative care, with more than 20 of those working in children's palliative care and internationally in Uganda, Africa, Eastern Europe and globally. She is an experienced palliative care nurse, advocate, educationalist and researcher. She is the Chief Executive of the International Children's Palliative Care Network (ICPCN) and has various visiting and honorary contracts at universities in Uganda, Serbia and the UK. She was part of the Children's Palliative Care Education and Training Action Group (CPCET), supporting the development of the Standards for Education and the Standards for Advanced Care Planning, as well as the Global Paediatric Standards. She has extensive experience in global palliative care, research and education, and is on the editorial boards of *eCancer*, *APM* and the *IJPN*. She serves on the boards of several international organisations, is regularly invited to speak at conferences and has an extensive publication history on global palliative care and nursing.

**Dr Susan Neilson** has over 30 years' experience in children's palliative nursing care, research and teaching. She is a qualitative methodologist and supervises research students. Sue teaches across undergraduate and post-graduate programmes and also leads interprofessional palliative care workshops. She is Chair of the Royal College of Nursing Children's Palliative Care Community. Her work focuses on education, recently coordinating the Children's Palliative Care Education and Training Action Group and Young Person's Advance Care Plan Collaborative's work on the Education Standard Framework and Standard Framework for Advanced Care Planning.

**Dr Duncan Randall** has over 20 years' experience in delivering, researching and teaching children's palliative nursing. He has worked on projects such as the Spectrum of Children's Palliative Care, the Involve to Evolve database project, founding the first data group on children's palliative care in the UK. He has also worked extensively with the Children's Palliative Care Education and Training Action Group (CPCET) on the Standards for Education and the Standards for Advanced Care Planning. Duncan has an extensive publication history including his theoretical work using Pragmatics to set out a theory of children's nursing for children and their childhoods.

## CONTRIBUTORS

**Dr Maha Atout,** the Philadelphia University of Jordan. She is an Associate Professor at the Philadelphia University of Jordan. Maha completed her PhD at the University of Nottingham in 2017. Her PhD work focused on investigating communication in the care of children with palliative care needs from different perspectives. Maha has over 16 years' experience in delivering, researching and teaching paediatric palliative care nursing. She has worked on projects such as the Guideline Development Group Meeting: Chronic Pain in Children (WHO). Maha has an extensive publication history including, "A narrative inquiry into the communication experiences of mothers caring for children with cancer in Jordan".

**Bernadette Basemera,** Makerere/Mulago Palliative Care Unit (MPCU), Palliative Care Education and Research Consortium (PcERC), Uganda. Bernadette trained in general palliative care for both children and adults. She is trained in end-of-life care (EPEC) and has over 27 years' experience in both clinical palliative care and education. Bernadette has strong skills in patient care, counselling, training and mentorship of healthcare professionals. She has worked with various palliative care institutions in Uganda and other African countries in different capacities including palliative care nurse, Senior Clinical Trainer and programme officer. Bernadette has a strong passion for the suffering patients and their families, especially children. She continues to support and advocate for the need for palliative care integration in Uganda and other African countries.

**Dr Karen Carr,** Ulster University Belfast, Northern Ireland. Karen has nursed children in acute care and community settings, in rural and urban areas for over 30 years. Children's palliative care has been Karen's speciality for more than 20 years with responsibilities which include care of the ill child and family alongside specialist education of many health professionals. Initiation of advance care planning conversations for children was the focus of Karen's PhD which has resulted in a number of publications. In her current lecturing role Karen has responsibility for community children's specialist nursing education which includes a focus on palliative care. Karen is a member of the Palliative Care Research Society and has an avid interest in furthering education and research in children's palliative care.

**Professor Hicran Çavuşoğlu,** Hacettepe University, Türkiye. Hicran has been working in the field of children's nursing for 42 years. She has worked in the clinical field with children who have long-term and terminal diseases in Turkey. She has over 40 years of graduate and undergraduate teaching experience in children's nursing. Her publications include pain management and critical care in children with cancer and ethical issues in the terminal period in the field of palliative care. She has been the president of the Ankara Office of the Paediatric Nurses Association for more than 15 years and has chaired three international paediatric nursing congresses and many national symposiums. She is also a member of the editorial board of JPN.

**Professor Jane Coad,** Nottingham University/University Hospitals Coventry and Warwickshire, UK. Jane has over 35 years in nursing, drawing on her arts background and as a Registered Children's Nurse. Jane uses co-creation participatory and complex mixed methods in national and international research to transform care inequalities, services and outcomes. She specifically focuses her cross-disciplinary programme on babies, children and young people with complex and life-limiting conditions. In terms of professional recognition, Jane was awarded a Royal College of Nursing Fellowship in 2013 for lifetime research and leads a number of local, national and international groups/committees holding substantive posts.

**Dr Lucy Coombes,** Royal Marsden Hospital, UK. Lucy Coombes is the Lead Nurse for the paediatric palliative and symptom care team at the Royal Marsden Hospital, UK, and has extensive clinical experience in the field. Her PhD research developed the UK Children's Palliative Outcome Scale (C-POS) and provided evidence of its face and content validity, as well as feasibility and acceptability of use. Lucy has experience of conducting qualitative research with children and young people with life-limiting conditions and their families. She was also a member of the Guideline Development Group for the first End of Life Care for Children NICE guidance. She has been a registered children's nurse for 24 years, working in paediatric palliative care for the past 16 years.

**Doris Corkin,** Queen's University Belfast, Northern Ireland. In her 40 years of nursing, Doris has delivered palliative and end-of-life care within hospital and community settings, facilitates learning opportunities using high-fidelity simulation within pre-registration and post-graduate nursing, with specific interests in the palliation needs of children and young people. She also welcomes parent perspective and public involvement (PPI) across approved curricula. Doris was invited to contribute to the Children's Palliative Care Education and Training Action Group (CPCET), agreeing core principles of practice and standardising children's palliative care. Doris has a diverse publication portfolio in healthcare education, and co-edited well-thumbed text-books.

**Alexandra Daniels,** International Children's Palliative Care Network, South Africa. Alex is an experienced children's palliative care nurse and educationalist, working with the International Children's Palliative Care Network, South Africa, since 2017. She has a Masters in Paediatric Palliative Care from the University of Cape Town.

Alex has been working in the field since 2007, initially facilitating bereavement training workshops, and then as a clinician and trainer in paediatric palliative care. Her work includes managing the ICPCN's e-learning programme, teaching on face-to-face courses, webinars and workshops on paediatric palliative care. Alex has experience in developing new courses and is involved in education internationally.

**Becky Davis**, Gloucestershire Health and Care NHS Foundation Trust, UK. Becky has over 22 years' experience in delivering palliative and end-of-life care to children at home as a community children's nurse (CCN), and children's outreach palliative care clinical nurse specialist. She is currently team leader for a CCN team, and part of the Southwest Regional Palliative Care Group, focused on developing children's palliative care services for the region. Becky contributed to the recent Southwest Neonatal Network guidelines for taking a baby home/to a hospice after death, and is currently helping to develop teaching packages for the South of England Paediatric Palliative Care Education Programme.

**Maraliza de Haan** is a South African-trained social worker and qualified as a nurse in the Netherlands. She has been involved with palliative care within the hospice movement in South Africa since 1999. Maraliza qualified and specialised in paediatric palliative care, loss/grief, trauma and play therapy. She was director of an organisation caring for abused and HIV/AIDS-infected/affected children in South Africa. Maraliza coordinated national paediatric palliative care programmes in South Africa, working for the hospice palliative care association in South Africa and was an international trainer in paediatric palliative care for the International Children's Palliative Care Network. Currently living in the Netherlands, she is the coordinator/teacher of five e-learning courses connected to the Dutch Centre of Expertise in Children's Palliative Care and the International Children's Palliative Care Network.

**Peter Ellis**, former Chief Executive, Richard House Children's Hospice, London, UK. Peter established Richard House as the first children's hospice in London. His experience taught him an enormous amount about children's palliative care, building on his former work as a nurse, and operations manager for cancer services. Peter also helped develop a UK plan proposing how the public health approach in children's palliative care should be organised. He was an advisor to the Belarussian Children's Hospice service. He also visited the Kerala Hospice service in India to gain an understanding of the public health approach. Since retirement, Peter has had a massive stroke leaving him severely disabled. However, he has the ability to write and speak about his own near-death experience and the consequences of his disability.

**Sara Fleming**, Flinders University/Palliative Care Australia, Australia, Sara is a nurse practitioner with 25 years of experience working in paediatric palliative care and a senior lecturer at Flinders University and topic coordinator of the postgraduate palliative care topic, Australia. She is currently working with Palliative Care Australia on Paediatric Projects and brings her clinical experience, love of teaching, and passion for the sector to the body of this work.

**Professor Marie Friedel,** University of Luxembourg, Luxembourg. Marie worked for several years as a paediatric palliative care nurse in Belgium. She is the founder of the unique interdisciplinary continuous education training in paediatric palliative care which has been offered at the Haute Ecole Léonard de Vinci in Brussels since 2014. Her PhD in public health at UC Louvain, Belgium, in 2020 explored children's and parents' quality of life in a paediatric palliative care context, while developing children's patient-reported outcomes measures. She was appointed in 2022 full professor in nursing sciences at the University of Luxembourg, where she implements with her team new bachelor's in nursing sciences degrees. Besides that, she is also actively involved in starting paediatric palliative care services, education and research in Luxembourg with ministries and healthcare professionals.

**Tara Kerr-Elliott,** Great Ormond Street Hospital, UK. Tara is a registered children's nurse with over 20 years' experience of working clinically in palliative care. She is also an educator, with a particular interest in communication and simulation-based education. Tara is currently completing a PhD, exploring the care of children who have died. She is a member of the Bioethics service at Great Ormond Street Hospital, UK, and an advisor to two UK-based children's palliative care charities.

**Jitka Kosikova,** Mobile Hospice, Czech Republic. Jitka is a lecturer in Paediatric Palliative Care, Communication and Management in Healthcare programs in the Mobile Hospice, in the Czech Republic. She works as a freelance mentor/coach/facilitator/mediator. Jitka has a nursing degree from Napier University, Edinburgh, and a degree in Management for Health and Social Services and Supervision from Charles University, Prague, in the Czech Republic. Jitka has international experience working for over 14 years for the humanitarian organisation, Doctors Without Borders in African, Asian and Middle Eastern countries. She has worked in the Czech Republic and abroad as a paediatric intensive care nurse, then in 2017 focused her interests on palliative care where she specialises in communication, team building, change and agile management, systems building and paediatric palliative care at home.

**Katrina McNamara-Goodger,** Fellow of the Association of British Paediatric Nurses, UK. Katrina is a children's nurse who has worked across the National Health Service, in the UK Department of Health and most recently in the NGO children's palliative care sector. She continues as a trustee for Acorns Children's Hospices, UK. Katrina was awarded the Elisabeth Kübler-Ross Award for Outstanding Contribution to the field of Children's Palliative Care from Children's Hospice International, following the development of the care pathway approach in children's palliative care. She led the development, launch and implementation of the Diana, Princess of Wales community children's nursing teams across England. She has also been linked to international activity to develop children's palliative care services in Belarus, Crimea, India and Norway.

**Florence Nalutaaya**, Makerere/Mulago Palliative Care Unit (MPCU), Palliative Care Education and Research Consortium (PcERC), Uganda. Florence has 37 years of professional engagement with patients, 14 years in curative settings and 23 years practising palliative care. She is the coordinator of Uganda Children Palliative Care Leadership Fellowship, advocacy officer, and a clinical mentor in Mulago Specialised Hospital. She majored in Palliative Care Medicine and has a Masters of Philosophy in Palliative Care from the University of Cape Town, a Bachelor's degree and a diploma in Palliative Care affiliated by Makerere University, a diploma in Palliative Care Clinical Practice and a diploma in Nursing. She is highly experienced in paediatrics palliative care and offers clinical services to children in five oncology wards in the Mulago National Specialised Referral Hospital in Uganda.

**Anna Oddy**, Northern Care Alliance Trust, UK. Anna has over 20 years of experience in delivering complex and palliative care to babies, children and young people and supporting their families. Anna is the co-chair of the Greater Manchester palliative care network and has worked on projects such as the Greater Manchester service mapping exercise and has developed advance care plan awareness teaching sessions across the North-West region. She has also worked with the Royal College of Nursing in updating the palliative care competency framework. Anna has previously contributed to the *Oxford Handbook of Children's and Young People's Nursing*.

**Dr Stacey Power Walsh**, University College Dublin, Ireland. Stacey is a Registered Intellectual Disability and Children's Nurse. Her clinical background is in nursing children and young adults with palliative and complex care needs, within the disability, acute, hospice and community setting. She has contributed to the development and delivery of the only Masters/Postgraduate Diploma in Health Sciences (Children's Palliative/Complex Care) in Ireland. Stacey is currently a member of the Board of Directors for the Irish Association of Palliative Care. Stacey's research influences policy and practice through her involvement on both the Advisory Group for the National Standards for Bereavement Care Following Pregnancy Loss and Perinatal Death and the Children's Palliative Care Strategic Advisory Group.

**Helen Queen**, Birmingham Women's and Children's Hospital, UK. Helen has 30 years' experience in palliative care, working as a Children's Macmillan Nurse while obtaining her first degree in palliative care. She has been a children's community nurse and an oncology outreach nurse, gaining her master's degree in clinical oncology., and is currently the lead nurse for palliative and bereavement care for Birmingham Women's and Children's Hospital. Helen has an honorary contract with the University of Birmingham teaching the paediatric palliative care Master's module and is a Nurse Representative for the APPM and Vice Co-Chair for the West Midlands Paediatric Palliative Care Network.

**Angela Rackstraw,** Paedspal, South Africa. Angela is a UK-trained Art Psychotherapist and a nurse currently working with Paedspal, South Africa. She also teaches and supervises Art Therapy trainees at the University of Johannesburg, and mainly works in a paediatric palliative care setting. She is a practising artist. Prior to training as an Art Therapist at the University of Hertfordshire, she had worked as a nursing sister for 13 years, three of these as a Paediatric Nursing Sister. Angela has worked with Paedspal, a paediatric palliative care non-profit organisation, for the past 8 years. In addition to working with her young patients, Angela supports nursing and other hospital staff members in these clinical settings, as well as the mothers/carers sitting alongside their children. She is passionate about play, and frequently teaches on the importance of play in clinical settings. Angela also offers support groups to mothers who are bereaved or experiencing anticipatory grief. At the moment she is exploring how needle and thread are often the material of choice for many of these women, and how stitching not only seems to mend, but also contains and soothes, especially during a time of bereavement.

**Dr Rima Saad Rassam,** St Jude Children's Research Hospital, USA. Rima is the Programme Co-ordinator at the St Jude Global Palliative Care Programme. Rima obtained her Master's and PhD degrees in Nursing Sciences from the American University of Beirut. She has more than 20 years' combined expertise in paediatric oncology nursing and palliative care practice, education, and research in Lebanon and the USA. She completed two research residencies at the University of Michigan and Harvard University in 2019. Her research focuses on parents' perspectives of paediatric palliative care, to uncover and implement potential improvement strategies in limited resource settings.

**Dr Maiara Rodrigues dos Santos,** University of São Paulo, Brazil. Maiara is an Assistant Professor in the School of Nursing, University of São Paulo, Brazil. She has been a leader and researcher in the Interdisciplinary Group for Research in Loss and Bereavement (NIPPEL). She has been a member of the family ethics subcommittee of the International Family Nursing Association and of the nursing committee of the National Academy of Palliative Care in Brazil. Maiara has experience in teaching paediatric palliative care. Her research focuses on the relationship between providers and families of children in the end-of-life care and family ethics.

**Zodwa Sithole,** the Cancer Association of South Africa. She is the Head of Advocacy for the Cancer Association of South Africa. Zodwa has worked in the health sector for a long time: general nursing, midwifery, community health and palliative care. She gained experience in private, government and community institutions. She is trained in Nursing, Midwifery, Primary Health Care, Nursing Administration and Education, Community Health Care and Palliative Care. She holds a B. Cur degree and a Master's degree in Nursing. She has participated in national and international conferences. She advocated for the integration of palliative care into the caring of inmates living with life-threatening illnesses in the South African prisons, palliative care with traditional healers and development of a palliative care curriculum for traditional healers. She is also a Board Member of the International Children's Palliative Care Network (ICPCN).

**Professor Regina Szylit,** University of São Paulo, Brazil. Regina was the Dean (2019–2023) and is a Professor at the School of Nursing, University of São Paulo USP, Brazil. She is a researcher at the USP Institute for Advanced Studies and a Fellow of the American Academy of Nursing. Founder and leader of the Interdisciplinary Group for Research in Loss and Bereavement (NIPPEL), she is also the founder of the International Palliative Care Nursing Network PAHO/WHO. She is also Vice-president of the International Work Group in Death, Dying and Bereavement (IWG). Regina has over 30 years' experience in teaching and researching children's palliative care, family nursing, family bereavement, and qualitative research methods.

**Anu Savio Thelly,** Mahatma Gandhi Medical College and Research Institute, India. Anu trained in Children's Palliative Care (CPC) and Education in Palliative and End-of-life Care (EPEC)-Paediatrics, and has over a decade of experience in paediatric palliative care. She founded two youth voluntary groups in South India to support children in palliative care and their families. In 2014, she received the "No Pain for Children, Young Researchers Award" in Rome. Anu has been instrumental in establishing paediatric palliative care services in Puducherry, organising training programmes, and contributing to the *Textbook of Pediatric Palliative Care*, published by Paras Medical Books. She has also integrated paediatric palliative care into Sri Balaji Vidyapeeth University's nursing curriculum.

**Alice Stella Verginia,** Indian Association of Palliative Care, India. Stella has worked as a clinical bedside nurse and faculty educator. She was commissioned as an army officer in 1986. Stella has contributed to several palliative care textbooks and the national programme of palliative care for the Government of India. She has delivered training programmes for doctors, nurses, volunteers, campus students, and for patients' informal caregivers. After retirement in 2020, she continues to deliver palliative care training. In 2020, she received an international award for excellence in leadership in palliative care from the Cancer Aid Society, for her work on the End of Life Nursing Education Consortium programmes, training nurses at the Ruhana University, Sri Lanka, and she is recognised as a national leader by ICPCN.

# Abbreviations

| | |
|---|---|
| ACP | Advance Care Planning |
| AIDS | acquired immunodeficiency system |
| ALCP | Asociación Latinoamericana de Cuidados Palliativos |
| APCA | African Palliative Care Association |
| APCA c-POS | African Palliative Care Association Children's Palliative Outcome Scale |
| APHN | Asia Pacific Hospice Palliative Care Network |
| APPG | All Party Parliamentary Group (UK) |
| APPM | Association for Paediatric Palliative Medicine |
| APRN | Advanced Practice Registered Nurse |
| BiPAP | bilevel positive airway pressure |
| BTF | breathing, thinking, functioning |
| CANSA | Cancer Association of South Africa |
| CEC | Clinical Ethics Committee |
| CNS | central nervous system |
| CoPPAR | Collaborative Paediatric Palliative Care Research Network |
| CPAP | continuous positive airway pressure |
| CPC | children's palliative care |
| CPCET | Children's Palliative Care Education and Training Action Group |
| C-POS | Children's Palliative Outcome Scale |
| CYP | child and/or young person |
| EAPC | European Association for Palliative Care |
| ECHO | Extension for Community Healthcare Outcomes |
| ELC | end-of-life care |
| EMRO | Eastern Mediterranean Region |
| FLACC | faces, legs, activity, cry and consolability |
| FMS | foetal medicine specialist |

| | |
|---|---|
| FNF | Florence Nightingale Foundation |
| GHAP | Global Health and Palliative Care |
| GI | gastrointestinal |
| GICC | Global Initiative for Childhood Cancer |
| GO-PPaCS | Global Overview – Paediatric Palliative Care Standards |
| GORD | gastro-oesophageal reflux disease |
| GPNN | Global Palliative Nursing Network |
| HFNC | high flow nasal cannula |
| HIE | hypoxic ischaemic encephalopathy |
| HIV | human immunodeficiency virus |
| IAHPC | International Association for Hospice and Palliative Care |
| ICN | International Council of Nurses |
| ICP | intracranial pressure |
| ICPCN | International Children's Palliative Care Network |
| IGAD | interview, gather, assess/achieve, decide/disclosure/discuss |
| IOM | Institute of Medicine |
| i-PARiHS | integrated-Promoting Action on Research Implementation in the Health Services |
| KEHPCA | Kenyan Hospice and Palliative Care Association |
| LMICs | low- and middle-income countries |
| LPI | Leadership Practices Inventory |
| MCCD | Medical Certificate of Cause of Death |
| NC | non-communicable disease |
| NEO-SPEAK | neonatal uncertainty, encounter, organisation, situational stress, processuality, emotional burden, attention to individuality, knowledge |
| NGO | non-governmental organisation |
| NGT | nasogastric |
| NHS | National Health Service (UK) |
| NMC | Nursing and Midwifery Council (UK) |
| NSAIDS | non-steroidal anti-inflammatory drugs |
| OPD | outpatient department |
| PallCHASE | Palliative Care in Humanitarian Aid Situations and Emergencies |
| PaPas | Paediatric Palliative Screening |
| PEG | percutaneous endoscopic gastrostomy |
| PEJ | percutaneous jejunostomy |
| PICU | paediatric intensive care units |
| PPC | paediatric palliative care |
| PPE | personal protective equipment |
| PROMs | patient-reported outcomes |
| RCN | Royal College of Nursing (UK) |
| SCORM | Sharable Content Object Reference Model |
| SHS | serious health-related suffering |

| | |
|---|---|
| SOGBPIE | situation, opinions/options, basics, parent's stories, information, emotions |
| SPIKES | setting, perceptions, invitation, knowledge, emotions, strategy and summary |
| S-P-w-ICE-s | setting, perception, what, communication, emotions, strategy and summary |
| TCA | tricyclic antidepressant |
| TPN | total parenteral nutrition |
| VUCA | volatile, uncertain, complex and ambiguous |
| WHO | World Health Organization |
| WHPCA | Worldwide Hospice Palliative Care Alliance |

# Introduction and categorisation of children's palliative care needs and prevalence

*Duncan Randall, Susan Neilson and Julia Downing*

## INTRODUCTION

It was not our idea to write this book. Grace McInnes from Routledge approached us looking for a book on children's palliative care. We had recently published the *Children's Palliative Care Education Standard Framework* (Neilson et al., 2021), so naturally we thought of producing a book to support learners on programmes aligned to the standards.

We understood why Grace wanted to publish a book on children's palliative care. Interest in palliative care has been growing and was particularly brought into focus by the 2020 COVID-19 pandemic. The lockdown and restrictions enforced by the COVID-19 response were particularly felt by those who were separated during the period of end of life and death. The provision of nursing care, particularly in community settings, was also irreparably changed by the pandemic experience. Prior to the pandemic, we had seen an increasing focus in recent decades on children's palliative care around the world. Of course, throughout human existence, children have died. However, in medicine, palliative care is a "young" medical sub-speciality dating from the 1960s. A social stigma which prohibits the discussion of children's palliative care and child death still exists today. As a result, the suffering of children and their carers (parents, families and communities), while often witnessed by nurses and other medical practitioners, has not been the focus of education, research, clinical management or publications. This is now changing with the World Health Organization (WHO) calling for the universal provision of healthcare to include palliative care for all people, including children (WHO, 2022). In addition, there is a renewed focus on children's palliative care with organisations such as the International Children's Palliative Care Network (ICPCN), the United Nations Children's Fund (UNICEF) and the World Health Organization highlighting the palliative care needs of children (Connor et al., 2020). In order for us to put this into context, we need to consider what we mean by children's palliative care, the need for such services, the prevalence and the existing provision.

DOI: 10.4324/9781003384861-1

We knew once we invited Julia to join the editorial team that the book was going to be a global endeavour. Julia was able to reach out to her global network, which is built and sustained by her work at the International Children's Palliative Care Network, her World Health Organization advocacy and activism in children's palliative care in many low- and middle-income countries, as well as her campaigning in high-income countries. Julia also brought an understanding of the very different approaches to children's palliative care seen in low- and middle-income countries, where public health approaches dominate care. We wanted a book that addressed both the Global North (generally high-income) country approaches and those from low-/middle-income Global South perspectives.

## WHAT DO WE MEAN BY CHILDREN'S PALLIATIVE CARE?

In order to understand what we mean by children's palliative nursing care, we need to first consider what we mean by children's palliative care. Palliative care is a relatively new concept in many countries, with a range of terms used (e.g. palliative care, hospice care, end-of-life care, terminal care) and a range of definitions applied. While it is recognised that there are variations in definitions and how they are applied in different parts of the world, we felt it was important to have a common understanding for the purposes of this book. Thus, we have used the umbrella term *palliative care* to allow for discussion of palliation from diagnosis (or even prior to diagnosis as some children may never receive a diagnosis due to the rarity of their condition, a lack of resources, or late presentation), throughout the disease trajectory through to end-of-life care and into bereavement. We consider children with both life-limiting and life-threatening conditions to be living with palliative care needs. We have broadly adopted Shaw et al.'s (2012) conceptions of the spectrum of children's palliative care needs, that children are considered to be living with varying degrees of palliative care needs if death before the age of 18 years is probable, or if people would not be surprised by their death at that age (UN Convention on the Rights of the Child, UN, 1989, Article 1). We also subscribe to the Together for Short Lives' definition of children's palliative care (Chambers, 2018) along with the globally followed WHO's definition (WHO, 2023) (see Box 0.1). While slightly different, their concepts and philosophies are similar.

---

**BOX 0.1 DEFINITIONS OF CHILDREN'S PALLIATIVE CARE**

**Together for Short Lives**

Palliative care for children and young people with life-limiting or life-threatening conditions is an active and total approach to care, from the point of diagnosis or recognition throughout the child's life and death. It embraces physical, emotional, social, and spiritual elements, and focuses on enhancement of quality of life for the child/young person and support for the family. It includes the management of distressing symptoms, provision of short breaks and care through death and bereavement.

(Chambers, 2018, p. 9)

---

**World Health Organization**

The active total care of the child's body, mind and spirit, and also involves giving support to the family. It begins when illness is diagnosed, and continues regardless of whether or not a child receives treatment directed at the disease. Health providers must evaluate and alleviate a child's physical, psychological and social distress. Effective palliative care requires a broad multi-disciplinary approach that includes the family and makes use of available community resources; it can be successfully implemented even if resources are limited. It can be provided in tertiary care facilities, in community health centres and even in children's homes.

(WHO, 2023)

## WHAT IS THE NEED FOR CHILDREN'S PALLIATIVE CARE?

Having an understanding of the local, national, regional and global need for children's palliative care can help us, as nurses, ensure that the care we are providing meets the needs of the children whom we are caring for. We believe that palliative care should be available for all children with a life-limiting or life-threatening condition and their families, from diagnosis throughout the course of their illness, wherever they are being cared for.

A number of studies have attempted to define and estimate the numbers of children requiring palliative care, however, this process is extremely challenging. In order to do this, we need to be clear as to what we mean by "children" and the life-limiting and life-threatening conditions that may lead to children needing palliative care. We also need to identify how many children will potentially need to access services, and where they are located.

We recognise that in different countries there are different legal definitions of a child, different ages at which maturity is achieved, according to individual state/country laws, and different arrangements for nursing services for babies, children, adolescents and young adults.

There is evidence of an increasing need for children's palliative care. Although based on UK prevalence, Lorna Fraser and her collaborators have shown an increase in conditions likely to require palliative and end-of-life care in childhood since 2001/2002. The national prevalence of children with life-limiting conditions aged 0–19 years in England increased from 26.7 per 10,000 in 2001/2002 to 66.4 per 10,000 in 2017/2018, and is set to increase to 84.2 per 10,000 by 2030 (Fraser et al., 2020).

Various studies have been conducted over the years to estimate the number of children globally who need palliative care. Estimates range from 2.5 million 0–14 year-olds needing end-of-life care (Connor and Sepulveda, 2014) to 21.1 million 0–19 year-olds (Connor et al., 2017). In 2017, Connor et al. conservatively estimated there were 21.1 million children in need of palliative care worldwide, with more than 8 million requiring some degree of specialist care. The Lancet

Commission on alleviating the access abyss in palliative care and pain relief (Knaul et al., 2018) estimated that one-third of the children who died in 2015 experienced Serious Health-related Suffering,[1] with >5.3 million children under the age of 15 years needing access to palliative care. These estimates have since risen, as reflected in the ongoing work to identify the number of children with Serious Health-related Suffering who need palliative care using a revised and updated methodology (Kwete Jiang et al., 2024). As a result the numbers are expected to be a lot higher than originally identified, as the methods for calculating need have been refined for children.

One of the misconceptions within palliative care is that it is mainly for children with cancer. Knaul et al. (2020), in the *Global Atlas of Palliative Care*, estimate that just over 5% of children in need of palliative care globally will have cancer, with the largest groups being those with HIV disease (29.6%), those born prematurely and experiencing birth trauma (17.7%), those with congenital malformations (16.2%) and those with injuries, poisoning and external causes (16.0%). However, work on global projections for the burden of Serious Health-related Suffering in both adults and children with cancer indicates that this is expected to double by 2060, with a larger and faster increase in low-income countries. Thus, more people will die with unnecessary suffering unless there is an expansion of palliative care to meet the need (Sleeman et al., 2021).

It should be borne in mind that there are large disparities in both the prevalence of palliative care needs for children between states and continents and the nature of children's life-limiting or life-threatening conditions. Africa, for example, with large populations affected by HIV/AIDS has a high prevalence rate (Connor et al., 2017; Knaul et al., 2020). It is estimated that 51.8% of children globally who need palliative care live in the African region, 19.5% in the Southeast Asia Region, 12% in the Eastern Mediterranean region, 7.7% in the Western Pacific Region, 6.2% in the Region of the Americas, and just 2.8% within the European Region (Knaul et al., 2020). Thus, while it is recognised that there is a global need for children's palliative care, the nature of the care required, the provision of care and the structure and resourcing of care provision vary widely in particular areas of the globe. The disparity can perhaps be best seen in two sets of statistics. The population rates for palliative care in children (per 10,000 child population) are highest in low-income countries, e.g. 113.3 per 10,000 in Zimbabwe, compared to high-income countries, e.g. 21.5 per 10,000 in the USA (Connor et al., 2017). Yet low- and middle-income countries only have access to 10% of the global opioid supply when pain is the most commonly experienced symptom worldwide for children, experienced on 22.6–34% of days (Cleary et al., 2020) (see Chapter 7).

Estimating the global provision of palliative care is also challenging. An estimated 5–10% of children globally needing palliative care currently have access to it. Knapp et al. (2011) support this inverse care law seen in opiate supply with high- and upper middle-income countries having much more developed children's palliative care services (Figure 0.1). In 2011, they estimated that 65.6% of countries had no known

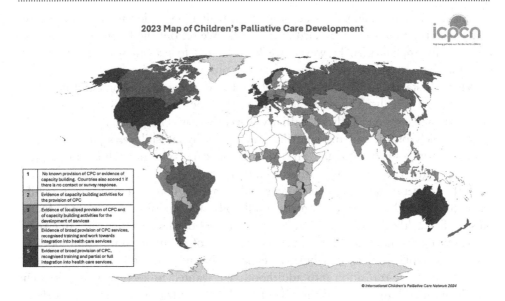

**FIGURE 0.1** Level of children's palliative care provision in 2019

Source: ICPCN (2023).

children's palliative care, 18.8% had capacity-building activities, 9.9% had localised provision and only 5.7% of countries globally had provision that was reaching mainstream providers. The International Children's Palliative Care Network has been tracking the development of children's palliative care over many years, estimating the provision of children's palliative care globally (Downing et al., 2017; ICPCN, 2023). While there has been an increase in the development of services, there are still a wide range of countries globally where there is little or no access to children's palliative care.

## THE CHILDREN'S PALLIATIVE CARE EDUCATION AND STANDARD FRAMEWORK

We should perhaps take a step back at this point and return to the impetus to develop this book. In 2018, there was a UK All Party Parliamentary Group inquiry into children's palliative care (Cooper, 2018). It was noted that although there were some excellent examples of education programmes, these were not universally accessible and, across the sector, education to inform practice was often fragmented or not available. In response to the report of the Parliamentary Group report, Susan Neilson with others set up a stakeholders group to review the existing education and professional guidance landscape of children's palliative care. The Children's Palliative Care Education and Training Action Group (CPCET Action Group) met in person prior to the COVID-19 pandemic and continued as an online forum, producing the standards for children's palliative care education in 2020 (Neilson et al., 2021).

This book was designed to accompany learning on children's palliative care mapped to the Education Standard Framework. We set out the Framework and the mapping in Appendix A. However, we first wanted to present some of the other thinking that set the course for this book with our author teams.

When we started to look at the sort of books out there already on children's palliative care, we realised that, while there were some contributions to texts and a literature by nurses on children's palliative care, there was no published book which focused solely on the nursing contribution. Naturally, as children's palliative care nurses we wanted to fill that gap. So early on we decided on a global book by and for children's nurses on children's palliative nursing care.

With the overall approach decided, we had to face the common dilemmas for children's nurses. Did we want to segment childhoods into stages? Did we want to focus on specific health conditions? We reflected that the Education Standard Framework is structured to allow application across the span of childhood into adulthood. It allows for application to new-borns, neonates, infants, etc., all the way to adolescents and their transition into adulthood. We wanted to keep that broad reach across childhood and adopted the World Health Organization's 0–18 years definition of childhood (UN Convention on the Rights of the Child, UN, 1989, Article 1). Throughout the book we are considering children as being under the age of 18, unless otherwise stated. We have in places used specific terms for periods of childhood, as appropriate, such as infants for children under 1 year old. However, unless otherwise stated, we use child, children and childhoods to refer to all children, irrespective of their age or the period of childhood they may be considered, by others, to be living through.

We wanted a global children's nursing book that addressed the palliative nursing of children across the socially designated span of childhood. Our aim was to produce a book which would assist learners to understand the full diversity of childhood, including the transition into young adulthood and the span of palliative care from diagnosis through the illness trajectory to end-of-life care and bereavement. Quite a task!

Thankfully, to keep us on task, we already had the Education Standard Framework, thus we were able to devise the structure of the book. The book has three Parts: Part I: Public Health and Universal; Part II: Core; and finally, Part III: Specialist. These reflect the four levels of the Education Standard Framework (Neilson et al., 2021), with public health and universal considered together in Part I. The division of these levels reflects that this book is aimed at nurses, so we have focused on the aspects of public health nursing and working with other formal and informal carers that we felt were pertinent to nurses. The Core level was designed to prepare nurses to deliver children's palliative care, aimed at those for whom such work is a part of their nursing work but not their only, or main, focus or specialism. Thus, the Core level is designed for all nurses who deliver nursing care to children with life-limiting and life-threatening conditions and where children may die, where palliative care may be required, but is not the sole focus of the nursing care. The Specialist level is for those nurses who specialise in children's palliative care nursing and for whom palliative care, including dying, death and bereavement support, is the focus of their work. Hence the Core and Specialist sections are longer, as the main focus is on nurses who work with children living with palliative care needs, albeit informed and underpinned by the public health nursing and interdisciplinary universal aspects.

The four levels of the Education Standard Framework were designed to be both stand-alone but also cumulative, so that practitioners wishing to attain Specialist level must build their skills and understanding in all the three other levels, in addition to meeting the Specialist level standards. In the Framework, the levels are defined as set out in Table 0.1. You are, of course, welcome to read the book either as stand-alone chapters or Parts or to study the chapters in sequence. We have cross-referenced the chapters and sections as we saw fit, to be true to the complex nature of children's palliative care, in which themes intersect and aspects echo between chapters and through the book.

**TABLE 0.1** Four levels of the Education Standard Framework (CPCET Action Group, 2020)

| | |
|---|---|
| **Public Health** | In this level children's palliative care as a public health issue will be addressed. Aspects such as social attitude to death and dying in childhood and bereavement following a child death are explored. This would be expected to be across education, health and social care and involve other stakeholder groups concerned with children, their experience of childhood, learning and support of children, siblings, parents and other family members as well as communities affected by child death (e.g. school communities). |
| **Universal** | In this level the needs will be addressed of all people working in institutions or facilities which provide care and support to children and their carers. It addresses what any person working in such environments is likely to need to understand about children's palliative care. This includes clinical and non-clinical staff. Where children's palliative care is everyone in the workplaces business. |
| **Core** | In this level the focus will be on the learning for people who deliver care to children and their carers. It includes everyone who delivers care to children in education, social and health care who might encounter a child living with a life limiting/threatening condition and or the child's carers (family and communities). The core programmes for sectors of health, education and social care might be different to address the needs of children accessing these types of care. In healthcare this level should include care of the dying child and their carers as well as supporting people with loss and bereavement following a child's death. |
| **Specialist** | In this level leadership and management of palliative and end of life care for children is the focus. It includes clinical, research, education and management leadership. As well as addressing the needs of children and carers with complex and or multiple palliative care needs it would prepare practitioners to be a resource for those learning and delivering care at the other levels. This level includes learning to deliver end of life care in complex situations or where symptom management is challenging. |

Each of the four levels has learning outcomes set in relation to four areas:

- *Learning Outcome 1* Communicating effectively
- *Learning Outcome 2* Working with others in and across various settings
- *Learning Outcome 3* Identifying and managing symptoms
- *Learning Outcome 4* Sustaining self-care and supporting the well-being of others

We have included a copy of learning outcomes in the Standard in Appendix A, and it is freely available on the International Children's Palliative Care Network website (https://icpcn.org/resources/education-framework-self-audit-tool/).

## THE STRUCTURE OF THE BOOK

Part I of the book contains three chapters (Chapters 1–3) that set out the children's palliative care and child death beliefs and attitudes common in communities and shared by nurses. In Chapter 1, the focus is on compassionate communities and the nurse's role in facilitating, constructing and sustaining communities' participation in children's palliative care. Beliefs, attitudes and values in children's palliative care, along with public perceptions of childhood dying and death, are then considered and the nurse's role in public health nursing relating to children's palliative care. In these chapters there is consideration of how nurses responded to and continue to (re)construct the COVID-19 pandemic, which had a profound effect on public understanding and nurses' provision of palliative care.

Part II contains five chapters (Chapters 4–8). In Chapter 4, nurses' communication in dealing with unwanted news is considered, relating to diagnosis and assessment of palliative care needs. Chapter 5 has a focus on the nurse and their self-care, recognising the need to find sustainable and nourishing ways to provide children's nursing care. Chapter 6 turns to children's coping through play and education, with consideration of the nurses' role in supporting children and their carers through living a childhood with palliative care needs. Chapter 7 is a very long chapter in which we discuss symptom management – both the assessment of symptoms and the nursing management. As symptoms are numerous and the management often complex, this chapter requires some space in which to consider the nursing interventions and practices. The final chapter in this Part, Chapter 8, is where we consider end-of-life care, including the care of children's bodies after death, carers and others, bereavement and the legal frameworks that pertain to the death of a child.

Part III also contains five chapters (Chapters 9–13) and here we focus on the specialist skills and understandings required to deliver palliative nursing care for children. Chapter 9 on managing complexity builds on Chapter 7 and considers the interaction of managing connected symptoms and also complex situations and contexts of palliative care, including the ethics of palliative and, specifically, end-of-life care for children. Chapter 10 is where we consider how nurses learn to design, deliver, and evaluate and lead children's palliative nursing care and Chapter 11 picks up the service improvement aspects to consider the nurse's role in leading and developing practice and policy. Chapter 12 has a focus on evaluation of services, including considering quality issues and the framing of performance evaluation for teams of nurses delivering care. Last, but not least, Chapter 13 is where we consider research specific to children's palliative care and what might be the new frontiers of children's palliative nursing care research.

This book could not have been written without the dedication, love and support of our contributing authors. We came together on Zoom from different time zones, cultures and contexts. We have to acknowledge that our conversation was mostly conducted in English and that this book is published in English. While recognising the imperialist history and the power differentials of an Anglicised approach, we also acknowledge the global disparity in academic publishing and the problems that the imposition of English as a global language pose. We are especially grateful to all the contributing authors whose native language is not English, and we wish to pay respectful homage to their additional work in interpreting their native languages, customs and culture for us to be represented in this work.

---

**AIM OF THE BOOK**

As we send this book out to nurses all over the world, it seems inappropriate to hope you will all enjoy the book.

We are sure that some of you will shed a few tears in reading this text, many of us shed quite a few tears in writing it. As a colleague once remarked:

> We are all scarred by palliative care, we accept these scars, we bear them for all the children and their carers that we have the privilege of helping during some of the most difficult times children, parents or any community can endure.

What we do hope is that this book informs and empowers your nursing care as we believe that nurses are the people who can help children and communities to live with their symptoms, experience childhoods and to facilitate good deaths for children which live on in the memories and bereavement of those who remain in our world.

---

## NOTE

1. According to Knaul et al. (2018):

> Suffering is health-related when it is associated with illness or injury of any kind. Suffering is serious when it cannot be relieved without medical intervention and when it compromises physical, social, or emotional functioning, Palliative care should be focused on relieving the SHS that is associated with life-limiting or life-threatening health conditions or the end of life.
>
> *(p. 15)*

## REFERENCES

Chambers, L. (2018). *A guide to children's palliative care: Supporting babies, children and young people with life-limiting and life-threatening conditions and their families. Together for Short Lives* (4th edn). Available at: https://www.togetherforshortlives.org.uk/app/uploads/2018/03/TfSL-A-Guide-to-Children%E2%80%99s-Palliative-Care-Fourth-Edition-FINAL-SINGLE-PAGES.pdf (accessed 12 June 2024).

Cleary, J., Hastie, B., Harding, R., Jaramillo, E., Connor, S., Krakauer, E. (2020). What are the main barriers to palliative care development? In S.R. Connor, (ed.), *Global atlas of palliative care* (2nd edn; pp. 33–44). Available at: https://www.iccp-portal.org/system/files/resources/WHPCA_Global_Atlas_FINAL_DIGITAL.pdf (accessed 12 June 2024).

Connor, S. R. et al. (eds) (2020). *Global atlas of palliative care at the end of life* (2nd edn). Available at: https://www.iccp-portal.org/system/files/resources/WHPCA_Global_Atlas_FINAL_DIGITAL.pdf) (accessed 8 February 2024).

Connor, S. R., Downing, J., Marston, J. (2017). Estimating the global need for palliative care for children: A cross-sectional analysis. *Journal of Pain and Symptom Management*, 53(2), 171–177. https://doi.org/10.1016/j.jpainsymman.2016.08.020

Connor, S. R., Sepulveda, C. (eds) (2014). *Global atlas of palliative care at the end of life.* World Health Organization/Worldwide Hospice Palliative Care Alliance. Available at: https://www.iccp-portal.org/system/files/resources/Global_Atlas_of_Palliative_Care.pdf (accessed 12 June 2024).

Cooper, J. (2018). *End of life care: Strengthening choice. An inquiry report by the All-Party Parliamentary Group (APPG) for Children Who Need Palliative Care.* Available at: https://www.togetherforshortlives.org.uk/app/uploads/2018/10/Pol_Res_181019_APPG_Children_Who_Need_Palliative_Care_inquiry_report.pdf (accessed 12 June 2024).

CPCET Action Group (Children's Palliative Care Education and Training Action Group, UK and Ireland). (2020). Children's Palliative Care Education Standard Framework. https://icpcn.org/resources/education-framework-self-audit-tool/ (accessed 8 February 2024).

Downing, J., Boucher, S., Nkosi, B., Daniels, A. (2017). Palliative care for children in low- and middle-income countries. In I. MacGrath (ed.), *Cancer control 2017: Cancer care in emerging health systems* (pp. 71–76). INCTR and Global Health Dynamics. Available at: http://www.cancercontrol.info/wp-content/uploads/2017/12/71-76-downing.pdf (accessed 12 June 2024).

Fraser, L. K., Gibson-Smith, D., Jarvis, S., Norman, P., Parslow, R. (2020). Make every child count: Estimating current and future prevalence of children and young people with life-limiting conditions in the United Kingdom. Available at: https://www.togetherforshortlives.org.uk/app/uploads/2020/04/Prevalence-reportFinal_28_04_2020.pdf (accessed 8 February 2024).

ICPCN. (2023). Our work: Advocacy. Available at: https://icpcn.org/our-impact/ (accessed 12 June 2024).

Knapp, C., Woodworth, L., Wright, M., Downing, J., Drake, R., Fowler Kerry, S., Hain, R., Marston, J. (2011). Pediatric palliative care provision around the world: A systematic review. *Pediatric Blood & Cancer*, 57(3), 361–368. https://doi.org/10.1002/pbc.23100

Knaul, F. M., Farmer, P. E., Krakauer, E. L., De Lima, L., Bhadelia, A., Kwete, X. J., Arreola-Ornelas, H., Gómez-Dantés, O., Rodriguez, N. M., Alleyne, G. A. O., Connor, S. R., Hunter, D. J., Lohman, L., Radbruch, L., del Rocío Sáenz Madrigal, M., Atun, R., Foley, K. M., Frenk, J., Jamison, D. T., …, on behalf of the Lancet Commission on Palliative Care and Pain Relief Study Group. (2018). Alleviating the access abyss in palliative care and pain relief – an imperative of universal health coverage: The Lancet Commission report. *The Lancet*, 391(10128), 1391–1454. https://doi.org/10.1016/S0140-6736(17)32513-8

Knaul, F., Radbruch, L., Connor, S., de Lima, L., Arreola-Ornelas, H., Mendez Carniado, O., Kwete Jiang, X., Bhadelia, A., Downing, J., Krakauer, E. L. (2020). How many adults and children are in need of palliative care worldwide? In S. R. Connor et al. (eds), *Global atlas of palliative care* (2nd edn; pp. 17–32). Available at: file:///Users/juliadowning/Downloads/WHPCA_Global_Atlas_DIGITAL_Compress.pdf (accessed 12 June 2024).

Kwete Jiang, X., Bhadelia, A., Arreola-Ornelas, H., Mendes, O., Rosa, W. E., Connor, S., Downing, J., Dean, J., Watkins, D., Calderon, R., Cleary, J., Freidman, J., de Lima, L., Ntizimira, C., Pastrana, T., Perez, P. C., Spence, D., Rajagopal, M. R., Enciso, V. V., ..., Knaul, F. M. K. (2024). Global assessment of palliative care need: Serious health-related suffering measurement methodology. *Journal of Pain and Symptom Management*, S0885-3924(24): 00708–5. Online ahead of print. https://doi.org/10.1016/j.jpainsymman.2024.03.027

Neilson, S., Randall, D., McNamara, K., Downing, J. (2021). Children's palliative care education and training: Developing an education standard framework and audit. *BMC Medical Education*, 21(1), 539. https://doi.org/10.1186/s12909-021-02982-4

Shaw, K. L., Brook, L., Mpundu-Kaambwa, C., Harris, N., Lapwood, S., Randall, D. (2012). The spectrum of children's palliative care needs: A classification framework for children with life-limiting or life-threatening conditions. *BMJ Supportive & Palliative Care*, 5(3), 249–258. https://doi.org/10.1136/bmjspcare-2012-000407

Sleeman, K. E., Gomes, B., de Brito, M., Shamieh, O., Harding, R. (2021). The burden of serious health-related suffering among cancer decedents: Global projections study to 2060. *Palliative Medicine*, 35(1), 231–235. https://doi.org/10.1177/0269216320957561

UN (United Nations). (1989). Convention on the rights of the child. Available at: https://www.unicef.org/child-rights-convention/convention-text (accessed 12 June 2024).

WHO (World Health Organization). (2022). Universal health coverage. Available at: https://www.who.int/health-topics/universal-health-coverage#tab=tab_1 (accessed 12 June 2024).

WHO (World Health Organization). (2023). Palliative care for children. Available at: https://www.who.int/europe/news-room/fact-sheets/item/palliative-care-for-children#:~:text=Palliative%20care%20for%20children%20is,treatment%20directed%20at%20the%20disease (accessed 12 June 2024).

# PART I

# Public health and universal

## CHAPTER 1

# Building and sustaining compassionate communities with children

......................................

*Anu Savio Thelly, Alice Stella Verginia,*
*Katrina McNamara-Goodger and Peter Ellis*

## INTRODUCTION

It takes a whole village to raise a child.

(Old African proverb)

The availability of children's palliative care services for children and their families varies across countries, with some having well-established programmes, including children's hospice facilities or palliative care programmes, children's hospitals, and community-based palliative care, yet many places remain without any organised children's palliative care services although professionals there endeavour to ensure that care is provided through the existing services.

Bluebond-Langner et al. (2007) described the psychological and social costs of caring for a child with life-limiting conditions, parents experience emotional strain, physical exhaustion, financial difficulties, social isolation, lack of support, along with the challenges of decision-making and end-of-life planning. Randall (2017) identified that caring for a child with palliative care needs places significant emotional, physical, and financial burdens on parents. Families caring for children with complex health conditions also report feeling isolated and strained due to the lack of knowledge and inadequate organisation of healthcare outside of hospitals. Tailored support, flexible care options, and access to psychosocial and sibling support are crucial to address their needs. Failure to provide these resources can lead to family breakdown and an increased need for additional support.

By building a compassionate community, we create an environment that promotes empathy, support, and understanding for children with palliative care needs and their families. It aims to enhance their quality of life, reduce isolation, and ensure that they receive the comprehensive care and support they require throughout their

DOI: 10.4324/9781003384861-3

palliative care journey. Globally, specialist palliative care services are not configured to provide for all of the needs of children and families but can supplement the support provided by compassionate communities for the child's needs, as well as the emotional and practical support of the other family members.

This chapter addresses how a community can create an environment that promotes care, empathy and understanding to support and accompany families with children living with palliative care needs during the child's journey through their life and through death, creating positive experiences along the way which become good memories for the future. We will also explore the nurse's role in building and sustaining compassionate communities to support children and families.

---

**LEARNING OBJECTIVES**

The reader will be able to do the following:

1.  Describe what a compassionate community is and how it can enhance the care of children and their families.
2.  Describe the nurse's role in facilitating the building and sustaining of compassionate communities.
3.  Discuss how to build and sustain compassionate communities.
4.  Describe how a holistic approach can be enhanced by inclusion of a community voice.
5.  Reflect on their own beliefs, attitudes and understanding of personal and community responses to death in childhood and how this might influence their approach to care and support.
6.  Identify relevant local, regional and national policies and practices which support, facilitate and sustain palliative and end-of-life care for children and their families.

---

## BACKGROUND

Children with life-limiting or life-threatening conditions and their families often experience isolation and exclusion from their communities, significantly impacting their quality of life. The complex care that is required to meet the needs of these children is often provided by parents at home and can be emotionally demanding (and is described further in Chapter 8). Parents are often responsible for their daily caregiving which exceeds that of healthy and typically developing children. This can encompass a wide range of tasks, including medical care, therapy sessions, administering medications, attending appointments with specialists, and providing assistance with daily activities such as feeding, bathing, and mobility. Parents may experience a range of intense emotions, including stress, anxiety, guilt, grief, and even depression, as they navigate the complex and often uncertain journey of caring for their child. Witnessing their child's struggles and facing the reality of their condition can be heartbreaking, and parents may grapple with feelings of inadequacy or helplessness. Caregiver fatigue is another significant challenge faced by parents of children with special needs. The relentless demands of caregiving, combined with the emotional strain and often disrupted sleep patterns, can lead to physical and emotional exhaustion over time. Parents may find themselves constantly juggling multiple responsibilities, sacrificing their own needs and well-being in the process (Kase, Waldman and Weintraub, 2019).

While some children may need specialised children's palliative care interventions and complex symptom management in a hospital setting, it is important to recognise that, where services are available, children can receive care and support from a children's palliative care team in the familiar surroundings of their own homes. Families often prefer to keep their child at home, especially during end-of-life care, to maintain a sense of normalcy (an ordinary life) for the child and their siblings, to reduce stress and improve comfort for the sick child. This responsibility takes a toll on the family's emotional, spiritual and physical well-being, adding to the already challenging situation they face. Sometimes they find the challenges overwhelming and the child is admitted to hospital during the final stages of their life.

Families providing care may experience social isolation due to the time and energy demands of caregiving, disruption of normal activities, financial strain, stigma, and emotional distress. These factors can lead to limited social connections and feelings of loneliness for parents and siblings.

Social isolation and loneliness are related but distinct concepts. Social isolation refers to having limited social contacts and interactions with few individuals on a regular basis, while loneliness is the subjective feeling of being alone, regardless of the amount of social contact one has (Dickens et al., 2011). It is possible for someone to live alone without feeling lonely or socially isolated, just as others can feel lonely even when surrounded by people. Social isolation and loneliness can increase poor health, psychological distress, sleep deprivation, exhaustion and lead to a lower quality of life (Fonseca, Nazaré and Canavarro, 2012). Research suggests that prolonged social isolation can have detrimental effects on health, comparable to smoking 15 cigarettes a day (Kroll, 2022).

Recognising and addressing these challenges through comprehensive support are crucial for parents. Supporting families in caring for children with life-limiting or life-threatening conditions, and in preparing for the death of a loved one, can significantly enhance their grieving journey. It is recommended that services should implement a model that specifically addresses this aspect, with a particular emphasis on the participation of community members. This may be an unfamiliar role for many nurses, but this chapter aims to help them change their practice to feel more confident in being able to change their roles. A multi-disciplinary and public health approach to a child's well-being addresses their physical, emotional, social and spiritual needs through collaboration among professionals, social workers, educators, family members and volunteers. Understanding these realities emphasises a need to build "compassionate communities" that involve community-led interventions, volunteer participation and naturally occurring networks to enhance care, support, and build and sustain social connections for children receiving palliative care at home and their families. Key to the development of compassionate communities is the public health approach to palliative care.

## PUBLIC HEALTH APPROACH TO PALLIATIVE CARE

Access to palliative care is a crucial global public health issue that affects millions of children and adults, leading to unnecessary suffering. A public health strategy for palliative care enables the translation of evidence-based knowledge and skills into cost-effective interventions that can reach the entire population. Active involvement of society through collective and social action is fundamental to the success of such a strategy. Palliative care services should not be limited to specific healthcare organisations but should be integrated at all levels of society, starting from the community level and extending throughout the healthcare system. This has the potential to make a real difference and have a sustainable impact.

Implementation of the enhanced WHO Public Health Model (Stjernswärd, Foley and Ferris, 2007) and addressing all elements of the strategy, including the provision of quality palliative care services, means population-based coverage can be achieved and lead to significant relief of suffering and improvement in the quality of life for patients with advanced illnesses and their families. Healthcare systems should collaborate closely with communities, including the involvement of relatives, friends and neighbours to enable more people to have a dignified home death and meet their unique needs. The importance of the community has been recognised in the revised WHO conceptual model for palliative care development (WHO, 2021), which expands the Public Health Model (Stjernswärd, Foley and Ferris, 2007) to include research which rests on the foundations of empowered people and communities and health policies. To date, the public health approach has focused mainly on adults, whereas this chapter addresses adapting the concept for children's palliative care, with the model starting to emerge in practice.

The medicalisation and institutionalisation of illness and death have led to a disconnection from the traditional practices of dying within the supportive networks of family and community, resulting in limited choices, reduced autonomy, and a lack of knowledge in navigating end-of-life care. The rising burden of non-communicable diseases, alleviation of suffering, promotion of equitable access to care, strengthening health systems, and upholding human rights and dignity need to be addressed. Additionally, the growing population of children with life-limiting and life-threatening conditions poses additional challenges. Equitable care, regardless of diagnosis, is necessary, along with the expansion of non-medical supportive services. Moreover, the increasing longevity of children with life-limiting and life-threatening conditions adds strain to already stretched health, education, and social care systems, compounded by a global shortage of nurses (WHO, 2020).

According to the perspective put forward by Abel and Kellehear (2022), palliative and end-of-life care should be viewed as a collective responsibility, emphasising the importance of compassionate communities that actively engage the public in end-of-life care (see Chapter 3).

By adopting a public health approach, living and dying become a matter of societal concern. This requires the collaboration and co-operation of various stakeholders, including healthcare systems, community members, and public institutions. This inclusive approach aims to address the physical, emotional, and social needs of individuals approaching the end of life, ensuring that they receive comprehensive support and compassionate care. Box 1.1 offers a good example.

---

**BOX 1.1 A GOOD PRACTICE EXAMPLE: THE KERALA MODEL**

The Centre for Empowerment & Enrichment (CEFEE) is a non-governmental organisation (NGO), in the Indian state of Kerala, for the benefit of people with special needs, working with the motto, "I AM DIFFERENT NOT LESS" (Centre for Empowerment & Enrichment, 2024). Figure 1.1 shows the three levels of application.

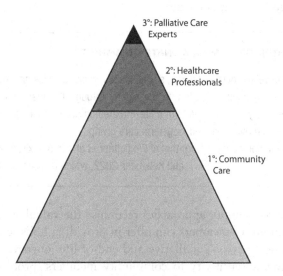

3°: Palliative Care Experts

2°: Healthcare Professionals

1°: Community Care

**FIGURE 1.1** The Kerala model

Since 2007, the organisation has initiated projects and ensured involvement of the public and college students as volunteers and, as a result, has seen an increase in compassion and empathy among them. Every year, around 2000 people improve their skills through interactive socialising projects. The Centre runs a range of projects, supported by volunteers to meet their aim of bringing people with special needs to the forefront of society.

The *Uniquely Me* project recognises that some children with special needs live in their own homes and need appropriate socialising skills. It aims to develop life skills through experience, e.g., experiencing different types of transport, their ticketing systems, how to seek help, visiting shops, cinemas, the hospital and the police station. The project works with small groups to give the participants time and attention to help their understanding of the experience. It also aims to build parental confidence and help children with special needs to participate in events in Kerala, by providing them with a secure space to do so. The project works with the District Administration to ensure support with the provision of necessary equipment and any need for hospitalisation.

The *Break the Silence* project is delivered with the support of the local police department and educates the children about abuse and how they can protect themselves.

---

## WHAT ARE COMPASSIONATE COMMUNITIES?

Compassion is difficult to quantify and objectively identify but many people (not all) know intuitively what this looks like. Compassion is the human and moral part of care, the philosophical foundation and centrepiece of the nursing profession. One definition of compassion by *Merriam-Webster Dictionary* (2024) is the "sympathetic consciousness of others' distress together with a desire to alleviate it". In a compassionate community, people are motivated by compassion to take responsibility for and care for each other. This offers an opportunity for nurses to support people to re-engage with compassionate interactions with one another and to embed this in activities to support children living with palliative care needs and their families. See also Box 1.2 for another definition.

---

**BOX 1.2 DEFINITION OF COMPASSIONATE COMMUNITIES**

Communities that develop social networks, social spaces, social policies and social conduct that support children, young people, adults and the elderly through the many hours, days, weeks, months and sometimes years of living with a life-threatening or life-limiting illness and dying in childhood, grief and bereavement, and long-term care giving.

(Definition adapted from that of Wegleitner et al. 2015 p. xiv, as discussed in Abel and Kellehear, 2022, which focuses on supporting elders)

---

Compassionate community approaches recognise the valuable contributions and expertise that community members can offer in providing holistic and compassionate care throughout a person's palliative and end-of-life journey. Compassion in a community involves a sensitivity to community members' problems and concern for social justice for all. As compassion declines, so do the core values of caring for the welfare and respecting the dignity of others. Kellehear (2005) discusses a compassionate city charter, which includes the principles of public health practice, of community engagement and development, prevention, harm reduction and early intervention. The charter sets out an example of the social changes to key institutions and activities that can underpin the development of a compassionate city or community and may be useful to adapt for local use. This can help identify policies that are useful to the development of a compassionate community and identify gaps in policy provision and a need to influence the policy agenda.

There are several different public health approaches that can support the development of compassionate communities. The implementation of such approaches can empower communities to identify strengths, set priorities, and develop strategies within their local contexts. Community development, a proven and cost-effective public health practice, offers a commitment to equity and meaningful participation. By recognising community assets and respecting community-defined priorities, community development empowers people to address shared concerns through participatory action.

Reaching community members through existing neighbourhood groups, faith organisations, workplaces, schools, local government agencies, sports clubs, and cultural institutions, among others, helps to build community capacity and participation and promote understanding and equity in accessing palliative care across diverse populations. Communities become everyday settings where people can access and provide care through active partnerships with palliative care services.

Acknowledging and appreciating the existing strengths within diverse communities help palliative care services explore and offer expert support that aligns with the wishes and social context of these communities and help to address inequitable access to palliative care. To reimagine access to children's palliative care, and promote more equitable outcomes, it is essential to prioritise public health partnerships and community participation (Mills et al., 2021). This requires strengthening community action and creating supportive environments, as outlined in the World Health Organization's 1987 Ottawa Charter for Health Promotion (WHO, 1987).

## What are compassionate communities in children's palliative care?

Compassionate community initiatives in children's palliative care aim to build partnerships between children's services and communities, leveraging the strengths and skills present within the community instead of relying solely on professional care. By engaging the community, these initiatives empower children, families, caregivers, and community members to actively participate in the care and support of children living with palliative care needs.

By creating a safe and supportive environment, professionals, various organisations, and society contribute to the child's higher quality of life, respect their rights and dignity, and enable them to live fully. Community-led models aim to meet social and practical needs, build community capacity and resilience, and normalise the process of care, dying, death, and bereavement as well as improving death literacy and addressing stigma and cultural barriers related to palliative care. Death literacy is defined by Graham-Wisener et al. (2022) as the knowledge and skills that people need to make it possible to gain access in order to understand and make informed choices about end-of-life and death care options.

Initiatives in children's palliative care aim to ensure that children have access to the same childhood activities and education opportunities as their peers. Advocacy and direct support from community members, including nurses, can provide emotional and practical assistance to both the child and their family members.

Compassionate communities in children's palliative care can also help to reawaken compassion and transform the way society views and responds to the needs of children living with palliative care needs, recognising the significance of the home and family environment. They promote community engagement, education, and the establishment of supportive networks to ensure comprehensive physical, emotional, and psychosocial care and support is accessible within the community, providing comfort and assistance during difficult times.

A child with a life-limiting or life-threatening condition and the death of a child in any society have a profound impact on their family, friends, neighbours and community (Collins et al., 2016). This impact will last for many years; and as Bowlby's (1980) work on attachment identified, for the siblings, this may affect them for the rest of their lives. Dying and death, loss and grief are everyone's business yet some people, including some professionals, may find it uncomfortable to talk about and acknowledge the death of an adult, and even more so of a child.

---

**LEARNING ACTIVITY**

Reflect on your own beliefs about dying and death, and how they may impact on the care that you provide.

---

In children's palliative care, stakeholders working together can ensure that children living with palliative care needs receive equitable access to care, educational opportunities and social inclusion. Non-medical supportive services such as respite care, counselling and bereavement support play a crucial role in alleviating the physical, emotional and practical burdens experienced by families.

Many children can live for years with a life-limiting or life-threatening condition and compassionate communities can raise community awareness of the issues facing families following such a diagnosis. This promotes participation in the ongoing care and support of children and their families, as well as helping families access services they may not be aware of. Additionally, it underscores the need for collaborative and child-centred care that involves healthcare professionals, patients, families, and the broader community. In the specific context of palliative care for children and young people, compassionate communities through a public health approach aim to bring necessary support directly into their homes by building a network of community support (Carter et al., 2014). By leveraging community resources and fostering collaboration, this approach strives to meet the diverse needs of these children and their families. It recognises the significance of the home environment and works to ensure that comprehensive care and support are accessible within the community, providing comfort and assistance during difficult times.

In a compassionate community for children needing palliative and end-of-life care, it is recognised that the following conditions are needed:

1. *Dying and death are everyone's concern*: The community recognises that dying and death impact individuals, families, friends, the wider community and professionals. Open conversations and education about death are promoted to support those going through these experiences.
2. *All children have equal value and equal rights*: Compassionate communities understand that every child, regardless of their condition or circumstances, has inherent value and rights that should be respected.

3. *A community-wide approach*: Communities understand the importance of creating solidarity in a sense of belonging, understanding and empathy. They encourage individuals, families, neighbours and various organisations to offer to provide a network of support that goes beyond medical interventions. This includes emotional support, compassion, spiritual care and practical assistance to children and their families throughout illness, death, or bereavement, creating positive experiences along the way.

4. *Complementing professional support*: Compassionate communities recognise that professional support is most effective when combined with the involvement of the wider community. Community members and professionals work collaboratively to ensure the provision of care that is additional to the family care, for example, offering social connections and practical help, to enhance the overall well-being of children and their families. Community support (from professionals and community members) supplements the care given by families, it does not replace the key parental roles and responsibilities in caring for their children. This approach also helps to empower parents to ask for help and support.

5. *Understanding of the social determinants of health*: Beaune et al. (2013) suggest that there should be an assessment of the socio-economic and demographic characteristics of communities to improve access to care, exploring the impact of physical and social environments on health and well-being and the social determinants of health. This recognises the social aspects of illness and dying and will underpin the work of nurses in preventing suffering and illness within the community. Compassionate communities actively involve community members in decision-making processes to contribute to the design and delivery of supportive services.

6. *Collective and social action for positive, sustainable change*: Compassionate communities take collective action to address systemic issues and create sustainable change. They advocate for radical changes in policy, infrastructure and societal norms to create improved social justice, policy reforms, raise awareness about the importance of children's palliative care, and support initiatives that promote community well-being. Training programmes cater to the specific needs of children, young people and adults. By working together, individuals and organisations can shape societal attitudes and structures to foster a more compassionate and supportive community for children needing end-of-life care. Box 1.3 presents a good practice example from Brazil.

---

**LEARNING ACTIVITY**

Reflect on how you would discuss this approach with families as you seek to involve the wider community.

---

**BOX 1.3 A GOOD PRACTICE EXAMPLE FROM BRAZIL**

In 2018, palliative care was introduced in the Rocinha and Vidigal favelas (slum areas) in Rio de Janeiro, led by Alexandre Silva, from the Federal University of São João del-Rei in Minas Gerais, Brazil.

Silva emphasised the importance of a multi-disciplinary team approach, involving healthcare professionals from various specialties during monthly patient visits. The initiative goes beyond healthcare professionals and actively involves community members who receive training and resources to serve as volunteer caregivers. The initiative is built upon strong community bonds, with active participation from community members who receive training and resources to serve as volunteers. These caregivers provide comprehensive support to patients (including children), addressing their physical, psychological, social, and spiritual needs. They also act as intermediaries with the local public healthcare system, ensuring access to necessary medication, food and hygiene materials (Silva et al., 2021).

Successful experiences in Rocinha and Vidigal have encouraged the expansion of the project to other communities. Notably, a project has been underway since September 2021 in the Cabana do Pai Tomás favela in Belo Horizonte.

---

## THE ROLE OF NURSES IN BUILDING A COMPASSIONATE COMMUNITY

The child who is not expected to live until adulthood has the right to live life fully enjoying the benefits of relationships and fulfilment. This entails recognising the social aspects of illness and dying, prioritising the child within the community, and valuing the knowledge and contributions of local communities alongside professional expertise. These principles require nurses to do the following:

- Acknowledge that illness and dying have social dimensions and implications beyond the individual.
- Place a focus on the child within the context of their family and community.
- Recognise the significance of local knowledge from communities in addition to the specialised knowledge of professionals in areas such as healthcare, social care and education.

Nurses play a multi-faceted, pivotal role in implementing a public health approach to children's palliative care, contributing to the improvement of care quality, accessibility, and the establishment of a supportive environment for children and families facing life-limiting conditions. Through their expertise, advocacy and collaborative efforts, nurses shape policies, raise awareness and ensure comprehensive care for children in need. For a nurse caring for children with palliative care needs, applying a public health approach involves:

1. *Facilitating understanding and support*: by helping society better understand the unique needs of children with life-limiting conditions and their families,

raising awareness and advocating for these children, nurses help foster a sense of recognition and support for them as valued members of the community.

2. *Mitigating social isolation*: Nurses work to reduce the social isolation faced by children with life-limiting conditions and their families by connecting them with supportive resources, networks and community services. By facilitating social connections and providing emotional support, nurses contribute to creating a more inclusive environment for these children and their families.

3. *Promoting normalisation of dying and death*: Dying and death are natural processes. Nurses help individuals and communities develop a more realistic and compassionate view of these experiences and understanding of death through education, open discussions and addressing misconceptions. By normalising these topics, nurses empower individuals to approach them with greater resilience and understanding.

4. *Empowering skills development*: The development of necessary skills to navigate the challenges of palliative care through education, open discussions and addressing misconceptions, helps to empower and safeguard children and families, sometimes the nurse may be the primary trainer, other times the nurse can collaborate with other professionals and community members to implement training programmes. Nurses' expertise and support ensure that the training aligns with the specific needs of children living with palliative care needs and their families.

5. *Safeguarding*: While appropriate safeguards should be in place, this should not become a barrier that prevents a valuable and potentially considerable level of support to be offered to families. At the same time, compassionate communities provide nurses with a unique opportunity to work within local communities, and this can help identify those who are at risk of abuse and neglect, but the changed nature of professional-public relationships may also present barriers if the community is afraid to share information or feel that they are being scrutinised. In all cases, the nurse must ensure that the child's welfare is paramount. Other family members may also be vulnerable to abuse and exploitation and may need help and support to protect themselves.

It is important to note that while there is limited evidence on the application of the public health approach in palliative care for children and young people nurses can play a crucial role in exploring and advancing this field. They can contribute to the development of knowledge, research and best practices, ensuring that the public health approach is tailored to meet the specific needs of children and their families.

We propose a systems-level model framework (see Figure 1.2) for the different layers of public health approaches for a child requiring palliative care and their family. A systems-level model framework for the delivery of palliative care for children integrates different layers of public health approaches, namely the micro, meso and macro levels (Hasselaar and Payne, 2016):

- *Micro-level* care is focused on the individual child and their family, providing tailored support and addressing their physical, emotional and spiritual needs.

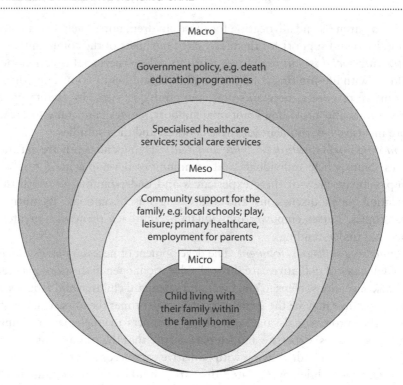

**FIGURE 1.2** Systems levels, micro to macro

Source: adapted from Fulop and Roberts (2015).

- *Meso-level* involves co-ordination and collaboration among organisations and community-based services to ensure comprehensive care and smooth transitions.
- *Macro-level* addresses policy development, system-level interventions, and public health approaches to promote equitable access and quality care (Hasselaar and Payne, 2016).

The public health approach integrates palliative care principles into broader strategies, while compassionate communities emphasise community support and holistic care. By combining these approaches, attempts can be made to improve access, enhance community engagement and promote well-being for children and families facing serious illnesses. This approach recognises that friends, family and social networks play a significant role in providing care during end-of-life and grief.

## Micro level

Nurses directly interact with children receiving palliative care and their families, by providing personalised nursing care and co-ordinating services. Nurses ensure that families have access to the necessary support and resources by serving as case managers and helping them navigate the healthcare system. By conducting thorough assessments, they identify physical, emotional, social and spiritual needs and develop comprehensive care plans. Throughout the palliative care journey, nurses offer ongoing support and interventions to address these needs and provide education and guidance to families.

Linebarger et al. (2022) identified that prevention and early intervention are important aspects of children's palliative care, and nurses actively engage in these areas. They educate families about healthy lifestyle choices, disease prevention and early signs of health problems. By identifying risk factors and potential health issues early on, nurses can intervene promptly and provide appropriate support and resources.

Grief and bereavement support is a significant aspect of compassionate communities, and nurses play a crucial role in providing emotional support and guidance to families during the end-of-life phase and beyond. By offering comfort, reassurance and age-appropriate explanations, nurses help children process their feelings and develop coping mechanisms. In addition, nurses offer creative activities to children in palliative care, such as art, music or drama, to promote their social and emotional development. These activities provide opportunities for self-expression, boost self-esteem, and help children explore their emotions in a positive and therapeutic way.

## Meso level

Nurses contribute to building compassionate communities by promoting education and awareness. They raise awareness about children's palliative care, dispel misconceptions and provide age-appropriate education to children, helping them understand illness and death in a supportive manner. Nurses also work towards normalising dying and death by engaging in conversations about end-of-life care and facilitating discussions within the community. They empower individuals by helping them develop coping skills and navigate challenging situations associated with palliative care

Nurses can also create supportive environments such as organising events, supporting groups and activities that foster social connections and understanding within the community. By reducing social isolation and promoting inclusivity, nurses help build a network of support for families facing children's palliative care. Nurses also amplify the voices of children living with palliative care needs, ensuring their perspectives are heard and valued. They collaborate with community leaders and stakeholders to raise awareness about the unique needs of these children and advocate for their inclusion in community activities and services.

## Macro level

Nurses expand their role in building compassionate communities by engaging in public health and policy initiatives. They actively participate in policy development by sharing their expertise and insights, advocating for the inclusion of children's palliative care in public health policies, and contributing to the creation of guidelines that support quality care. Nurses can collaborate with stakeholders from various sectors, including healthcare professionals, policymakers, researchers, educators and community leaders. By working together, they address complex healthcare challenges, develop innovative solutions, and contribute to the development of comprehensive and patient-centred care models.

Research and evidence-based practice are important aspects of nursing at the macro level. Nurses contribute to generating new knowledge, conducting research studies, and evaluating the effectiveness of interventions. By utilising research findings, they advocate for evidence-based practices and contribute to the improvement of healthcare services for individuals with palliative care needs. Nurses also raise awareness by providing education and training to healthcare professionals, community leaders and the public.

Nurses with strong leadership skills play a crucial role in engaging colleagues, identifying policy levers, and leveraging available resources. Standardising intervention and data collection processes is important, but nurses should also consider individual experiences in their evaluation methods. To prevent palliative care from becoming solely a technical specialty, nurses must actively acknowledge and address these challenges, promoting transparency and collective moral responsibility.

Research indicates that there are strategic challenges associated with translating community forums into action, including the establishment of community partnerships, the collection of local information, and the adaptation of frameworks to suit local contexts (Kothari and Armstrong, 2011). These challenges highlight the complexities involved in implementing interventions within communities and reinforce the need for careful attention to how partnerships are formed, for knowledge gathering, and for changes to ensure successful adoption and integration of interventions within community-based settings.

---

**LEARNING ACTIVITY**

While understanding the concept of public health palliative care, do you feel uncomfortable about this approach for children and young people? If so, how would you manage your anxiety?

---

## COPING WITH THE CHALLENGES IN BUILDING COMPASSIONATE COMMUNITIES

Nurses also face various challenges when engaging the community in compassionate communities for children's palliative care. These challenges include limited community participation, power imbalances, trust issues, communication barriers and resource constraints. To overcome these challenges, nurses need to facilitate open dialogue, demonstrate cultural sensitivity, and respect diverse perspectives on death. They must also address complexities related to data collection, sustainability and finding the right balance between top-down and community-driven approaches.

Nurses need to cultivate a range of key skills and qualities to provide compassionate support to children and families living with palliative care needs These include empathy, active listening, effective communication, collaboration and teamwork, advocacy, self-awareness, emotional resilience, cultural competence and sensitivity, education and teaching, flexibility and adaptability, and a commitment to respect and dignity.

It is important that nurses continuously reflect on their own biases, values, and beliefs to ensure they provide unbiased and patient-centred care. Self-awareness is crucial for palliative care nurses when reflecting on their beliefs, attitudes and understanding of personal and community responses to death in childhood. By exploring their cultural, religious and societal influences, nurses can provide more empathetic and culturally sensitive care. This helps nurses navigate potential conflicts and tailor their approach to meet the unique needs of each child and family.

Emotional resilience allows nurses to support families through challenging situations while maintaining their own well-being and staying updated with advances in the field.

Nurses can also take advantage of existing community development programmes and modules available globally and virtually (e.g. https://www.elearnicpcn.org/, https://thewhpca.org/resources/ and https://hospicecare.com). These resources can enhance nurses' skills in working with communities and further support efforts in promoting a public health approach to children's palliative care.

In palliative care, it is important to recognise that cultural norms and traditions can significantly influence decision-making processes, especially when it comes to healthcare choices. For example, in certain cultures, the responsibility of making important healthcare decisions may rest solely with designated family members, often the eldest male. This dynamic can sometimes lead to communication breakdowns within the context of the examination room. It is crucial for nurses to be aware of these cultural dynamics. They should understand that a female family member who appears hesitant or resistant to accepting treatment might be deferring the decision-making process to a husband or son who is not present at that moment. Without this understanding, a nurse might misinterpret the situation and fail to effectively address the patient's needs.

To provide optimal children's palliative care, nurses must approach these situations with cultural sensitivity and open-mindedness. They should strive to create a safe and inclusive environment where patients feel comfortable expressing their concerns and discussing their cultural beliefs and values. By actively listening and engaging with both the patient and their family, nurses can gain a deeper understanding of the decision-making dynamics at play and ensure that all voices are heard and respected.

Collaboration with interpreters or cultural mediators, if available, can also be beneficial in bridging communication gaps and facilitating discussions between healthcare providers and patients from diverse cultural backgrounds. By embracing cultural competence and being mindful of cultural norms and values, nurses in palliative care can navigate these challenges and work towards providing patient-centred care that respects the individual's autonomy and dignity while honouring their cultural traditions and preferences.

Effective communication skills allow nurses to convey information, educate and engage with various audiences. Collaboration and teamwork are essential for working with interdisciplinary teams to develop comprehensive care plans. Nurses should prioritise education and continuous professional development to stay updated with advances in their field, enabling them to provide accurate and evidence-based information. Flexibility and adaptability are essential traits as they recognise and address the unique needs and preferences of each individual and family. Upholding principles of respect and dignity, they ensure that patients and families are treated with compassion and maintain their autonomy.

Children who are experiencing the illness or loss of a loved one need emotional support to help them process their feelings and cope with their grief. Creating safe spaces is an important strategy to promote their emotional and social well-being and can help them to develop the resilience they need to navigate difficult circumstances. Nurses should recognise the important role that families play in safeguarding their children, but the families may need support and information to be able to make safe choices for their children, for example, how to ensure access to virtual platforms and activities.

This is a considerable expectation, but it is important to remember that it does not have to be one individual carrying out all activities. Many of the ways that nurses can respond to these challenges, and the challenges themselves, are discussed throughout this book.

---

**LEARNING ACTIVITY**

How can you use your skills and experience to enable and empower children, young people and their families, to be involved in developing compassionate communities?

---

## APPROACHES TO BUILDING A COMPASSIONATE COMMUNITY

Building a compassionate community should ensure that those whose voices are less often heard are sought out and listened to, so that children have a voice and a viewpoint. Even if they struggle with language, it is important to listen to their words, watching their actions and provide opportunities to hear their views, such as through play or creative activities.

Nurses play a crucial role in creating a compassionate community, particularly in the healthcare sector. Their unique position as caregivers and advocates, ensuring that the voices and preferences of individuals and communities are heard and respected within the healthcare system, positions them to contribute significantly to the four-phase process of creating a Compassionate Community (Armstrong, 2009) (see Table 1.1).

**TABLE 1.1** Nurses' contribution to the four phases of creating a compassionate community (Armstrong, 2009)

| Phase | Definition |
| --- | --- |
| 1. Discover and Assess | • Nurses can actively engage with patients, families, and community members to understand their healthcare needs, challenges and concerns. They can gather data, conduct assessments, and participate in community health needs assessments to identify gaps and areas for improvement. <br>• Recognise existing assets and efforts: Nurses can collaborate with other healthcare professionals and community organisations to identify existing healthcare resources, programmes and initiatives. They can acknowledge the successes and contributions made by individuals and organisations in addressing healthcare needs in the community. |
| 2. Focus and Commit | • Narrow down focus areas: Nurses can participate in interdisciplinary teams and community forums to discuss and prioritise healthcare issues that require compassionate action. Their clinical expertise and understanding of community needs can help inform the selection of priority areas for intervention. <br>• Set goals and define priorities: Nurses can contribute to the goal-setting process by providing insights and evidence-based recommendations on healthcare interventions. They can advocate for the inclusion of healthcare access, equity and patient-centred care as core components of the compassionate community's objectives. |
| 3. Build and Launch | • Develop and implement initiatives: Nurses can collaborate with other healthcare professionals, community organisations and policymakers to develop programmes that focus on prevention, health promotion, and improving healthcare access. <br>• Engage the community: Nurses can engage through health education programmes, outreach activities and support networks. They can provide health screenings, preventive care services and counselling to promote well-being and foster a compassionate healthcare environment. <br>• Build partnerships: Nurses can foster collaborations between healthcare institutions, community organisations and social service agencies to create a network of support that addresses the healthcare needs of the community. They can actively participate in interdisciplinary teams and community-based organisations to ensure comprehensive and co-ordinated care. |

*(Continued)*

**TABLE 1.1** Nurses' contribution to the four phases of creating a compassionate community (Armstrong, 2009) *(Continued)*

| Phase | Definition |
| --- | --- |
| 4. Evaluate and Sustain | • Evaluate effectiveness: Nurses collect and analyse healthcare data, monitor health outcomes, and assess the impact of healthcare interventions. They can identify areas of improvement and propose changes to ensure the effectiveness of compassionate healthcare initiatives. <br> • Reflect and adjust: Nurses can engage in reflective practice and continuous learning to enhance their own compassionate care skills and practices. They can share their experiences and insights with colleagues and contribute to the development of best practices in compassionate healthcare. <br> • Establish sustainability systems: Nurses advocate for policies that prioritise healthcare access, equity, and quality, and contribute to the development of guidelines and protocols that foster compassionate care. |

## WHAT IMPACT DO COMPASSIONATE COMMUNITIES HAVE ON CHILDREN, YOUNG PEOPLE AND FAMILIES?

Compassionate communities can help provide the support and safe spaces the child needs to live a full life, as well as emotional and practical support for family members to help navigate the complex challenges associated with specialist palliative care services, as and when required. The prioritisation of the well-being and care of children with life-limiting or life-threatening conditions and their families, raising community awareness about palliative care, dying, death and bereavement, and encouraging the community's active participation in their care and support will enable the nurse to perform the following:

- The normalisation of conversations about dying, death and bereavement, removing the taboo around these subjects within society (this is considered further in Chapter 3).
- Improved management and support for children.
- Re-orienting palliative care to co-production, with health and social care staff working with children and families, carers and communities in equal partnership at all stages of service design, development and evaluation.

Compassionate communities empower individuals and families by involving them in decision-making processes and respecting their preferences, promoting a sense of agency and control. Inclusion is a vital aspect of compassionate communities, fostering acceptance and openness for every community member, including marginalised groups, and combating stigma and misconceptions surrounding children's palliative care.

Volunteers and community organisations play a crucial role in compassionate communities, offering practical assistance, emotional support, and companionship to children and their families. They can bridge gaps in service provision and provide respite for families. These communities also recognise the needs of the entire family unit, providing emotional and practical support to siblings and parents who face significant challenges. By fostering connections and creating a sense of belonging, compassionate communities allow families to connect, share experiences, and draw strength from one another.

By implementing the compassionate communities' approach, professionals shift from sole responsibility to shared responsibility with the community, strengthening the healthcare system and improving care for children living with palliative care needs. This collaborative approach uses the resources and expertise of both professionals and community members, leading to more personalised and effective care. It also creates sustainable frameworks for compassionate and supportive care, ensuring that children and their families receive comprehensive support throughout their journey. Holistic and compassionate care becomes a reality for children and families facing serious illness and bereavement.

Compassionate communities can organise support groups, provide counselling services, and facilitate access to specialised healthcare resources. Recognising and valuing the expertise and experiences of community members enables the care provided to be more responsive to the specific needs and challenges faced by children and families. Studies have shown that community-based palliative care can lead to cost savings by reducing hospital admissions, emergency department visits, and unnecessary medical interventions. Providing proactive management of symptoms and timely interventions can help avoid costly crisis-driven care and improve the efficient use of healthcare resources (Yosick et al., 2019).

Actively involving the community ensures that families are supported not only practically but also emotionally and spiritually. The community can provide a network of understanding, empathy and companionship, offering comfort and solace during difficult times. They can also support families to navigate complex decisions, offer guidance on available resources, and advocate for their needs within the broader healthcare system. The involvement of faith groups and religious establishments or civil society organisations enhances emotional, psychological and spiritual support for families.

Views held by communities about children with life-limiting or life-threatening conditions and end-of-life care, including spiritual and religious perspectives, may vary widely. They may be long standing, possibly highly controversial and even potentially violent. Negotiating spiritual and religious beliefs may be challenging and complex but the beliefs often play a significant role in how communities approach end-of-life care, providing comfort, guidance and rituals. Negotiation will involve actively listening, promoting open communication, and understanding and respecting diverse cultural and religious backgrounds. Collaborating with faith leaders and spiritual counsellors, incorporating meaningful rituals and practices, and providing access to supportive resources are essential. Education and training, interdisciplinary collaboration and ensuring continuity of care contribute to addressing the spiritual needs of individuals and families. By integrating spiritual care into the fabric of a compassionate community, meaningful support can be provided during challenging times.

Creating a compassionate community in palliative care requires collaboration and partnership among healthcare providers, community organisations, and individuals and families. This includes engaging and involving everyone in the community, including marginalised groups who may face barriers to accessing care. The inclusion of a community voice is crucial in fostering a compassionate community where empathy, understanding, and collaboration thrive. Community members can be involved in participatory decision-making, shaping policies and programmes, needs assessment and asset mapping to identify community strengths and resources.

## THE ESSENTIAL COMPONENTS REQUIRED TO ESTABLISH COMPASSIONATE COMMUNITIES FOR CHILDREN

Establishing a compassionate community for children with palliative care needs involves working closely with care providers and integrating various essential components to provide comprehensive, responsive and dynamic support and care. The following are essential components in establishing compassionate communities for children:

1.  *Specialised children's palliative care programmes and home-based services* that address the unique needs of children and their families. These programmes offer medical care, pain and symptom management, psychosocial and spiritual support, and respite care, ensuring holistic care and maintaining a sense of normalcy for the children. Financial assistance schemes, where they exist, help alleviate the financial burden on families, covering medical expenses and necessary resources.
2.  *Emotional and social support.* Counselling, psychosocial services and support groups play a crucial role in helping children and families cope with the challenges of palliative care. Sibling support programmes recognise the needs of siblings, while bereavement support services provide essential assistance after the loss of a child.
3.  *Advocacy campaigns* raise awareness, reduce stigma, and advocate for improved access to palliative care services. While many individuals express compassion and a desire to support these children and their families, others may experience fear or discomfort and may avoid the topic.
4.  *Promote education, understanding, and empathy* within communities to create a compassionate and inclusive environment for these children and their families. Addressing fears, challenging stigmas, and providing necessary resources and support are essential in honouring the unique needs and beliefs of these children during their end-of-life journey.
5.  *Practical assistance and community connections.* Respite care offers temporary relief to parents and caregivers, while educational support ensures continuity in the child's education.
6.  *Spiritual support.* When facing an existential crisis, such as having a child with a life-limiting or life-threatening condition, spirituality often comes to the fore. This can either come as a challenge to an existing faith or as a prompt to explore a deeper meaning of life. Spiritual grief crosses many faith traditions and rituals

(typically in diverse communities). Faith communities can offer support through spiritual guidance, counselling, and support to individuals and families based on their cultural and religious beliefs. Those with no faith require equal support and this could also be offered through other community networks (e.g. death cafés).

7. *Effective communication* facilitates the sharing of knowledge, critical thinking, and informed decision-making, enabling individuals to take an active role in their own care and well-being.

8. *Safeguarding children* requires collaboration among healthcare professionals, social workers, educators, family members, and other relevant stakeholders. Information sharing and joint decision-making are essential for effective care provision.

9. *Death literacy* is an essential component of compassionate communities, as it equips individuals with the knowledge and skills necessary to understand and act upon end-of-life and death care options. It enables people to make informed decisions, engage in meaningful conversations, and provide support to those nearing the end-of-life while fostering a culture that embraces compassionate care and empowers individuals to navigate the complexities of dying and death.

10. *Empowering marginalised individuals and communities* through education, capacity-building, and advocacy can help amplify their voices and enhance their participation. For example, children and families affected by HIV/AIDS face socio-economic challenges such as poverty, limited employment opportunities, educational barriers and housing instability. Comprehensive support is needed, including access to healthcare, education and income-generating opportunities, reducing stigma and discrimination, providing counselling and mental health support, spiritual support and fostering supportive communities. Collaboration among healthcare providers, social workers, and community organisations is essential in addressing these challenges.

## SOME IMPORTANT THEMES TO BE CONSIDERED IN TRAINING PROGRAMMES

- Resilience and taking care of yourself
- Effective communication
- Emotional intelligence
- Safeguarding children and young people and vulnerable adults
- Confidence
- End-of-life care
- Death literacy
- Nursing aspects of caring
- Grief and bereavement
- Available public, social and spiritual support systems
- Cultural awareness and appreciation
- Learning to express empathy, when appropriate.

Box 1.4 presents two good practice examples from the UK.

---

**BOX 1.4 GOOD PRACTICE EXAMPLES FROM THE UK**

*Cannock Chase's Compassionate Communities Network* includes individuals from the National Health Service, voluntary and community sector and Local district and county council working with the community to provide and facilitate support for those affected by life-threatening illness, chronic disability, grief and bereavement (ehospice, 2023).

Some of the highlights of the projects were:

- Two bereavement charities for children, young people and parents and bereavement training for schools.
- The Places of Welcome network – drop-in cafés where people can feel safe, belong and contribute (see https://www.lichfield.anglican.org/about-us/strengthening-communities/).
- Inspiring Healthy Lifestyles, which offers sports, outdoor recreation and creative activities to support physical health and wellbeing (see https://inspiringhealthylifestyles.org/about-us/).
- Memorials, memorial services and gardens, which give people a private space to reflect and grieve.
- Fiveways Ramblers, a group which encourages friendship and reduces isolation by meeting weekly for walks and social activities.

*Good Life, Good Death, Good Grief* is a project in Scotland that is addressing how to create a country where everyone knows how to help when someone is dying or grieving. A number of resources and a toolkit have been developed to support practice (Scottish Partnership for Palliative Care, 2011).

---

Box 1.5 presents a good practice example from India.

---

**BOX 1.5 A GOOD PRACTICE EXAMPLE FROM INDIA**

The Children's Palliative Care Project of the Department of Palliative Medicine, Tata Memorial Centre, Mumbai, has started a collaborative project at three general hospitals for children with life-limiting conditions (Indian Association of Palliative Care, 2021).

A needs assessment survey identified the number of children requiring children's palliative care by visiting the children's outpatients departments at the hospitals. It also identified that the families had huge social and financial needs in addition to medical needs, and most of the families are from lower socio-economic backgrounds.

The team at each centre networks with non-governmental organisations (NGOs), special schools, women's groups and local organisations. They have conducted short awareness programmes to help the community recognise children needing support, to create a system to get social and financial help to families in need and to introduce the concept of palliative care.

---

Some NGOs provide free skill-development programmes such as tailoring, beautician courses and auto-rickshaw driving to empower female caregivers of children with chronic conditions. One has started free tuition classes for children in slums and another has agreed to appoint a speech therapist so that the families do not have to pay fees for private provision. College students collect toys and books for the children and participate in support group meetings and diversion activities.

As patients come from faraway places, the projects have networked with the local NGOs and community leaders to help the families to access medicines, blood transfusions and urgent medical intervention. They also help in finding children to follow up cases and help school dropouts to re-join their studies. Local networking seems to work as they understand the communities better and can help in a more effective manner.

In the rural tribal area of Jawhar, situated in the Maharashtra region of India, local communities were able to help special needs children with basic education and other social needs.

## SUMMARY

Compassionate communities prioritise empathy, kindness, and compassion towards others. Adopting a compassionate communities' approach in children's palliative care requires recognition of the importance of collective involvement and shared responsibility by professionals and community members. It acknowledges that everyone has the capacity to play active and supportive roles when children are living with palliative care needs. By fostering a compassionate and supportive environment within the community, the burden on a few individuals, such as family members or healthcare professionals, is lessened. This approach encourages community members to provide emotional support, practical assistance, and companionship to children and their families. The active engagement of the community creates a holistic and comprehensive approach to children's palliative care, enhancing the well-being of children and their families.

## KEY POINTS

- Dying, death, loss and grief are everyone's business, but sometimes we over-professionalise palliative care.
- Everyone has the capacity to play an active and supportive role within compassionate communities.
- Nurses have important skills and knowledge to share with compassionate communities in children's palliative care.
- Compassionate communities in children's palliative care promote an understanding that dying and death are normal and empower people to develop the skills they will need to deal with these issues as they go through life.
- Compassionate communities can help society to better understand the needs of children who live with palliative care needs and their families and help communities "see" these children and support them as part of the community and help to reduce the social isolation of the children and their families.

## SUGGESTED READING

Abel, J., Kellehear, A. (2016). Palliative care reimagined: A needed shift. *BMJ Supportive & Palliative Care*, 6(1), 21–26. https://doi.org/10.1136/bmjspcare-2015-001009

Abel, J., Kellehear, A. (eds) (2022). *Oxford textbook of public health palliative care*. Oxford University Press.

Community Tool Box (n.d.). Other models for promoting community health and development | Section 16. building compassionate communities. Available at: https://ctb.ku.edu/en/table-of-contents/overview/models-for-community-health-and-development/building-compassionate-communities/main (accessed 10 June 2024).

Heaps, K., Shaw, N., Richardson, H., Devlin, J. (2021). P-228 Compassionate neighbours sharing power and resources with communities to drive better end-of-life care. *BMJ Supportive & Palliative Care*, 11(Suppl. 2), A91–A92. Available at: https://doi.org/10.1136/spcare-2021-Hospice.243

Kellehear, A. (2005). *Compassionate cities: Public health and end-of-life care* (1st edn). Routledge.

Sallnow, L. (2016). The impact of a new public health approach to end-of-life care: A systematic review. *Palliative Medicine*, 30(3), 200–211. https://doi.org/10.1177/0269216315599869

Sallnow, L., Paul, S. (2015). Understanding community engagement in end-of-life care: Developing conceptual clarity. *Critical Public Health*. http://dx.doi.org/10.1080/09581596.2014.909582

## REFERENCES

Abel, J., Kellehear, A. (eds) (2022). *Oxford textbook of public health palliative care*. Oxford University Press.

Armstrong, K. (2009). The Charter for Compassion. Available at: https://charterforcompassion.org/ (accessed 10 June 2024).

Beaune, L., Morinis, J., Rapoport, A., Bloch, G., Levinn, L., Ford-Jones, L., Chapman, L. A., Shaul, R. Z., Ing, S., Andrews, K. (2013). Paediatric palliative care and social determinants of health: Mitigating the impact of urban poverty on children with life-limiting illnesses. *Paediatric Child Health*, 18(4), 181–183. https://doi.org/10.1093%2Fpch%2F18.4.181

Bluebond-Langner, M., Belasco, J. B., Goldman, A., Belasco, C. (2007). Understanding parents' approaches to care and treatment of children with cancer when standard therapy has failed. *Journal of Clinical Oncology*, 25(17), 2414–2419. https://doi.org/10.1200/JCO.2006.08.7759

Bowlby, J. (1980). *Attachment and loss*. Vol. 3: *Loss, sadness and depression*. Basic Books.

Carter, B., Bray, L., Dickinson A., Edwards, M., Ford, K. (2014). *Child-centred nursing: Promoting critical thinking*. Sage Publications Ltd.

Centre for Empowerment & Enrichment. (2024). Welcome to New Hope of Life. Available at: http://cefee.org/ (accessed 8 February 2024).

Collins, A., Hennessy-Anderson, N., Hosking, S., Hynson, J., Remedios, C., Thomas, K. (2016). Lived experiences of parents caring for a child with a life-limiting condition in Australia: A qualitative study. *Palliative Medicine*, 30(10), 950–959. https://doi.org/10.1177/0269216316634245

Dickens, A. P., Richards, S. H., Greaves, C. J., Campbell, J. L. (2011). Interventions targeting social isolation in older people: A systematic review. *BMC Public Health*, 11, 647. https://doi.org/10.1186/1471-2458-11-647

ehospice (2023). Cannock Chase District Council is celebrating being awarded Compassionate Community status. Available at: https://ehospice.com/uk_posts/cannock-chase-district-council-is-celebrating-being-awarded-compassionate-community-status/ (accessed 8 February 2024).

Fonseca, A., Nazaré, B., Canavarro, M. C. (2012). Parental psychological distress and quality of life after a prenatal or postnatal diagnosis of congenital anomaly: A controlled comparison study with parents of healthy infants. *Disability and Health Journal*, 5(2), 67–74. https://doi.org/10.1016/j.dhjo.2011.11.001.

Fulop, N., Roberts, G. (2015). Context for successful quality improvement. The Health Foundation. Available at: https://www.health.org.uk/sites/default/files/ContextForSuccessfulQualityImprovement.pdf (accessed 10 June 2024).

Graham-Wisener, L., Nelson, B., Byrne, A., Islam, I., Harrison, C., Geddis, J., Berry, E. (2022). Understanding public attitudes to death talk and advance care planning in Northern Ireland using health behaviour change theory: A qualitative study. *BMC Public Health*, 22(1), 906. https://doi.org/10.1186/s12889-022-13319-1

Hasselaar, J., Payne, S. (2016). Moving the integration of palliative care from idea to practice. *Palliative Medicine*, 30(3), 197–199. https://doi.org/10.1177/0269216315626039

Indian Association of Palliative Care. (2021). Children's palliative care projects in Maharashtra and Goa. Available at: https://www.palliativecare.in/childrens-palliative-care-projects-in-maharashtra-and-goa/ (accessed 8 February 2024).

Kase, S. M., Waldman, E. D., Weintraub, A. S. (2019). A cross-sectional pilot study of compassion fatigue, burnout, and compassion satisfaction in pediatric palliative care providers in the United States. *Palliative & Supportive Care*, 17(3), 269–275. https://doi.org/10.1017/S1478951517001237

Kellehear, A. (2005). *Compassionate cities: Public health and end-of-life care* (1st edition). Routledge.

Kothari, A., Armstrong, R. (2011). Community-based knowledge translation: unexplored opportunities. *Implementation Science*, 6, 59. https://doi.org/10.1186/1748-5908-6-59

Kroll, M. M. (2022). Prolonged social isolation and loneliness are equivalent to smoking 15 cigarettes a day. Available at; https://extension.unh.edu/blog/2022/05/prolonged-social-isolation-loneliness-are-equivalent-smoking-15-cigarettes-day (accessed 11 June 2024).

Linebarger, J. S, Johnson, V., Boss, R. D. (2022). Guidance for pediatric end-of-life care. *Pediatrics*, 149(5), e2022057011. https://doi.org/10.1542/peds.2022-057011

*Merrian Webster Dictionary*. (2024). Compassion. https://www.merriam-webster.com/dictionary/compassion#:~:text=%3A%20sympathetic%20consciousness%20of%20others'%20distress,a%20desire%20to%20alleviate%20it (accessed 10 June 2024).

Mills, J., Abel, J., Kellehear, A., Patel, M. (2021). Access to palliative care: The primacy of public health partnerships and community participation. *The Lancet Public Health*, 6(11), e791–e792. https://doi.org/10.1016/S2468-2667(21)00213-9

Randall, D. C. (2017). Two futures: Financial and practical realities for parents of living with a life-limited child. *Comprehensive Child and Adolescent Nursing*, 40(4), 257–267. https://doi.org/10.1080/24694193.2017.1376360

Scottish Partnership for Palliative Care. (2011). Good life, good death, good grief. Available at: https://www.palliativecarescotland.org.uk/content/good-life-good-death-good-grie/ (accessed 8 February 2024).

Silva, A. E., Coelho, F. B. P., Pereira, F. M. S., de Castro, I. C., Braga, L. S., Menezes, M. F., Mesquita, P. S., Martins, R. M. R., Riberio, S. A., Carvalho, T. V. (2021). Cuidados paliativos em favelas no Brasil: Uma revisão integrativa. *Research, Society and Development*, 10(6), e55110616183–e55110616183. https://doi.org/10.33448/rsd-v10i6.16183

Stjernswärd, J., Foley, K. M., Ferris, F. D. (2007). The public health strategy for palliative care. *Journal of Pain and Symptom Management*, 33(5), 486–493. https://doi.org/10.1016/j.jpainsymman.2007.02.016

Wegleitner, K., Heimerl, K., Kellehear, A. (2015). *Compassionate communities: Case studies from Britain and Europe*. Routledge.

WHO (World Health Organization). (1987). Ottawa Charter for Health Promotion, first International Conference on Health Promotion, Ottawa, 21 November 1986. https://www.who.int/publications-detail-redirect/WH-1987 (accessed 10 June 2024).

WHO (World Health Organization). (2020). State of the world's nursing 2020: Investing in education, jobs and leadership. Available at: https://iris.who.int/bitstream/handle/10665/331677/9789240003279-eng.pdf?sequence=1 (accessed 9 February 2024).

WHO (World Health Organization). (2021). Assessing the development of palliative care worldwide: A set of actionable indicators. Available at: https://www.who.int/publications-detail-redirect/9789240033351 (accessed 9 February 2024).

Yosick, L., Crook, R. E., Gatto, M., Maxwell, T. L., Duncan, I., Ahmed, T., Mackenzie, A. (2019). Effects of a population health community-based palliative care program on cost and utilization. *Journal of Palliative Medicine*, 22(9), 1075–1081. https://doi.org/10.1089/jpm.2018.0489

## CHAPTER 2

# Beliefs, attitudes and values in children's palliative care

......................................

*Alexandra Daniels and Maha Atout*

## INTRODUCTION

In this chapter we discuss the important considerations for all healthcare providers caring for children and families with palliative care needs at the public health level. Education and training are well-established key components of high-quality children's palliative care service provision and aim to provide nurses with essential skills and knowledge, while eliciting a favourable shift in their attitude towards children's palliative care (Downing et al., 2013; WHO, 2014; CPCET, 2020). Nonetheless, meaningful engagement and exploration through skilful communication with the child and family around their beliefs, attitudes and values are required for nurses to deliver care that is respectful and culturally sensitive (Kongnetiman et al., 2008; Semlali et al., 2020; Rapa et al., 2023).

Culture and religion play a significant role in shaping individual and family beliefs, attitudes and values around serious illness and/or the death of a child. In an evolving multicultural society, it is important for nurses working in children's palliative care to understand how these perceptions influence the experience of the child and their informal carer throughout the disease trajectory (Kongnetiman et al., 2008). Thus, cultivating cultural competency in nurses serving culturally diverse communities is vitally important to ensure they respond appropriately to those in their care and improve the quality of care they provide (Monette, 2021).

In this chapter, we address core beliefs, attitudes and values encountered in a children's palliative care context and the reader is encouraged to reflect on their own beliefs, attitudes and values in an attempt to understand how this influences the care they provide. Furthermore, the implications for practice of these perceptions for nurses and informal carers in a children's palliative care context are discussed. The final focus of the chapter discusses ways nurses may support informal carers to overcome these perceptions with the aim of framing care in a positive way that enhances

DOI: 10.4324/9781003384861-4

the quality of life of children and their families. Learning is enhanced through the inclusion of several learning activities to encourage the reader to examine their own behaviour and practices.

---

**LEARNING OBJECTIVES**

The reader will be able to do the following:

1. Discuss the general public's beliefs, attitudes and values in relation to children's palliative care at the public health level.
2. Reflect on the implications of these perceptions on the child's care for informal carers and nurses.
3. Explore how nurses can engage with informal carers to understand carers' perceptions of palliative care in order to promote positive cultures of communication and practices.

---

## GENERAL PERCEPTIONS OF CHILDREN'S PALLIATIVE CARE AND END-OF-LIFE CARE

Children's palliative care is a care approach that aims to enhance the well-being of children with life-limiting and life-threatening conditions and addresses the challenges faced by their families from diagnosis to the end of life. It involves early detection, thorough evaluation, and strategic interventions to alleviate the physical, psychological and spiritual distress experienced by children and their families (Doherty and Thabet, 2018; Vig et al., 2021).

The terms "children's palliative care" and "end-of-life care" on occasion are used by some nurses interchangeably. This confusion may lead to children's palliative care being incorporated late in the progression of the disease, for example, during the end-of-life stages of the child's illness (Salins et al., 2022). The disparity between the concept of children's palliative care and practice has led to unfavourable perceptions of children's palliative care alongside frequently identified obstacles to its prompt integration.

While initially the concept of palliative care focused on reducing end-of-life suffering, the concept of palliative care, and in particular children's palliative care, has evolved to address the requirements of individuals who may not be considered terminally ill, but for whom the relief of suffering and enhancement of quality of life are essential (Winger et al., 2022). However, this association of palliative care with death has contributed to parents and healthcare professionals perceiving children's palliative care negatively since it could indicate that the child's death is imminent (Wallerstedt et al., 2019). This was highlighted in a recent study that explored the concept of children's palliative care from the viewpoint of healthcare professionals in three paediatric settings in Norway. Children's palliative care was seen to be a frightening concept, unfamiliar and not meaningful by the health professionals. Moreover, the concept of children's palliative care was seen as connected to the concept of dying and death rather than quality of life (Winger et al., 2022).

Healthcare practitioners have seen that parents hold misconceptions about children's palliative care, perceiving it as mutually exclusive to treatment aimed at cure. Consequently, informal carers often link children's palliative care with giving up (Thompson et al., 2009; Dalberg et al., 2013). Healthcare professionals frequently identify parents' viewpoints as obstacles to the incorporation of children's palliative care, for example, in the management of paediatric cancer (Haines et al., 2018). In their study, Knapp and Thompson (2012) surveyed 303 paediatricians to examine the factors linked to perceived barriers to children's palliative care. The findings indicated that the primary obstacles to referring children for palliative care were the families' reluctance to accept hospice or palliative care and a perception among informal carers that hospice or palliative care implies that healthcare workers are "giving up" on their child. Similarly paediatric oncologists in Switzerland identified operational difficulties in timely integration of children's palliative care, differentiating it from end-of-life care. Participants related these difficulties to the strong stigma associated with the term "children's palliative care" by informal carers, the hesitancy of healthcare professionals to commence counselling at an early stage of the condition, and the cultural and religious backgrounds of patients and their families (De Clercq et al., 2019).

Thus, it is important that these misconceptions of both family members and health professionals are addressed. Twamley et al. (2014) found that the likelihood of referring children and young people with life-limiting and life-threatening conditions to children's palliative care teams can be increased by addressing misconceptions and educating healthcare and social care professionals and families about the benefits that palliative care can provide. Saad et al. (2022) also highlight the importance of providing education and formal assistance for healthcare professionals in order to address misconceptions and improve access to children's palliative care. Alongside formal training, cultivating positive experiences with palliative services can enhance healthcare professionals' positive attitudes and match their practices with the broader philosophy of palliative care, which extends beyond end-of-life care. Moreover, as per the World Health Assembly Resolution (WHO, 2014), it is important that healthcare providers receive comprehensive education and training in the fundamental principles of children's palliative care at the onset of their professional journeys, as well as through continuing and specialist education. It is also essential for services to establish guidelines that guarantee the prompt incorporation of children's palliative care into the comprehensive care strategy for all children with life-limiting and life-threatening conditions. By establishing a connection between the philosophy of children's palliative care, its practical application and the impact on quality of life for both the child and their family, healthcare practitioners will see the clear benefit of early integration of palliative care and have the potential to enhance the quality of life of children and their families, thus enhancing their overall experience at a challenging period.

Alongside the attitudes and beliefs of health professionals it is also essential to address the misconceptions of family members. Some families may resist early explorations or discussions of palliative care, advance decisions regarding the use of life-support interventions and other preparations for a child's anticipated mortality (Saad et al., 2022). Although evidence suggests that most children are aware that they are dying, they may not express their anxieties and concerns to their parents. This could be a result of the message they have received from their parents and society as a whole that discussing such sensitive topics is undesirable or taboo (Atout et al., 2019).

## DYING AND DEATH IN CHILDHOODS

The death and impact of the death of a loved one are distressing for anyone, however, the impact of the death of a child may be perceived as more traumatic and painful than that of an adult. This can be attributed to the concept of reversing the order of our lives (Riches and Dawson, 1996) where parents do not expect their children to die before them. The experience of the death of children can be seen as being unspeakable, which reflects the trauma that occurs before, during and after the death of a child (Campbell et al., 2022).

Work has been undertaken with regards to children's understanding of dying and death and this is discussed in Chapter 3. However, there are many influencing factors on the development of a child's understanding. For example, Bluebond-Langner (1978) contends that even if their patents attempt to conceal it, children are typically aware of their terminal illness and are capable social actors due to the additional experience they have gained from being critically unwell. Ironically, however, children may try to conceal the knowledge of their impending death to protect their parents and therefore conform to societal expectations of dying children.

The research of Bluebond-Langner (1978) has since been supported by a range of studies, including Goldman and Christie, 1993, Clarke et al., 2005, Patenaude, 2005, and Van der Geest et al., 2015, which assert that increasing age alone does not necessarily explain cognitive development. There are several factors, including the child's individual life experiences, that influence their ability to comprehend. Therefore, a more recent perspective concludes that children develop an understanding of death by combining biological reasoning with information from their cultural environment, including religious and spiritual contexts (Harris, 2018). Therefore, children's understanding of death emerges as a result of an interaction between their biological reasoning, spiritual information, experiences with death-related rituals and parental socialisation (Menendez et al., 2020), and they frequently incorporate religious and spiritual beliefs into this perception of death (Astuti and Harris, 2008; Watson-Jones et al., 2017). For example, although children acknowledge the end of physiological and mental processes at death, they nonetheless believe in an afterlife (Harris, 2018; Superdock et al., 2018). This suggests that children may have two views of death: a biological view of the deceased as a corpse and a religious view of the deceased as someone who has passed on but lives on in some form.

To provide optimal palliative care for children, it is important to understand not only their views of death, but also their perspectives about their illness and the significance of diagnosis. Not just their understanding of the medical reality but the meaning of it in their lives. Consequently, it is essential to evaluate not only the cognitive and psychological abilities of children but also their cultural and religious/ spiritual beliefs about illness. What it means for them. This is crucial in order to communicate with them effectively (Wiener et al., 2013). For example, a recent study examined the end-of-life experiences and perspectives of Chinese adolescents with cancer. They felt a loss of control over their bodies and futures after receiving a diagnosis and expressed a fear of being forgotten and being alone. Despite this, they understood that their mortality was something that they would have to face alone in the future. Lin et al. (2023) also noted that they are frightened by the prospect of being isolated from their loved ones.

---

**LEARNING ACTIVITY**

1.  Engage in a conversation with your colleagues to explore the challenges associated with implementing children's palliative care and the potential contributions of healthcare providers, including nurses, in overcoming these challenges.
2.  Reflect on what you have heard from children and young people about their illness and their views of dying and death. How does this link in with what is written above and also in Chapter 3?

---

## NURSES' PERCEPTIONS OF CHILDHOOD DEATH

Caring for children differs from caring for adults due to the development of children's physiological, psychological and cognitive characteristics, as well as their legal, ethical and social status. Therefore, nurses face several challenges when they care for children with palliative care needs. For example, the increased uncertainty associated with situations filled with fear, anxiety and desperation complicates the ability of health professionals and families to evaluate and weigh up the potential risks and benefits of available treatment options, and this can lead to differences of opinions (Field and Behrman, 2003). In addition to discrepancies between healthcare staff and the family in terms of treatment goals, a lack of understanding of the concept of palliative care can delay the introduction of children's palliative care services, not only prolonging physical suffering, but also emotional and psychological suffering among children, their parents and the treatment team (Davies et al., 2008; Mack and Wolfe, 2006). Moreover, in the minds of many parents, physicians and nurses, end-of-life care for a child seems inherently unnatural and they struggle to believe that nothing more can be done for a child in terms of a cure or prolonging life. This presents a unique challenge for nurses in children's palliative care services (Wiener et al., 2013).

Furthermore, nurses indicate that the death of a child they are caring for affects them emotionally and professionally and some report that they can clearly recall the tragic fatalities of children that occurred over a decade ago. In addition, nurses felt anger, weakness, helplessness and remorse following the deaths of children, while witnessing a sorrowful, grieving family evoked unwelcome emotions. Shimoinaba et al. (2021) studied emergency nurses' experiences with the deaths of children, as well as their coping strategies and support requirements. They found that most participants were traumatised by the death of a child, more so than the death of an adult. All the nurses described longer attempts at resuscitation in children than adults and some recounted painful memories of children's deaths from over 10 years earlier. The death of a child affected the nurses emotionally and professionally, particularly if their own children were the same age as the child who had died. Some of them had temporarily left their jobs after such experiences. Although the experience of witnessing children dying was terrible in itself, they also felt unsupported and lacked the training to deal with this situation (Shimoinaba et al., 2021).

---

**LEARNING ACTIVITY**

1. Reflect on the major challenges you experience when a child dies.
2. How are you and your colleagues supported when a child you are caring for dies?
3. How might the experience be different within a palliative care environment to that described by Shimoinaba et al. (2021) with nurses working in the emergency setting?

---

## SPIRITUALITY AND FAITH

Spirituality and faith are two important factors that influence our attitudes, beliefs and understanding of caring for children living with palliative care needs. Puchalski (2012) defines spirituality *as* 'the aspect of humanity that refers to the way individuals seek and express meaning and purpose and the way they experience their connectedness to the moment, to self, to others, to nature, and to the significant or sacred'. For some people, spirituality will incorporate elements of faith and religion, however it is a broader concept that affects the way that we think, feel and behave.

Faith includes having trust, assurance and belief in something that we are anticipating but have not yet obtained. Having faith can be important for parents of children living with palliative care needs. For example, faith can offer parents a feeling of optimism and comfort during challenging periods when their children are confronted with a terminal disease (Meyer et al., 2006; Superdock et al., 2018). Faith may involve religious practices, or it may be more personal. Engaging in religious practices can assist individuals in building resilience to effectively manage the emotional and physical difficulties associated with tending to an ill child. Parents describe how their faith has helped them face existential challenges and find meaning in challenging situations. It assisted them in understanding the inscrutable (Cornelio et al., 2016). Faith can also serve as a source of purpose and significance, aiding parents in navigating the unpredictable and apprehensive circumstances that frequently accompany such situations. Moreover, faith can provide a sense of social belonging and assistance, fostering connections among parents who possess comparable convictions and encounters. Faith may also provide comfort and strength for parents as they deal with the challenges of caring for a child with a life-threatening disease.

While some people will not have any specific faith or religion, some may also have faith that no matter what occurs, God always has their best interests in mind (Higgs et al., 2016). In a study conducted in the US, researchers examined the influence of religion and spirituality on parental decision-making in 16 cases involving children with complex life-threatening conditions. Religion and spirituality were essential to all parents and influenced their decision-making, with some parents believing that their child is in a better place because they have become one of 'God's little angels' (Superdock et al., 2018). Studies with families of different religions in different cultures have also found the presence of faith to be either supportive – bringing comfort, or challenging as they question "why God has allowed this to happen". Mothers and fathers with a faith also reinforced their confidence in God's control. This concept can enable parents to make decisions (citing God as in control) or motivate them to abstain from decision-making (quoting God as the decision-maker). Thus, an exploration of a family's spirituality, faith or religion is important in helping us to understand how they cope with their child's illness.

---

**LEARNING ACTIVITY**

Think about an example from a family you have cared for and of how their spirituality, faith or religious beliefs may have affected their response to their child's illness.

---

## MAINTAINING HOPE

Hope is a feeling of expectation and desire for a particular thing to happen, the feeling of wanting something to happen and thinking that it could happen. It can be defined as "to cherish a desire with anticipation: to want something to happen or be true". It is a "desire accompanied by expectation of or belief in fulfilment" (*Merriam Webster Dictionary*, 2024). As a spiritual resource, hope is an important concept that allows parents to cope with the suffering they face because of their child's illness. It is a term that we use often in children's palliative care, for example, we "hope for the best but prepare for the worst". As nurses, we often use the term "hope" in our communication with a family about their child's condition and prognosis.

Hope is so important to families, with parents encouraged by the hope they derive from seeing the positive, such as having good days, or their child living longer than expected (Lotz et al., 2017). Hope enables parents to concentrate on their child's care and provide them with the highest quality of life (Misko et al., 2015). It also increases the ability of parents of children with life-threatening conditions to cope with the suffering they and their child face due to their child's illness. Parents did not lose hope that their child would survive (Superdock et al., 2018). As choices became more difficult or consequential, parents spoke with greater emphasis on the significance of retaining optimism and faith (Superdock et al., 2018).

Parents recognise the significance of maintaining hope for both their own well-being and that of their children. As their child's condition progresses, it becomes necessary for them to redefine hope, for example, from "hoping for a cure" to "hoping that they will be symptom-free". They acknowledge that by redefining hope, they may derive resilience and adaptability in the face of suffering. Rather than fixating on the adverse consequences or most unfavourable situations, they choose to concentrate on the positive possibilities. By adopting this new viewpoint, they are able to maintain resilience and provide ongoing assistance to their child under challenging circumstances. Through redefining hope and its significance, parents can successfully navigate the forthcoming obstacles related to their child's condition. It is also important to note that parents are able to balance the reality of the situation that they are going through, but still choose hope (Groopman, 2005). They can cling on to the "hope for a cure" while being realistic and "hoping that their child will not suffer".

On the other hand, if they are unable to reframe their hope, losing hope can be devastating to a parent. This can engender intense feelings of hopelessness, agony, grief, fear and rage along with other negative emotions (Higgs et al., 2016; Schaefer et al., 2021). Thus parents express their need for nurses and other health professionals to support them by keeping their hope alive (Taib et al., 2021), concentrating on the positive, taking things one day at a time, wishing for the best each day and exhibiting positivity (Smith et al., 2018). Thus, enabling families to maintain and/or reframe their hope in the context of children's palliative care is an important role of the nurse.

---

**LEARNING ACTIVITY**

Reflect on how you may support families to achieve a balance between maintaining hope and accepting the reality of the prognosis for children with palliative care needs.

---

## THE IMPLICATIONS OF BELIEFS, ATTITUDES AND VALUES ON THE CHILD'S CARE

Our beliefs, attitudes and values as nurses, as parents and family members and as members of the public can all have implications on the care provided to a child living with palliative care needs and their families. These can include, but are not limited to, the following:

1. *Delay in the diagnosis of life-limiting or life-threatening illness* will impact negatively on the disease trajectory, prognosis and the quality of life of children and their families, and this is particularly challenging in childhood cancer. Several factors account for this delay in diagnosis including a lack of understanding of childhood cancer, including that it impacts all ages, misinterpretation of early

symptoms, perceptions of serious illness in children and lack of access to an efficient and affordable health system (Abdelmabood et al., 2017; Gardie et al., 2023). For example, in Bangladesh, a study that examined the relationship between delay in the diagnosis of malignancy and the child's age found that older children experienced more of a delay in being diagnosed than children under the age of 2 years (Begum et al., 2016). During the COVID-19 pandemic, fear from exposure to infection as well as co-infection contributed to delays in diagnosis and treatment of children with cancer (Dvori et al., 2021).

2. *Delay in referral to palliative care services* has potential negative consequences that may lead to increased suffering, impacting on the child's and family's quality of life. Opportunities to integrate targeted referral and interventions through early palliative care services and resources for children and families are missed (Kaye et al., 2018). In one study, doctors identified several parent-related factors as a considerable barrier to referral, raising the concern that despite palliative care being demonstrated to be highly effective, doctors themselves tended to associate palliative care with dying and death and this association can influence their perception of the parents' reluctance to include a palliative care approach (Twamley et al., 2014). Therefore, professionals may in principle support the idea of a palliative care referral, but may delay acting on this due to the strong association with end-of-life care. Hence, if a child is not perceived as 'actively dying', referral may not be actioned. This lack of distinction between end-of-life care or hospice care and palliative care is common among both healthcare professionals and the public (Twamley et al., 2014).

3. *The misconception that palliative care is synonymous with "giving up"* accompanies a general lack of understanding of the benefits of integrating a palliative care approach from the time of diagnosis through the course of the disease trajectory alongside aggressive treatment, e.g. chemotherapy. Hence, an opportunity to implement early palliative care interventions is missed and the child suffers unnecessarily. In addition, referral to specialist children's palliative care services has been shown to reduce hospital admissions during end-of-life care for paediatric oncology patients, which is beneficial for the child and their family (Fraser et al., 2013).

4. *Stigma.* Sharing accurate information, addressing and eliminating the misconception that palliative care is associated with end-of-life care through advocacy and education are key steps in breaking down some of the barriers that prevent children and families from accessing timely and high-quality palliative care. When professionals and communities were provided with accurate information about children's palliative care, a positive shift in attitude was observed (Twamley et al., 2014).

5. *Perceptions* about children's palliative care matter and are of great significance as they influence how families understand and utilise services. In addition, these perceptions affect how families and children are cared for and ultimately shape how palliative care services for children are supported and funded (eHospice, 2022).

## THE IMPACT OF BELIEFS, ATTITUDES AND VALUES ABOUT CHILDREN'S PALLIATIVE CARE ON COMMUNICATION AND DECISION-MAKING

Informal carers may serve not only as the child's legal decision-makers, but also their emotional guardian and spokesperson. In addition, some children may have cognitive deficits and are unable to speak and/or communicate for themselves, in which case the informal carer's role, as a vital partner in the decision-making process, becomes essential.

Effective communication with children and young people requires skill and compassion and a range of developmental ages and stages need to be taken into consideration, ensuring that communication with children is consistently clear, honest and age-appropriate. The impact of beliefs, attitudes and values on communication with informal carers in a children's palliative care context is particularly significant due to the range of sensitive information covered, requiring skilful discussion including issues relating to: disclosure around diagnosis, prognosis, treatment options, advance care planning and decision-making around end-of-life care.

However, these discussions may be compromised if the healthcare professional is reluctant to share information with the child and/or family due to lack of confidence/experience/expertise or in the belief it will cause emotional distress or the child and family will lose hope. It is important to understand that children living with palliative care needs are generally wise beyond their years and withholding critical information about them is said to contribute to feelings of anxiety and fear in the child (Winger et al., 2022).

Furthermore, in settings where discussions on serious illness and/or death are culturally frowned upon, opportunities for advance care planning-related discussions may be missed. These discussions serve as important milestones in the child's journey and help prepare the child, family and healthcare providers for disease progression, symptoms at the end-of-life care, prognostication, etc. Most importantly, these discussions create an opportunity to tease out and integrate the child's and the family's wishes. The outcome of effective advance care planning discussions and compilation of a good comprehensive advance care plan contributes to the concept of seamless supportive care and ultimately results in an improved experience not only for the child and the family but also for nurses providing support across locations.

---

**LEARNING ACTIVITY: A NURSE'S EXPERIENCES OF WORKING WITH CHILDREN RECEIVING PALLIATIVE CARE**

The degree of emotional involvement with the child and family you are caring for can be a controversial issue. Nurse Rania described her psychological suffering due to frequent contact with children receiving palliative care. Rania mentioned that she finds it very difficult to control her feelings and she finds it emotionally distressing to care for them as she knows that the child has a high chance of dying. She describes the effect of her suffering on her private life and how she sometimes becomes very concerned about the health of her own children; she imagines that her son could be in the same position as the children she cares for. She says that the nature of her work affects her communication with her own family.

Reflect on how Nurse Rania feels, have you ever been in a similar situation, or seen colleagues in the same situation? How do you cope with it? How does it make you feel now?

## The implications for nurses

In a context where children's palliative care is not recognised as a discipline, it can be especially challenging to integrate palliative care into the public healthcare system and champions in the field might encounter resistance when attempting to introduce children's palliative care to their colleagues, the families they care for and key stakeholders. While adult palliative care services are generally more established, services for children tend to lag behind in many places (Downing et al., 2024) with more "buy-in" and commitment from strategic stakeholders required to deliver palliative care services for all children in need. This phenomenon is compounded by the fact that children dying from serious illness goes against the natural rhythm of life; as discussed at the start of this chapter, children are not meant to die before their parents (Riches and Dawson, 1996). Thus, recognising and responding to the enormous global need for children's palliative care requires a significant shift in attitude, particularly, but not exclusively, among healthcare professionals. As nurses make up the largest proportion of healthcare professionals globally, this is a particularly relevant and necessary shift for nurses to undertake.

As discussed, palliative care may be misconstrued as "giving up", hence, healthcare professionals may be reluctant to "switch" to palliative care as this may not be aligned with their image of themselves as "good" healthcare professionals. For nurses working in an acute cure focused setting, for example, on a paediatric oncology ward, where the focus is largely on cure, it may be challenging to shift the goal of care from cure to palliative care. Thus, we again highlight the need for education, yet historically, undergraduate teaching has not included a palliative care approach and chapters on disease outlines in conventional medical/nursing textbooks generally ended with treatment options and complications. However, this is changing with increased uptake of palliative care educational programmes at both undergraduate and postgraduate levels globally.

## ADVOCACY AS A TOOL TO "SET THE RECORD STRAIGHT"

The need to advocate for equitable children's palliative care services across the globe has been well documented and flagged as a priority (Downing et al., 2012; Rosa et al., 2022). Advocacy includes clear messaging of what children's palliative care is and how it may be integrated into generalist and specialist paediatric services. More specifically, there is a pressing need to highlight the potential benefits of early palliative care initiation that includes ease of suffering and improvement in quality of life and death for children and their families. In addition, advocacy for and integration of, early introduction of a palliative care approach pose no risk of harm to the patient (Doherty et al., 2020). Palliative care advocacy is most effective when the voices of those who deliver and receive services attest to the unmet need for palliative care (Pettus and de Lima, 2020).

1. *The nurse as advocate*: During the undergraduate years, nurses are primed as patient advocates and often assume a mediatory role between the patient/family and the healthcare environment. In this "go-between" role, nurses might be

prone to being involved in conflict management situations in clinical as well as organisational environments. However, due to their strategic position, level of engagement and expertise, nurses are well placed to advocate for patients and services, impacting on the quality of care provided to children and families locally and globally (Agrawal et al., 2023).

2. *Informal carers as advocates*: Parents often have an important advocacy role to play in children's palliative care. The informal carer of a child living with palliative care needs often spends protracted lengths of time at their child's bedside, attends countless hospital appointments and gains extensive knowledge and insights into their child's condition. Normally parents are intimately involved in their child's journey, with home often being identified as the preferred place of care and therefore they can offer unique perspectives as they navigate the public/private healthcare system (Winger et al., 2020). Through the process of sharing their stories, informal carers make meaning of their experiences and bereaved parents may proceed to inspire and support other families on their journey (Lord et al., 2021). Hence, important lessons can be learnt from informal carers and including their voice is vital in terms of providing perspectives of the impact of serious illness in childhood on the whole family.

3. *Children and young people as advocates*: Many children and young people will need palliative care over many years and are able to speak out and advocate for access to children's palliative care services. Hearing the voice of the children themselves is a powerful advocacy tools. One such example is that of Lucy Watts MBE (2018), a young person from the UK who received palliative care for many years. With her lived experience she became a strong and passionate advocate for access to palliative care services for children and young people globally. She met the Director General of the World Health Organization, Dr Tedros Adhanom Ghebreyesus, on several occasions, to promote and raise awareness of children's palliative care. As a young adult living with palliative care needs she was able to achieve much more than many of us as nurses and care providers.

## Stories as advocacy tools

Stories are powerful advocacy tools and form part of an essential strategy to address misconceptions of children's palliative care across society broadly to help improve public understanding and promote public support for children's palliative care. It may be helpful for a range of storytellers to relay a story; the child him/herself, an informal carer or a healthcare provider so that various perspectives may be considered. A child, depending on their age and level of cognition, may undertake the task of storytelling with or without support from an adult.

Stories offer unique insights into the child and family's lived experiences at various points along the child's disease trajectory, i.e. from time of diagnosis, throughout the illness to the end-of-life phase as well as into the bereavement period. In addition, stories across age and location of care need to be showcased, i.e. from neonates to young adults, acknowledging differences in needs across developmental ages, stages, and locations, e.g. home, hospital and hospice. However, it is important that stories to promote children's palliative care services reflect the difference good quality palliative care interventions can make to the lives of children and their families across the broad spectrum of childhood illness.

Stories that highlight the difference palliative care interventions make to the quality of the child and their family's life must be encouraged (Lord et al., 2021). When a child living with a life-limiting illness has had quality added to their days and is living well; free of distressing symptoms, free of suffering and able to enjoy meaningful engagements with their family and peers, this is a powerful motivator for palliative care. This is important because children who receive palliative care are primarily children and have the same needs as other children; universal connections and relationships are important to them and they want to play and engage with their peers, family and their environment, just like all children do. Equally important are stories that reflect on 'good death' experiences as these stories form an important part of the child's legacy. Moreover, sharing the child's story may be therapeutic for the author and integrating narrative medicine into children's palliative care education invaluable (Lanocha, 2021).

It is important that what good quality care looks like is modelled through these stories so that the gaps may be identified to actively lobby for greater support for children and families in need, wherever they may be. In addition, stories need to reflect the value of and collaborative nature of the team, a pivotal feature in children's palliative care. A range of professionals work together across locations of care to provide the best care possible and, most importantly, the child and their family are central to the team (Riiser et al., 2022).

## IMPORTANCE OF LANGUAGE AND IMAGERY

Language is a powerful and important tool that can help shift public perceptions around palliative care. A communications kit has been developed to help change the narrative and public perceptions about the field (Heard, 2022). It can be helpful to use language such as supportive care, all-encompassing care, care offered alongside medical care, emphasising that support extends to the whole family, including siblings (Heard, 2022).

It is equally important when advocating for palliative care services to create opportunities for children to be children, making sure that children with palliative care needs get the things all children need: access to their peer group, time to chill, engaging in fun activities, play and stimulating activities, etc. (see Chapter 6).

When showcasing the range of people providing supportive care, it is important to highlight partnerships, forming strong relationships, working collaboratively and that the team includes the children themselves, their parents, siblings, peers and healthcare and social care professionals (Heard, 2022).

## CULTURAL COMPETENCY IN CULTURALLY RESPONSIVE CARE

Cultural competence within a healthcare context implies that the nurse and other providers deliver effective healthcare services that meet the social, cultural and linguist needs of the community they serve. Relevant training for healthcare professionals on cultural competence, cross-cultural issues and creating appropriate policies are essential strategies for health systems to implement in order to move towards a culturally competent system.

Self-awareness is a key step in cultivating culturally competent care. Self-awareness is described as a basic understanding of how we feel and why we feel that way and the more we are aware of our feelings, the easier they are to manage and dictate how we might respond to others.

Nurses need to be culturally competent if they are to successfully navigate the textured landscape of the communities they serve and, most importantly, be equipped to support informal carers by respecting their beliefs and values (Wiener et al., 2013).

## SUMMARY

This chapter highlights critical issues for all healthcare professionals delivering palliative care to children and families to consider. In an evolving multicultural society, nurses working in a children's palliative care context must comprehend how culture, religion and spirituality influence individual and family beliefs, attitudes, and values in relation to serious illness and death in childhood. These misconceptions of palliative care vs end-of-life care have serious implications, including the delay in diagnosis and referral to palliative care services. Thus, nurses working in ethnically diverse populations must gain cultural competency to respond appropriately to their patients if they are to provide the best possible quality of care across the entire disease trajectory. Advocacy, through storytelling, the correct use of language and imagery, holds the key to promoting a better understanding of the experiences of families and a more balanced view of children's palliative care broadly.

## KEY POINTS

- Attitudes, beliefs and values about children's palliative care have a profound impact on the quality of care children living with life-threatening illnesses and their families receive.
- Nurses are well placed to support informal carers as well as their colleagues in addressing these perceptions and improve the quality of care.
- Nurses need to be equipped through training and appropriate policies to optimise their responses to these perceptions to deliver care that is culturally competent.
- Advocacy that includes stories, appropriate language and images, is helpful to address misconceptions about children's palliative care.

## REFERENCES

Abdelmabood, S., Kandil, S., Megahed, A., Fouda, A. (2017). Delays in diagnosis and treatment among children with cancer: Egyptian perspective. *Eastern Mediterranean Health Journal*, 23(6), 422–429. https://doi.org/10.26719/2017.23.6.422

Agrawal, U. S., Sarin, J., Garg, R. (2023). Nursing perspective of providing palliative care to the children: A narrative review. *Journal of Health and Allied Science*, 14, 157–162. https://doi.org/10.1055/s-0043-1769081

Astuti, R., Harris, P. L. (2008). Understanding mortality and the life of the ancestors in rural Madagascar. *Cognitive Science*, 32(4). 713–740. https://doi.org/10.1080/03640210802066907

Atout, M., Hemingway, P., Seymour, J. (2019). The practice of mutual protection in the care of children with palliative care needs: A multiple qualitative case study approach from Jordan. *Journal of Pediatric Nursing*, 45, e9–e18. https://doi.org/10.1016/j.pedn.2018.12.004

Begum, M., Islam, M. J., Akhtar, M. W., Karim, S. (2016). Evaluation of delays in diagnosis and treatment of childhood malignancies in Bangladesh. *South Asian Journal of Cancer*, 5(4), 192–193. https://doi.org/10.4103/2278-330x.195343

Bluebond-Langner, M. (1978). *The private world of dying children*. Princeton University Press.

Campbell, S., Moola, F. J., Gibson, J. L., Petch, J., Denburg, A. (2022). The unspeakable nature of death and dying during childhood: A silenced phenomenon in pediatric care. *Omega (Westport)*, 89(1), 88–107 https://doi.org/10.1177/00302228211067034

Clarke, S. A., Davies, H., Jenney, M., Glaser, A., Eiser, C. (2005). Parental communication and children's behaviour following diagnosis of childhood leukaemia. *Psychooncology*, 14(4), 274–281. https://doi.org/10.1002/pon.843

Cornelio, S.J., Nayak, B. S., George, A. (2016). Experiences of mothers on parenting children with leukemia. *Indian Journal of Palliative Care*, 22(2), 168–172. 10.4103/0973-1075.179608. https://doi.org/10.4103/0973-1075.179608

CPCET Children's Palliative Care Education and Training UK and Ireland Action Group. (2020). Education Standard Framework. ICPCN. Available at: https://icpcn.org/wp-content/uploads/2022/10/CPCET-Education-Standard-Framework.pdf (accessed 14 May 2024).

Dalberg, T., Jacob-Files, E., Carney, P. A., Meyrowitz, J., Fromme, E. K., Thomas, G. (2013). Pediatric oncology providers' perceptions of barriers and facilitators to early integration of pediatric palliative care. *Pediatric Blood & Cancer*, 60(11), 1875–1881. https://doi.org/10.1002/pbc.24673

Davies, B., Sehring, S. A., Partridge, J.C., Cooper, B. A., Hughes, A., Philp, J. C., Amidi-Nouri, A., Kramer, R. F. (2008). Barriers to palliative care for children: Perceptions of pediatric health care providers. *Pediatrics*, 121(2). 282–288. https://doi.org/10.1542/peds.2006-3153

De Clercq, E., Rost, M., Rakic, M., Ansari, M., Brazzola, P., Wangmo, T., Elger, B. S. (2019). The conceptual understanding of pediatric palliative care: A Swiss healthcare perspective. *BMC Palliative Care*, 18(1), 55. https://doi.org/10.1186/s12904-019-0438-1

Doherty, M., Okhuysen-Cawley, R., Chambers, L. (2020). Children's palliative care across a range of conditions, settings and resources. In J. Downing (ed.), *Children's palliative care: An international case-based manual*. Springer.

Doherty, M., Thabet, C. (2018). Development and implementation of a pediatric palliative care program in a developing country. *Frontiers of Public Health*, 16(6), 106. https://doi.org/10.3389/fpubh.2018.00106

Downing, J., Birtar, D., Chambers, L., Gelb, B., Drake, R., Kiman, R. (2012). Children's palliative care: A global concern. *International Journal of Palliative Nursing*, 18(2), 109–114. https://doi.org/10.12968/ijpn.2012.18.3.109

Downing, J., Ling, J., Benini, F., Payne, S., Papadatou, D. (2013). *EAPC core competencies for education in paediatric palliative care*; Report of the EAPC Children's Palliative Care Education Task Force; European Association for Palliative Care. Available at: https://www.ordemenfermeiros.pt/arquivo/colegios/Documents/2017/MCEESIP_PNAE_09_eapcnet_ppc_core_competencies.pdf (accessed 12 June 2024).

Downing, J., Namukwaya, E., Nakawesi, J., Mwesiga, M. (2024). Shared-decision-making and communication in paediatric palliative care within Uganda. *Current Problems in Pediatric and Adolescent Health Care*, 54(1), 101556. https://doi.org/10.1016/j.cppeds.2024.101556

Dvori, M., Elitzur, S., Barg, A., Barzilai-Birenboim, S., Gilad, G., Amar, S., Toledano, H., Toren, A., Weinreb, S., Goldstein, G., Shapira, A., Ash, S., Izraeli, S., Gilad, O. (2021). Delayed diagnosis and treatment of children with cancer during the COVID-19 pandemic. *International Journal of Clinical Oncology*, 26(8), 1569–1574. https://doi.org/10.1007/s10147-021-01971-3

eHospice. (2022). Shifting public perceptions and moving media reporting about children's palliative care. Available at: https://ehospice.com/inter_childrens_posts/shifting-public-perceptions-and-moving-media-reporting-about-childrens-palliative-care/ (accessed 13 June 2024).

Field, M., Behrman, R. (2003). *When children die: Improving palliative and end-of-life care for children and their families*. National Academy of Sciences.

Fraser, L.K., van Laar, M., Miller, M., Aldridge, J., McKinney, P. A., Parslow, R. C., Feltbower R. G. (2013). Does referral to specialist paediatric palliative care services reduce hospital admissions in oncology patients at the end of life? *British Journal of Cancer*, 108(6), 1273–1279. https://doi.org/10.1038/bjc.2013.89

Gardie, Y., Wassie, M., Wodajo, S., Giza, M., Ayalew, M., Sewale, Y., Feleke, Z., Dessie, M. T. (2023). Delay in diagnosis and associated factors among children with cancer admitted at pediatric oncology ward, University of Gondar comprehensive specialized hospital, Ethiopia: A retrospective cross-sectional study. *BMC Cancer*, 23(1), 469. https://doi.org/10.1186/s12885-023-10873-8

Goldman, A., Christie, D. (1993). Children with cancer talk about their own death with their families. *Pediatric Hematology and Oncology*, 10(3), 223–231. https://doi.org/10.3109/08880019309029488

Groopman, J. (2005). *The anatomy of hope: How people prevail in the face of illness*. Random House Trade.

Haines, E. R., Frost, A. C., Kane, H. L., Rokoske, F. S. (2018). Barriers to accessing palliative care for pediatric patients with cancer: A review of the literature. *Cancer*, 124(11), 2278–2288. https://doi.org/10.1002/cncr.31265

Harris, P. L. (2018). Children's understanding of death: from biology to religion. *Philosophical Transactions of the Royal Society of London. Series B, Biological Science*, 373(1754), 20170266. https://doi.org/10.1098/rstb.2017.0266

Heard. (2022). How to talk about children's palliative care. Available at: https://heard.org.uk/articles/childrens-palliative-care-project-page/ (accessed 13 June 2024).

Higgs, E. J., Mcclaren, B. J., Sahhar, M. A., Ryan, M. M. Forbes. R. (2016). 'A short time but a lovely little short time': Bereaved parents' experiences of having a child with spinal muscular atrophy type 1. *Journal of Paediatrics and Child Health*, 52(1), 40–46. https://doi.org/10.1111/jpc.12993

Kaye, E. C., Jerkins, J., Gushue, C. A., DeMarsh, S., Sykes, A., Lu, Z., Snaman, J. M., Blazin, L., Johnson, L. M., Levine, D. R., Morrison, R. R., Baker, J. N. (2018). Predictors of late palliative care referral in children with cancer. *Journal of Pain and Symptom Management*, 55(6), 1550–1556. https://doi.org/10.1016/j.jpainsymman.2018.01.021

Knapp, C., Thompson, L. (2012). Factors associated with perceived barriers to pediatric palliative care: A survey of pediatricians in Florida and California. *Palliative Medicine*, 26(3), 268–274. https://doi.org/10.1177/0269216311409085

Kongnetiman, L., Lai, D., Berg, B. (2008). Cultural competency in paediatric palliative care: A literature review. *Alberta Health Services*. Available at: http://fcrc.albertahealthservices.ca/publications/cultural/Cultural-Competency-in-Palliative-Paediatric-Care-Literature-Review.pdf (accessed 11 June 2024).

Lanocha, N. (2021). Lessons in stories: Why narrative medicine has a role in pediatric palliative care training. *Children*, 8(5), 321. https://doi.org/10.3390/children8050321

Lin, N., Lv, D., Hu, Y., Zhu, J., Xu, H., Lai, D. (2023). Existential experiences and perceptions of death among children with terminal cancer: An interpretative qualitative study. *Palliative Medicine*, 37(6), 866–874. https://doi.org/10.1177/02692163231165100

Lotz, J. D., Daxer, M., Jox, R. J., Borasio, G. D., Führer, M. (2017). 'Hope for the best, prepare for the worst': A qualitative interview study on parents' needs and fears in pediatric advance care planning. *Palliative Medicine*, 31(8), 764–771. https://doi.org/10.1177/0269216316679913

Lord, B. T., Morrison, W., Goldstein, R. D., Feudtner, C. (2021). Parents as advocates for pediatric palliative care. *Pediatrics*, 148(5), e2021052054. https://doi.org/10.1542/peds.2021-052054

Mack, J. W., Wolfe, J. (2006). Early integration of pediatric palliative care: For some children, palliative care starts at diagnosis. *Current Opinion in Pediatrics*, 18(1), 10–14. https://doi.org/10.1097/01.mop.0000193266.86129.47

Menendez, D., Hernandez, I. G., Rosengren, K. S. (2020). Children's emerging understanding of death. *Child Development Perspectives*, 14, 55–60. https://doi.org/10.1111/cdep.12357

*Merriam Webster Dictionary*. (2024). Hope. Available at: https://www.merriam-webster.com/dictionary/hope (accessed 13 June 2024).

Meyer, E. C., Ritholz, M. D., Burns, J. P., Truog, R. D. (2006). Improving the quality of end-of-life care in the pediatric intensive care unit: parents' priorities and recommendations. *Pediatrics*, 117(3), 649–657. https://doi.org/10.1542/peds.2005-0144

Misko, M. D., Dos Santos, M. R., Ichikawa, C. R., De Lima, R. A., Bousso, R. S. (2015). The family's experience of the child and/or teenager in palliative care: Fluctuating between hope and hopelessness in a world changed by losses. *Revista Latino-Americana de Enfermagem*, 23(3), 560–567. https://doi.org/10.1590/0104-1169.0468.2588

Monette, E. M. (2021). Cultural considerations in palliative care provision: A scoping review of Canadian literature. *Palliative Medicine Reports*, 2(1), 146–156. https://doi.org/10.1089/pmr.2020.0124

Patenaude, A. F. (2005). Psychosocial functioning in pediatric cancer. *Journal of Pediatric Psychology*, 30(1), 9–27. https://doi.org/10.1093/jpepsy/jsi012

Pettus, K. I., de Lima, L. (2020). Palliative care advocacy: Why does it matter? *Journal of Palliative Medicine*, 23(8), 1009–1012. https://doi.org/10.1089/jpm.2019.0696

Puchalski, C. M. (2012). Spirituality as an essential domain of palliative care: Caring for the whole person. *Progress in Palliative Care*, 20(2), 63–65. https://doi.org/10.1179/0969926012Z.00000000028

Rapa, E., Hanna, J., Pollard, T., Santos-Paulo, S., Gogay, Y., Ambler, J., Namukwaya, E., Kavuma. D., Nabirye, E., Kemigisha, R., Namyeso, J., Brand, T., Walker, L., Neethling, B., Downing, J., Ziebland, S., Stein, A., Dalton, L. (2023). Exploring the experiences of healthcare professionals in South Africa and Uganda around communicating with children about life-threatening conditions: A workshop-based qualitative study to inform the adaptation of communication frameworks for use in these settings. *BMJ Open*, 13(1), e064741. https://doi.org/10.1136/bmjopen-2022-064741

Riches, G., Dawson, P. (1996). 'An intimate loneliness': Evaluating the impact of a child's death on parental self-identity and marital relationships. *Journal of Family Therapy*, 18(1), 1–22. https://doi.org/10.1111/j.1467-6427.1996.tb00031.x

Riiser, K., Holmen, H., Winger, A., Steindal, S. A., Castor, C., Kvarme, L. G., Lee, A., Lorentsen, V. B., Misvaer, N., Früh, E. A. (2022). Stories of paediatric palliative care: a qualitative study exploring health care professionals' understanding of the concept. *BMC Palliative Care*, 21(1), 187 https://doi.org/10.1186/s12904-022-01077-1

Rosa, W. E., Ahmed, E., Chaila, M. J., Chansa, A., Cordoba, M. A., Dowla, R., Gafer, N., Khan, F., Namisango, E., Rodriguez, L., Knaul, F. M., Pettus, K. I. (2022). Can you hear us now? Equity in global advocacy for palliative care. *Journal of Pain and Symptom Management*, 64(4), e217–e226. https://doi.org/10.1016/j.jpainsymman.2022.07.004

Saad, R., Abu-Saad Huijer, H., Noureddine, S., Sailian, S. D. (2022). Pediatric palliative care through the eyes of healthcare professionals, parents and communities: A narrative review. *Annals of Palliative Medicine*, 11(10), 3292–3314. https://doi.org/10.21037/apm-22-525

Salins, N., Hughes, S., Preston, N. (2022). Palliative care in paediatric oncology: An update. *Current Oncology Reports*, 24(2), 175–186. https://doi.org/10.1007/s11912-021-01170-3

Schaefer, M. R., Kenney, A. E., Himelhoch, A. C., Howard Sharp, K. M., Humphrey, L., Olshefski, R., Young-Saleme, T., Gerhardt, C. A. (2021). A quest for meaning: A qualitative exploration among children with advanced cancer and their parents. *Psychooncology*, 30(4), 546–553. https://doi.org/10.1002/pon.5601

Semlali, I., Tamches, E., Singy, P., Weber, O. (2020). Introducing cross-cultural education in palliative care: Focus groups with experts on practical strategies. *BMC Palliative Care*, 19(1), 171. https://doi.org/10.1186/s12904-020-00678-y

Shimoinaba, K., McKenna, L., Copnell, B. (2021). Nurses' experiences, coping and support in the death of a child in the emergency department: A qualitative descriptive study. *International Emergency Nursing*, 59, 101102. https://doi.org/10.1016/j.ienj.2021.101102

Smith, N. R., Bally, J. M. G., Holtslander, L., Peacock, S., Spurr, S., Hodgson-Viden, H., Mpofu, C., Zimmer, M. (2018). Supporting parental caregivers of children living with life-threatening or life-limiting illnesses: A Delphi study. *Journal for Specialists in Pediatric Nursing*, 23(4), e12226. https://doi.org/10.1111/jspn.12226

Superdock, A. K., Barfield, R. C., Brandon, D. H. Docherty, S. L. (2018). Exploring the vagueness of religion and spirituality in complex pediatric decision-making: A qualitative study. *BMC Palliative Care*, 17(1), 107. https://doi.org/10.1186/s12904-018-0360-y

Taib, F., Beng, K. T., Chee Chan, L. (2021). The challenges, coping mechanisms, and the needs of the in hospital parents caring for children with life-limiting neurological disorders: A qualitative study. *Indian Journal of Palliative Care*, 27(4), 483–489. https://doi.org/10.25259/ijpc_3_21

Thompson, L. A., Knapp, C., Madden, V., Shenkman, E. (2009). Pediatricians' perceptions of and preferred timing for pediatric palliative care. *Pediatrics*, 123(5), e777–e782. https://doi.org/10.1542/peds.2008-2721

Twamley, K., Craig, F., Kelly, P., Hollowell, D. R., Mendoza, P., Bluebond-Langner, M. (2014). Underlying barriers to referral to paediatric palliative care services: knowledge and attitudes of health care professionals in a paediatric tertiary care centre in the United Kingdom. *Journal of Child Health Care*, 18(1), 19–30. https://doi.org/10.1177/1367493512468363

van der Geest, I. M., van den Heuvel-Ebrink, M. M., van Vliet, L. M., Pluijm, S. M., et al. (2015). Talking about death with children with incurable cancer: Perspectives from parents. *The Journal of Pediatrics*, 167, 1320–1326. https://doi.org/10.1016/j.jpeds.2015.08.066

Vig, P. S., Lim, J. Y., Lee, R. W. L., Huang, H., Tan, X. H., Lim, W. Q., Lim, M., Lee, A. S. I., Chiam, M., Lim, C., Baral, V. R., Krishna, L. K. R. (2021). Parental bereavement: Impact of death of neonates and children under 12 years on personhood of parents: A systematic scoping review. *BMC Palliative Care*, 20(1), 136. https://doi.org/10.1186/s12904-021-00831-1

Wallerstedt, B., Benzein, E., Schildmeijer, K., Sandgren, A. (2019). What is palliative care? Perceptions of healthcare professionals. *Scandinavian Journal of Caring Sciences*, 33, 77–84. https://doi.org/10.1111/scs.12603

Watson-Jones, R. E., Busch, J. T. A., Harris, P. l., Legare, C. H. (2017). Does the body survive death? Cultural variation in beliefs about life everlasting. *Cognitive Science*, 41(suppl. 3), 455–476. https://doi.org/10.1111/cogs.12430

Watts, L. (2018). Taking palliative care to the top: My meeting with Dr Tedros. Available at: https://eapcnet.wordpress.com/2018/04/09/taking-palliative-care-to-the-top-my-meeting-with-dr-tedros/ (accessed 13 June 2024).

WHO (World Health Organization). (2014). WHA67.19. Strengthening of palliative care as a component of comprehensive care throughout the life course. Available at: https://apps.who.int/gb/ebwha/pdf_files/wha67/a67_r19-en.pdf (accessed 19 June 2024).

Wiener, L., McConnell, D. G., Latella, L., Ludi, E. (2013). Cultural and religious considerations in pediatric palliative care. *Palliative and Supportive Care*, 11, 47–67. https://doi.org/10.1017/s1478951511001027

Winger, A., Fruh, E. A., Holmen, H., Kvarme, L. G., Lee, A., Lorentsen, V. B., Misvaer, N., Riiser, K., Steindal, S. A. (2022). Making room for life and death at the same time: A qualitative study of health and social care professionals' understanding and use of the concept of paediatric palliative care. *BMC Palliative Care*, 21, 50. https://doi.org/10.1186/s12904-022-00933-4

Winger, A., Kvarme, L. G., Løyland, B., Kristiansen, C., Helseth, S., Ravn, I. H. (2020). Family experiences with palliative care for children at home: A systematic literature review. *BMC Palliative Care*, 19(1), 165. https://doi.org/10.1186/s12904-020-00672-4

# CHAPTER 3

# Public perceptions and participation in children's palliative care

## Promoting positive cultures of communication

..............................................

*Duncan Randall and Hicran Çavuşoğlu*

## INTRODUCTION

In the last few years, we have seen how important it is to understand that we do not provide nursing care to children in a social, political, or cultural vacuum. It matters to nurses what people in the communities we serve think about children, childhoods, parenting, the role of being a sibling, grandparents' participation and how we educate and care for our children. In this chapter we discuss the social and cultural public perceptions of death in childhood, because to deliver children's palliative nursing care we have to understand what people, including children, think about dying and death during childhood. The public understanding, as expressed through media reactions to high profile cases, will be explored. In recent years we have seen an increasing trend for such media reporting to fuel sometimes highly confrontational reactions which have direct impact on nurses and nursing. The public conception of palliative care is related to conceptions of dying and death and these too have recently been highlighted in the global COVID-19 pandemic. However, this is not the first pandemic to affect children and we explore how child death has been understood in times of epidemic and pandemics in the past.

The public understanding of childhood death is a vital component of promoting children's palliative nursing care as a public health concern. We discuss the theories and practices of nurses and nursing that facilitate nurses promoting positive public and community approaches, and patterns of communication which can enhance the nurses' work in addressing the public health issues of children's palliative care.

One aspect of this work is the support and care for those who have lost a child, or where children experience loss through death in their childhoods. In the final section of the chapter, we discuss the ways in which nurses can promote positive cultures that help people to express grief and live with bereavement.

DOI: 10.4324/9781003384861-5

**LEARNING OBJECTIVES**

The reader will be able to do the following:

1. Describe the historical and social/cultural public understanding of death and dying as it occurs and affects children and their childhoods.
2. Discuss how public health theories and practices are conceived and enacted in children's palliative nursing care.
3. Discuss nursing actions that promote positive cultures to facilitate public understanding and participation in dying and death in childhood, including positive cultures of communication and loss, grief and bereavement support.

## DEATH AND DYING: CHILDREN, CHILDHOOD AND THE MEDIA

Our conceptions of death are shaped by our experiences and the context in which we find ourselves (Cox et al., 2005). This is also true for children. Those who live in societies where dying and death are experienced more often, or where rituals and practices that surround dying and death are publicly acknowledged and recognised will perceive death differently from those living in societies where children do not encounter dying or death so frequently. We see that the fear of death is felt more acutely in children living in violent communities. Also, children who have direct experience of living with life-limiting or life-threatening conditions, and who have experienced their peers also living with such conditions, have a much more sophisticated understanding of death (Bonoti et al., 2013).

Bearing this in mind, it can be helpful to have some conception of how the understanding of dying and death develops in children, albeit perhaps only a rough guide. Four concepts are often agreed to be instrumental to children's understanding of death. These are outlined in Table 3.1 with some indications of when we think these concepts develop.

**TABLE 3.1** Children's development of the concepts of death (based on work by Nguyen and Gelman, 2002; Cox et al., 2005; Yang, 2013; Vázquez-Sánchez et al., 2019)

| Concept | Description | Estimated ages* |
|---|---|---|
| Universality | That all living things will die | Approximately from age 5 |
| Irreversibility | That once dead, things and people cannot return to being alive | Approximately from age 5 |
| Non-function/ cessation of life | That dying and death involve loss of function and eventually cessation of life | 5–9 years. Culturally dependent but firm by 10 years old |
| Causality of death | That death has a cause which can be determined | 5–9 years. Culturally dependent but firm by 10 years old |

Note: *These are estimates for healthy children as the studies were conducted with healthy participants, i.e. not with children with known life-limiting or life-threatening conditions.

While it is estimated that by age 16 only 4–7% of children will have experienced the death of a relative (Talwar et al., 2011), we can see the influence of exposure to violent death in films and games in the over-representations of this type of death along with accidental death in drawings of children living in high-income, democratic cultures in the Global North (Vázquez-Sánchez et al., 2019). It is suggested then that children's perceptions of death can be influenced by literature, schooling, where they live, family rituals and high use of smartphones (Vázquez-Sánchez et al., 2019). For example, African American children in the USA understand that, in their communities, people who look like them are more likely to die (Jenkins et al., 2014).

With children under 8 spending on average 2–3 hours a day on screens, television and other forms of media are perhaps as influential as cultural or religious influences in children's understanding of death. Children are exposed to various types of loss and death experiences through TV programmes, movies and games and this exposure can influence their understanding of death (Yang and Park, 2017).

There are a few studies that examine the influence of animated films on children's concept of death (Longbottom and Slaughter, 2018; Bridgewater et al., 2021). The findings of these studies showed that media portrayals of death provide children with valuable experiences about death which can be as important as first-hand experience, albeit that some of the films reflect cultural beliefs which run counter to biological understandings. However, as Bluebond-Langner and Clemente (2021) point out, adults too can hold contradictory ideas about death which can be based on "magical" thinking, often expressed in cultural or religious/spiritual beliefs.

There are also carefully and accurately crafted portrayals of death in the media and animated films and these can have a positive effect on children's understanding of death. Studies have shown that children often ask their parents about death scenes, especially in animated films (King and Hayslip, 2002; Longbottom and Slaughter, 2018). These findings suggest that animated films can serve as a valuable tool in initiating conversations about death between children and parents.

Thus, while we might think of children's conception of death following a developmental stepped course (as in Table 3.1), the development of understanding about death may be more accurately described as a continuous progression. This, in turn, is heavily influenced by social/cultural exposure leading towards a more adult conception of death. In addition, personal experiences of life-limiting and life-threatening conditions and dying/death also influence a child's development of their own conceptions of death.

Personal experiences of living with illness, including life-limiting or life-threatening conditions are not exclusive to children diagnosed with such conditions. Healthy siblings of children with these conditions may also be said to be living with a life-limiting or life-threatening condition, not in themselves but in their sibling (Wilkins and Woodgate, 2005; Knecht et al., 2015; McPoland et al., 2023). Again, such experiences will shape healthy siblings' perceptions of death and will facilitate their understanding of dying and death. Healthy children who have a parent or carer who has a life-limiting or life-threatening condition may also have a more developed sense of dying and death as they too, in a sense, are *living with* such conditions (Bonoti et al., 2013; McPoland et al., 2023).

---

**LEARNING ACTIVITY**

1.  Take a moment to write down what you believe about death. This might be your personal ideas or reflect your spiritual/religious or cultural background.
2.  From this personal reflection on your own understanding about dying and death, what are your beliefs or thoughts about childhood death?
3.  It might be useful to keep these reflections and come back to them after reading more of this book.

---

## THE INFLUENCE OF CULTURE AND RELIGION ON CHILDREN'S UNDERSTANDING OF DEATH

The development of the concept of death in children is influenced by their life experiences related to death and also their religious experience. Cultural factors and religious beliefs can dramatically shape the child's understanding of death (McPoland et al., 2023).

In a study involving Korean, Chinese and Chinese American children, children's feelings and concepts about death and loss were examined (Yang and Park, 2017). It was found that most children in all these cultures have negative feelings such as anxiety, sadness and fear about death and loss. However, in East Asia, due to the belief in shamanistic traditions, there is a tendency to avoid talking about death and loss in case it brings bad luck (Lee et al., 2014). Death is considered a taboo subject in Korea and China. Therefore, parents in both countries are reluctant to discuss topics related to death with their children.

Lane et al. (2016) compared the explanations about death held by religious American and secular Chinese children aged 4–12. They found that secular Chinese children believe in supernatural ideas (such as people continue to exist after life) about death less than religious American children. Supernatural beliefs about death are more frequently observed in children from religious cultural backgrounds (Rosengren et al., 2014).

Many studies have shown that religious belief in the family and in school can shape the understanding of death among American and Spanish children (Bering et al., 2005; Rosengren et al., 2014). These children believe that biological and psychological processes will continue after death. Findings of these studies indicated that a family's religious ideas affect the child's understanding of death. In Turkey, most of the people are Muslim, however, attitudes towards religious practices are different according to the regions, socio-economic levels and ethnicity of the family (Bilge and Öztürk, 2021). Children who have religious beliefs more often think that bodily functions continued after death than the ones who are secular. Similarly, in a study on Spanish children attending Catholic schools, aged 4–12, it was found that they believed biological and mental functions continue after death (Bering et al., 2005).

In another study (Panagiotaki et al., 2015), understanding of death by British and Pakistani children between the ages of 4 to 7 was examined. Three groups of children: White British, British Muslim living in London and Pakistani Muslim living in rural Pakistan were compared. It was observed that both British groups had similar understanding of the sub-concepts of death, while Pakistani Muslim children who were living in rural areas grasp the irreversibility of death earlier than the other groups. Additionally, in a further study conducted by Panagiotaki et al. (2018), it was seen that socio-economic level is an important factor in a child's understanding of the biological aspect of death. All these studies showed the importance of socio-cultural studies for understanding of the children's concept of death.

McPoland et al. (2023) spoke to children in Uganda, America and Haiti and found that children ages 5–18, mostly of Christian background, had a sophisticated and nuanced understanding of dying and death. These children living with dying and death had rich cultural understanding of their situation, showing understanding of loss of normalcy and relationships, but also resilience, altruism and spiritual lives. Children living with serious illness, including siblings of those in Uganda and America with serious illness, demonstrated both a rich spiritual life with appreciation of the comfort religion can provide but also the dilemmas and dissonance between spiritual and religious narratives and their own lived experiences.

In the African traditional societies in Nigeria, people have superstitious belief about death in general. The children who die after their birth (infant mortality) are seen as spirits that come to torment the family or died because of the anger of the gods against the family. Lack of information about the interpretation of death among those in Nigeria leads to these beliefs that spiritual phenomenon and enemies are responsible for the death. It is the responsibility of health personnel to inform the people about the realities of death as a natural phenomenon (Ekore and Abass, 2016; Okechi, 2017).

Having looked at children's views of dying and death, let us now turn to social, often adult, views of childhood death.

## HISTORICAL PERSPECTIVES OF DYING AND DEATH IN CHILDHOOD

At first, we might assume that death is timeless. We have evidence of child death throughout recorded historical periods and some evidence of child death in archaeological findings from the prehistorical period (Spellman, 2014; Graeber and Wengrow, 2021).

However, many of the certainties we once relied upon to determine death, such as a cessation of breathing or the arresting of a heartbeat, are now no longer definitive conditions of death. Technology means we can ventilate a child who is not breathing. We can place a child on bypass or use a pacemaker to ensure cardiac output (Alexander et al., 2021). Conditions once seen as fatal are now potentially survivable into adulthood (e.g. cystic fibrosis, see McBennett et al., 2021), while others that once were "uncurable" are now being cured (National Disease Registration Service, 2021).

These technologies and the associated nursing care are expensive. Access to specialist nursing and to the technical equipment required is not universal. These conceptions of the prevention of death through technology are often only available in middle- to high-income countries (Connor, 2020). Even in such economies, access is often not universal, so we might say death can only be redrawn in this way for some children, in some countries, depending on the funding structures of the healthcare systems in that country.

As well as the technical changes of the twentieth and twenty-first centuries, we can perhaps trace a history of public perceptions of child death. As Spellman (2014) points out, prior to the Industrial Revolution child death was common, particularly in infancy and early childhood, with perhaps between a third and a half of all children dying before they were aged 2. This high early childhood mortality gave rise to a fatalistic acceptance of child death, often with little ceremony being attached to a child's death and practices such as the withholding of naming children until they were older and more likely to survive (Spellman, 2014, p. 147).

In the painting reproduced in Figure 3.1, we see the Graham children painted by William Hogarth (1742), a commissioned painting of the Graham's family's children, in which Hogarth highlights the social issues of childhood of his time. Circled top left is a clock with the figure of death, equipped with his scythe, and circled right a cat threatens to kill the caged young bird. Also note the fruit in the picture, fruit that will spoil and decay. The child on the left of the picture in a gilded carriage is Thomas Graham who had already died when Hogarth painted the picture, on the floor are crossed carnation flowers, often used in funerals at the time, and his older sister holds out cherries – the fruit of paradise. Here Hogarth is pointing to the precarious nature of childhoods in the eighteenth century when child death was common.

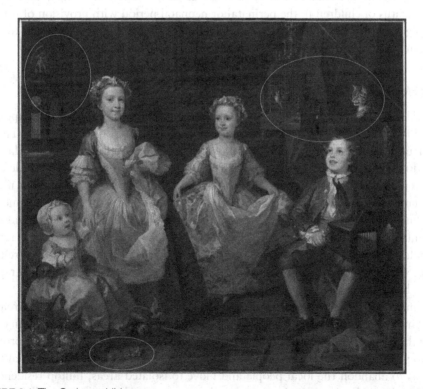

**FIGURE 3.1** The Graham children

Source: Hogarth, painted in 1742 @The National Gallery, London with permission.

Children's nursing was not immune to this history. A case in point is the Coram Foundling Hospital where, between 1756 and 1760, over 10,000 children died, mostly from infectious disease in a period known as the Grand Reception (Howell, 2014). This episode created a fear that, in an age before antibiotics, children would bring infectious disease that would kill adult patients, rather than a concern for children's lives or health. This may be why we see the development of the fever hospital where children were separated from adults and nursed in isolation (Kendrick, 2023).

This gendered history of separating adult care and children's care is also seen in a separation of adult palliative care and children's palliative care that persists in many parts of the world. Indeed, the development of children's palliative care has lagged behind that for adults (Connor, 2020) with initial developments focused on high-income countries. While the WHO have considered children's palliative care for many years (WHO, 2014; WHO and UNICEF, 2018), more recently they have emphasised the need for equity of access (WHO, 2022). There have also been recent developments in a wider acceptance of neonatal and perinatal palliative care (Leong Marc-Aurele and Nelesen, 2013; Mancini et al., 2020; Girgin et al., 2022), where previously public and professional perceptions led to a lack of recognition of perinatal and neonatal death (Currie et al., 2019). This led to a lack of support for parents who had suffered a perinatal or neonatal loss, and to practices that did not recognise the foetus or newborn as living people. In high-income countries there has been a more recent recognition of the person status of children in the perinatal or neonatal period with provision of funeral rites, legal registration of births and official naming as well as nursing practices to support families and communities (Kavanaugh et al., 2010; Currie et al., 2019).

## EPIDEMICS AND PANDEMICS

As we have already highlighted, experiences of death in childhood and exposure to childhood death influence the conception and perception of child death. This is also true for public perceptions of children's dying and death where populations have direct experience of, or exposure to, narratives of epidemics and pandemics. Children's dependence on adults due to physical and cognitive development places children at a structural social and political disadvantage in times of epidemics or pandemics. There is also the historical record of how children are often abandoned by adults in times of social and economic difficulty. There is now a more recent example of COVID-19 in which we can see the patterns of behaviour being (re)produced, where responses to previous infectious or disease outbreaks are both reproduced, but also produced in a new context, in a different age.

Farmer (2020) has pointed out that we can see colonial behaviours being (re)produced in the responses to epidemics. When epidemics broke out in the past, as in cholera outbreaks in colonial India, western colonialists could have attempted to provide care to people, care that they understood and had the resources to provide. What they did was to abandon the local people and move to isolated areas, hilltop residencies, allowing the epidemic to run its course, killing many people, until eventually the disease left no vector for transmission (so many people had died that the disease could no longer spread) or that the population developed herd immunity and the infectious agent was deprived of its means of transition or hosts. Normally both mechanisms were active concurrently. Once the danger was past, the colonial wealthy would return to govern and profit from the local population. A system of abandonment and containment. This same strategy was used to contain the Ebola virus in West Africa in 2014–2016. Rather than a global effort to treat people with Ebola, the population was advised to go home and isolate to stop the transmission of the disease (Farmer, 2020).

We see then the return of previous perceptions. For children, this arguably means that in epidemics and pandemics there is the return of a fatalistic acceptance that children will disproportionally be affected due to their inherent vulnerability. There is a public expectation and acceptance that children will be more likely to die in an epidemic or pandemic. However, this was not the case in COVID-19 despite much apprehension and concern in the early stages of the pandemic. What transpired was that COVID-19 was more deadly in older populations rather than in younger populations (Odd et al., 2022; Rodriguez Velásquez et al., 2022).

The vulnerable structural position of children and their dependence on adults may be thrown into focus by epidemics and pandemics. However, this may also reflect a more ambiguous framing of child death. The deliberate killing of infants or infanticide has been a common historical phenomenon (Spellman, 2014, pp. 149–153). In the pre-contraception and family planning era, infanticide was often used as a form of population control and family management. The inability to provide for a child, the censure of peers and shame over illegitimate children were the most often cited reasons for infanticide. However, the practice of abandoning children, which in effect was certain to kill them, was widespread and socially sanctioned, and facilitated in some cultures by the social and cultural practices surrounding a child's birth. Where a delay between birth and naming or registering a child as a person allowed for it, fathers would normally decide if the child was to be accepted or not. In ancient China, for example, a child's birth was not registered until the third day, thus allowing the opportunity to reject the child (Spellman, 2014).

Social and cultural understanding of personhood, and children's position in relation to being considered a person, were often key to the practices of infanticide and child murder. If a child was not deemed to be a person, or to have reached socially constructed maturity, then killing it could be overlooked. As Spellman (2014, p. 150) comments, in ancient Greece, children were seen as an investment, so often children with perceived disability or deformities were abandoned, and left to perish. There is also a gendered aspect, with infanticide of girls much more common, particularly in cultures with dowry practices, where girls pose a possible future financial burden. We might also consider the view of women as persons in cultures to be a factor. So, in cultures where women's status as people is contingent or refuted, girls are at much higher risk of abandonment and infanticide (Patel, 2007; Sharma, 2007).

The decision as to whether to accept or reject a child lay in pre-modern times with the fathers. As in some cultures today, children have traditionally been seen as the property of fathers. However, as Spellman points out, often while men would make the decision, the acts of murder and abandonment were often expected to be carried out by mothers (Spellman, 2014, p. 150). Despite increasing legal and social disapprobation in the eighteenth and nineteenth centuries and into the modern era, child murder and abandonment continue, albeit at vastly reduced rates. The growth of the provision of social support through institutions, such as the Coram Foundling Hospitals and other religious institutions, meant that abandonment could be mitigated. Children were abandoned by mothers, but the institution reduced the chances of death. However, mortality in such institutions was high and many children that were not admitted were consigned to unknown fates. Indubitably, child abandonment and murder have been reduced in the modern era by increasing social support, particularly for lone female parents and by the medicalisation of contraception and abortion (Spellman, 2014, pp. 152–153).

What we can say is that we can see the (re)production of previous social attitudes to children in epidemics or pandemics. In some societies we see the abandonment of children. However, social disapprobation, reflected in stringent legal sanctions and incarceration, together with social insurance or social support, family planning and contraception have led to a reduction in child murder. Yet, it still persists in communities, is gendered, ableist, economic and still reflects misperceptions of children as persons and the role of children in societies.

## PRESS MEDIA NARRATIVES AND PUBLIC DEBATES

In recent years there have been narratives created by press media reporting on public debates around certain cases of child death. We should recognise that these are "high profile" cases, in that many children, their carers and healthcare teams might face very similar ethical, moral and clinical dilemmas in palliative care and at the end of life, but these are not the subject of intense media press reporting. A small number of cases become a touchstone for public debates and can provoke extreme public responses which feed into the press and media narratives (Wilkinson and Savulescu, 2017).

---

**LEARNING ACTIVITY**

1.  With some work colleagues, identify a high profile or controversial case from your country. Perhaps it is just a case that you feel raised ethical or moral dilemmas for you.
2.  Gather some colleagues together, perhaps with some food and a drink! Present the case in brief (15–20 minutes). After the case presentation, allow colleagues to discuss initial thoughts (10 minutes). Then ask some reflective/open questions (20 minutes).

    *   How does this case make us feel?
    *   What has been the response of state/country officials and professional carers?
    *   What has been the response of the community?
    *   What might be the effect on our care of the public debates about this case?

3.  Allow some time to sum up and draw your own conclusions (10 minutes).

In the UK, the cases of Charlie Gard and Alfie Evans demonstrate such media narratives created around two particular cases (Wilkinson and Savulescu, 2017; 2018). Arguably these cases occurred in the context of the Liverpool Care Pathway and in a time of declining deference to medical expertise. The Liverpool Care Pathway was used in a media narrative that, rather than nurses managing end-of-life care, they were, in effect, practising euthanasia on some elders. The pathway and its use prompted a public enquiry (Neuberger et al., 2013) which was highly critical of nurses' implementation of the pathway, which some families felt was used to justify euthanasia. Neuberger et al. (2013) recognise that aspects of the pathway were helpful and that it could help teams to manage the end-of-life stage, but that the end-of-life phase was poorly defined and that often a lack of candour and poor communication led to a public perception that the pathway was not helpful.

Perhaps adding to the context was a focus in media narratives on the advancement of science and the struggles of the National Health Service (NHS). Particularly in the Charlie Gard case, there was a debate in the media about the availability of treatments which were experimental and expensive that were available in the USA, but not in the UK. The public perception was that the NHS, or healthcare professionals in particular, were not making such treatments available because of cost. Counter-arguments were presented about the likely success of the treatments but were not reflected in many popular press narratives (Das, 2017; Triggle, 2017). While focused in the UK, these cases were discussed and the implications felt internationally.

In both the Gard and the Evans cases, there were physical attacks and verbal assaults on nurses including threatening behaviour via social media (Triggle, 2017). As is often the case with violence directed at nurses, some of it had a sexual gendered aspect (Jakobsson et al., 2023). Nurses in both cases felt intimidated and some left the profession.

What we see in these high-profile cases is an extreme expression of tensions in the public debates on children's palliative and, in particular, end-of-life care. These appear to be highly contextual and influenced by media narratives which are also influenced by the recent and current public/political debates about healthcare and professional power dynamics.

Such "high profile" cases and the media narratives that surround them might be seen as expressions of the public disquiet about end-of-life decisions (Wilkinson and Savulescu, 2018). In the debates on neonatal and child euthanasia, some argue that the legalisation of euthanasia is a legalising of clinical decisions often taken by medical teams and nurses about children's quality of life (Verhagen and Sauer, 2005).

## Childhood Euthanasia

Euthanasia in childhood has been legalised in the Netherlands, Colombia and in Belgium, where in 2014 the existing 2002 euthanasia law for adults was updated to include children (Verhagen and Sauer, 2005, Raus, 2016; Benavides, 2018). The legislation highlights two aspects of the debate around euthanasia in childhood: that of euthanasia in neonates and for conditions arising during the prenatal or neonatal periods and, separately, the consideration of euthanasia for all children across the duration of childhood and the point at which children can and should make their own decisions. It should be noted that two of these countries are in Europe where the history of the Nazis' child death programmes is well known (Benedict et al., 2009). These programmes, which started well before targeting of other minority groups, were based on ideas of eugenics and led to disabled children being killed in attempts to "purify" the Arian population of unwanted people (Benedict et al., 2009). While the Nazi regime was rightly condemned, the narratives of eugenics could be heard in medical textbooks and practice well after the Second World War, particularly in relation to children with learning disabilities (Tredgold, 1952). It should also be noted that none of the main religions of the world condone euthanasia for any age group.

In the Netherlands, the debate centres on the neonatal period. In response to the clinical decision-making for neonates, in which a physician's report was scrutinised by criminal prosecutors and physicians could be interviewed by police relating to offences of murder, Verhagen and his colleagues developed the Groningen Protocol (Table 3.2).

The protocol reflects a number of the debates in the public perceptions of euthanasia. First, that suffering which may be akin to torture should be avoided, particularly suffering which has little or no perceived benefit in terms of health outcome and prognosis (Deak and Saroglou, 2017). That there are concerns about the effect that these end-of-life decisions have on the relationship between physician and the child and their carers. By extension, this concern also affects the nurses who are part of a healthcare team approach where decisions are taken following team consultation (Kavanaugh et al., 2010). This concern is sometimes expressed as worry that medical practitioners are "playing god", making decisions on life and death without reference to the child's family, community or other colleagues. Ensuring a second opinion is perhaps a way to ensure that individual practitioners cannot be deemed to have made decisions based solely on their own judgements.

In countries without the Groningen Protocol, it could be argued that the same steps are adhered to. End-of-life decisions are made in consultation with parents and, in some communities, with children, and that the healthcare team would be consulted, including nurses. In addition, that controversial decisions are scrutinised by hospital ethical committees and are subject to medical negligence legislation. As Verhagen and Sauer have commented, the Groningen Protocol may simply provide a formalised and legally recognised way to structure the decisions made by medical teams (Verhagen and Sauer, 2005).

**TABLE 3.2** The Groningen Protocol for neonates with severe illness (adapted from Verhagen and Sauer, 2005)

| Requirements |
| --- |
| • The diagnosis and prognosis must be certain |
| • Hopeless and unbearable suffering must be present |
| • The diagnosis, prognosis, and unbearable suffering must be confirmed by at least one independent doctor |
| • Both parents must give informed consent |
| • The procedure must be performed in accordance with the accepted medical standard |

The public perception of life at and around birth being precarious may make neonatal euthanasia more easily understood. The Belgium Act amendment (2014) and Colombian law that allow child euthanasia are more problematic in extending euthanasia to minors (children under 18 and, in Belgium, children who are not emancipated) (Raus, 2016; Benavides, 2018). Although, Raus points out that child euthanasia was part of the political and ethical debate in Belgium leading up to the original 2002 Act, and that amendments were suggested to allow for the inclusion of children, including amendments which would have been more radical than the eventual accepted amendment. The successful amendment was subject to public scrutiny via a public inquiry with many (but not all) experts being in favour of euthanasia for competent children. The legal position is somewhat confused in Belgium, in that the legal frameworks allow for emancipated minors. These minors were included in the original 2002 Act. A child over 15 can be emancipated, by a youth court or through marriage, and is deemed to have more capacity, mostly in financial rights, but not ascribed full adult status.

The main requirements of the amended Belgium Act as it applies to children are set out in Table 3.3. There are a number of important differences between the provision in Belgium and the Groningen protocol. Obviously, the requirement to have discernment and competence excludes neonates. The Belgian amendment requirements are not predicated upon parental ownership of children, but instead recognise the child's agency, albeit still requiring parental consent. The child's request has to be made free of influence, or coercion by others, thus precluding parental or other carers' wishes being expressed via the child. The Belgian amendment also makes other conditions which directly affect who can access euthanasia. As can be seen in Table 3.3, death has to be expected within a short period and this, together with the requirement that the competent request for euthanasia has to be sustained up to the point of death, means that advance care planning or advanced directives cannot be used. The only suffering that can be considered for children is physical suffering, while for adults and emancipated minors psychological suffering can be considered.

**TABLE 3.3** Amendment of the Belgian 2002 euthanasia law in 2014 (adapted from Raus, 2016)

| Requirements |
| --- |
| • The child, who must display a capacity of discernment, must request euthanasia repeatedly and the request must be current up to the moment of death |
| • Only for children who have "Medically futile condition of constant and unbearable physical suffering that cannot be alleviated and that will, within a short period of time, result in death, and results from a serious and incurable disorder caused by illness or accident" (*Belgian Official Gazette*, 2014) |
| • A second independent medical opinion must be secured, the child examined, and a check made that the legal criteria are met |
| • The child must be assessed by a paediatric psychiatrist or psychologist to evaluate if they are competent; the report of this assessment must be shared with the child and their legal representative (parents) |
| • Legal representative (normally parents) must give written consent |
| • The euthanasia has to be officially reported to the Federal Control and Evaluation Commission to determine if legal, with the option to refer to judicial authorities |

As Raus (2016) has pointed out, the legal framework does present some anomalies such that an emancipated 16-year-old could access and plan for euthanasia for a condition with a near-to-normal life expectancy, but which has physical and psychological distressing symptoms, while a non-emancipated child could not.

During the ICPCN International Conference on Children's Palliative Care in Mumbai, India, in February 2014, more than 250 experts from 35 countries decided to send a message to the Belgian government. They invited the government to reconsider their decision about child euthanasia (ICPCN, 2014; Devos, 2019). In their messages, they stated that they believe children with life-limiting diseases have the right to the best quality of life, and to receive high quality palliative care to meet their needs. They emphasised that euthanasia is not part of children's palliative care and is not an alternative to palliative care.

There is then a global public debate on children's right to life and their right to a dignified death. Arguably, much of the debate in general on euthanasia is applicable to children, the same concerns over choice and torture prevail (Deak and Saroglou, 2017). The same concerns are evident that the advances of medical science and supporting technologies make life possible for those living with conditions which previously often were fatal (Alexander et al., 2021). However, the cost may be pain and other distressing symptoms (Box 3.1) and/or the dependence on technologies and others. which may erode quality of life. These debates are influenced by religious doctrines, conceptions, practices and debates about the agency of children, the rights of different generations and about life, community and death. Social attitudes to disability and health and well-being also play into these public debates and influence the ideas about quality of life and social disability. Others make economic arguments that influence the debate as the highly technical and intensive nursing care are often expensive (Alexander et al., 2021; Currie et al., 2019). Ideas of deontology and utility clash in arguments over how limited resources might best be spent. Ideas on the duty owed to humans who suffer clash with those who argue that more social good could be achieved for a greater number of the general population, who can be helped to live productive longer lives, rather than for a very small number of children and their carers.

---

**BOX 3.1 EUTHANASIA CASE STUDY**

A 12-year-old girl with anoxic encephalopathy, who experienced a near-drowning at the age of 2, was admitted to the PICU because of viral meningitis. After she stayed three weeks in the intensive care unit, she remains on assisted ventilation. She has hypertension, hypoxemia, dystonia, seizure, respiratory failure and pain. Medical treatment did not improve any of these symptoms. Her parents said that watching their child suffering for 10 years was unbearable. They asked the intensive care team to "… Do whatever to stop her suffering, even if it shortens her life."

Discuss this case with a colleague and consider:

- What is your answer to the family's request?
- What legal arguments would you use to support your point of view and actions?
- Would your team agree, if not, why and how would you manage the conflict?

Source: adapted from Clement de Clety et al. (2016).

## CHILDREN'S PALLIATIVE CARE AS A PUBLIC HEALTH ISSUE: NURSING THEORIES AND PRACTICES

Both palliative care and public health are umbrella terms which contain often ill-defined sub-terms such as end of life, active dying and health promotion, or well-being (Dempers and Gott, 2017). To combine the terms into children's public health palliative care might seem counter-intuitive. However, as Kellehear (2007) has argued over a number of years, this is because of a professionalised view of both public health work and palliative care which ignores the social meaning of death and loss and the contribution of communities to supporting and helping people live with dying, death and loss (see Chapter 1). Furthermore, Kellehear suggests that these professional frames contribute to the negative perception of death and loss, where death and loss are characterised as a disappearance, nothingness, associated with embarrassment, isolation and a lack of social function or legitimacy (Kellehear, 2007; Higo, 2012). Nurses may reinforce these social stigmas and death anxiety (Bassah et al., 2014).

To oppose this negative view of death and loss, Kellehear (2007) points out that individuals and communities all live with death and loss. That the experience of loss through death is not resolved with "therapy", but that loss can inspire art, creativity and political and social change. Also, in many cultures and for many individuals, the dead are not absent, not gone, but remain connected to the living through remembrance, and observance of practices and rituals. Be these formalised social expressions such as the Day of the Dead (Día de los Muertos, celebrated in Mexico, 31 October till 2 November), or personal remembrance and experiences of "seeing" and or "talking" to the dead. Box 3.2 presents a public health approach to palliative care.

---

**BOX 3.2 DEFINITION OF A PUBLIC HEALTH APPROACH TO PALLIATIVE CARE**

A public health approach to palliative care is a health promotion approach to end-of-life care, one that views the community as an equal partner in the long and complex task of providing quality health care at the end-of-life. Just as health, according to WHO, is 'everyone's responsibility' so too is death, dying, loss and care.

(Public Health and Palliative Care International, 2023)

---

It is agreed that public health work is part of nursing, as it is agreed in the definitions of nursing that palliative and end-of-life care is also a part of nursing (see Meleis, 2012). What does not seem evident is how both these elements of nursing are accounted for in the theories and practice of children's nurses and nursing (Randall, 2016a). There are theories and approaches to public health nursing, to nursing that make mention of death and dying (King, Rogers and Roy, cited in Meleis, 2012, pp. 233, 313, 330) and to nursing children (Randall, 2016b; 2021). What appears to be missing is a unifying approach in which public health children's palliative nursing is reflected in the nursing theory. The literature describing nursing practice is also limited. Rowse (2006) provides an account from a community children's palliative team and Hexem and Feudtner (2012) give a broader account, including population health concerns, health promotion and social determinants.

While we see a growing awareness in professional nursing circles of public involvement and understanding of social relations and compassionate communities (see Chapter 1), this has not been articulated in any detail in nursing theories and seems underdeveloped in nursing practices. However, in 2024, an international collaboration came together to attempt to define and set out principles of children's palliative public health (Downing et al., 2024, in press) (Box 3.3). The group set out eight principles but also note the differing approaches to children's palliative care between high-income and low- and middle-income countries, while also noting that a public health approach has to balance the population needs, support to communities and professional carers' capacity.

---

**BOX 3.3 CHILDREN'S PALLIATIVE CARE AND PUBLIC HEALTH: POSITION STATEMENTS**

1.  Dying, death, loss and grief are *everyone's business*. Despite our anxieties in the professional world, we can empower the community.
2.  No matter how long or short a childhood is, children are all children who have the right to live full and fulfilling lives as children.
3.  The community and professionals supporting the child must complement each other, and offer regular, practical support, to enable children and their carers to continue living connected sustainable lives.
4.  Theories of children's palliative public health must be coproduced by health, education and social care professionals and children, carers and communities.
5.  Governments must incorporate children's palliative public health care into all levels of their health, education and social care systems. Communities must be involved through collective social action, and through co-design, co-creation and co- production.
6.  We must be the change we want to see. Everyone involved has a role to play in delivering a radical and transformational change to build more sustainable and robust models of care and services.
7.  Children's palliative public health must be embedded in all health and social care education curriculums, in particular in primary and community care.
8.  More research and co-evaluation into children's palliative public health care are needed to ensure the delivery of appropriate, individualised palliative care.

Source: Downing et al. (2024, in press)

---

## IS A GOOD CHILD DEATH POSSIBLE?

An assumption which underpins such public health approaches is that a healthy death is possible, that there are ways for children and their carers to experience a good death, one in which well-being is not entirely destroyed. The conception of a good childhood death being possible has gained acceptance (Hendrickson and McCorkle, 2008; Chong et al., 2019). In their literature review, Hendrickson and McCorkle (2008) identified seven overarching themes all with sub-themes as set out in Table 3.4. While this review was focused on children dying with an oncology condition and the

**TABLE 3.4** A good childhood death (children with oncology diagnosis) (adapted from Hendrickson and McCorkle, 2008)

| Themes | Sub-themes |
| --- | --- |
| Age-appropriate participation | Awareness of dying |
| | Autonomy |
| | Acceptance |
| | Personal ideal |
| | Timing |
| | Location |
| | Control |
| | Self-determination |
| | Self-image |
| | Independence |
| Personal style | Dignity |
| | Individuality |
| | Personal affirmation of whole person |
| | Privacy |
| Quality of life | Pain and symptom management |
| | Length of illness/dying |
| | Social relations/being present |
| | Survival goals |
| Preparation for death | Advance care planning |
| | Hope |
| | Resolution |
| | Completion |
| | Honesty |
| | Communication |
| Aspects of care | Continuity |
| | Cultural sensitivity |
| | Attributes of staff |
| | Addressing spiritual concerns |
| | Having someone present: relationships |
| Legacy | Contributing to others |
| | Establishing meaning |
| Impact on survivors | Importance of ritual or funeral |
| | Grief counselling |
| | Economic distress |
| | Emotional distress |

majority of studies were in medical journals rather than nursing (24 vs 12 respectively), it seems some important themes emerge which may be applicable to childhood death from other conditions. One of the most-represented themes in terms of papers featured was symptom management, followed by the desire for individuality. These themes are also reflected in many of the practices of nurses, in particular, guiding advance or future care planning, the facilitation of location of death, the participation in creating legacy and memories that can sustain the bereaved (Yang, 2013; Winger et al., 2020).

To construct a good death requires open communication, and to work directly with children on many of the aspects identified in Table 3.4 one will need candour and trust between nurse and child. As Cooke and Randall (2021) have pointed out, patterns of communication are not always open in this way. The approaches identified by Grinyer (2012) are used by children and nurses, but also by other carers and professionals (Box 3.4).

---

**BOX 3.4 RANGE OF AWARENESS APPROACHES**

- *Closed awareness:* Where children are not included and others who know about the illness/ death conceal it.
- *Suspected awareness:* The child is aware something is wrong, but not certain what is happening, and is not included by others who are aware.
- *Mutual pretence:* The child and others are all aware, but no one talks about the illness/ death or acknowledges it.
- *Open awareness:* Everyone knows and talks openly/acknowledges the illness and or death.

Source: adapted from Grinyer (2012).

---

Challenging such widespread conceptions and moving children and their carers to the open awareness approach, which is beneficial in constructing a good death (Box 3.5), can be difficult (Dunlop, 2008). As Cooke and Randall (2021) discuss, children and their carers may need time to process emotions and information and harm can be done in attempting to move people to open awareness before they are ready and have worked through cognitive and emotional responses.

---

**BOX 3.5 A GOOD CHILD DEATH?**

Maura, a beautiful girl, was born, perfect from the forehead down but with anencephaly and without the top of her head. Her parents learned about her anencephaly during an ultrasound before birth. After receiving much information at the hospital, they decided to continue the pregnancy. If Maura lived long enough after birth, her parents wanted to take her home. After a few days Maura was stable and discharged from the hospital with her mother. Her parents and their relatives cared for and loved her and sang to her at home. Their friends, pastor and the hospice team provided support to the family by visits. Maura peacefully took her last breath in her mother's arms without pain or distress at the age of 8 days.

- What is your suggestion to this family after the delivery of the baby?
- Using Table 3.4, reflect and discuss with a colleague on the aspects of this case that could make it a good death.

Source: adapted from Welch (2008).

---

## PERCEPTIONS OF LOSS, GRIEF AND BEREAVEMENT

### Being there, presence and remembrance

Ideas of grief, loss and bereavement have changed in the past few decades. When once grief was thought of in the classic Kübler-Ross (1970) staged fashion, as a process people moved through and which could be completed, there is now more recognition that bereavement and loss remain with people, and they live with their loss. This dual process model developed by Stroebe and Schut (1999; 2010) proposes that people process death, loss and grief alongside their continuing life activities.

This continual processing model suggests that nurses need to be ready to provide support on an ad hoc, ongoing basis, rather than providing interventions which resolve grief issues. Such support would seem to be more possible and reliable, developed through public health models in which social relationships, familial and friendship networks would seem more appropriate in providing such ad hoc and prolonged support, than the often brief and outcome-orientated professional interventions.

In addition, as discussed above, the perceptions of grieving as in those of death are influenced by factors such as religious beliefs, cultural values, social environment and what they have learned from the media, as well as the presence of social support (Downdey, 2000). Children express their grief reactions as both behavioural and verbal expressions. Therefore, identifying fears and concerns of children about death, using methods such as drawing, storytelling and play therapy can be more effective than conversation. The dual processing model is also seen in how children need to discuss their grief with others who have similar experiences (Rolls and Payne, 2007; McClatchey and Wimmer, 2012). Being with other bereaved children can help children feel less isolated. In addition to this, giving opportunities to remember the deceased one and talk about their memories, can facilitate growth and aid coping with loss.

## KEY POINTS

- Children develop their understanding of death between the ages of 5 and 10 but their understanding is influenced by culture, their environment and their exposure to dying and death.
- Childhood death changes over time, both in terms of the nature of death and the public perceptions and reactions to dying and death in childhood.
- Living with dying and death in childhood is not limited to children with a life limiting or life-threatening condition but extends to their siblings and to children with carers (parents) with palliative and end-of-life care needs.
- Pandemics and epidemics can alter public perceptions of death in childhood and social attitudes to child death are influenced by social attitudes to children and beliefs about children's agency, cognitive ability, and economic and social participation.
- There are tensions between public perceptions of medical science's ability to cure, the allocation of health resources and trust in nurses/healthcare professionals which can be heightened by media narratives and lead to confrontation.

- Nurses can help to reframe child death as "good" by working with children, their carers and communities and such a good childhood death approach can help people live with grief and bereavement.
- A new public health approach is emerging in which childhood death is everyone's business as it affects all generations, communities, and cultural/social/economic/ religious and political groups.

## SUGGESTED READING

These are some suggestions from colleagues in practice and we thank everyone who suggested a resource they use. We have not been able to include them all and your local team may have other suggestions.

### For younger children

*Pepper, Pooch and Little* by Caroline Jay. Illustrator: Catherine Swan (4 years plus).
*Badger's Parting Gifts* by Susan Varley (4–7 years old approximately).
*Missing Mummy* by Rebecca Cobb (5 years old and under).

### For older children

*Tough Stuff Journal: Someone Has Died* by Pete English (9–13 years old). This booklet by Ataloss.org is available at: https://www.ataloss.org/shop/tough-stuff-journal-someone-has-died
*Rory's Story*, by Anna Jacobs (teenagers). This is a story of an adolescent boy who experiences the death of his mother.

### For children with additional needs

*Finding Your Own Way to Grieve* by Karla Helbert (ages 5–18). A creative activity workbook for grieving children and teens on the Autistic Spectrum.
*Supporting Children with Autism to Manage Death, Loss and Grief: A Guide for Parents, Carers & Educational Settings* by Birmingham City Council Educational Psychology Service, available at https://edwardstrust.org.uk/wp-content/uploads/2020/07/Bereavement_and_autism_a_guide_for_parents.pdf

### Talking with children (for adults)

Jenni Thomas talks about child bereavement: through Jenni's website you can hear a range of podcasts, available at: https://www.jennithomas.com/podcasts

## REFERENCES

Alexander, D., Eustace-Cook, J., Brenner, M. (2021). Approaches to the initiation of life sustaining technology in children: A scoping review of changes over time. *Journal of Child Health Care*, 25(4), 509–522. https://doi.org/10.1177/1367493520961884
Bassah, N., Seymour, J., Cox, K. (2014). A modified systematic review of research evidence about education for pre-registration nurses in palliative care. *BMC Palliative Care*, 13, 56. https://doi.org/10.1186/1472-684X-13-56
*Belgian Official Gazette*. (2014). Act amending the Act of 28 May 2002 on euthanasia, sanctioning euthanasia for minors. *Belgian Official Gazette*, number 2014009093: 21053.

Benavides, L. (2018). The right to die with dignity in Colombia. *Forensic Research and Criminology International Journal*, 6, 426–429.

Benedict, S., Shields, L., O'Donnell, A. J. (2009). Children's "euthanasia" in Nazi Germany. *Journal of Pediatric Nursing*, 24(6), 506–516. https://doi.org/10.1016/j.pedn.2008.07.012

Bering, J., Hernandez, B. C., Bjorklund, D. (2005). The development of afterlife beliefs in religiously and secularly schooled children. *British Journal of Development Psychology*, 23, 587–607. https://doi.org/10.1348/026151005x36498

Bilge, A. R., Öztürk, R. (2021). Conceptualizing death: How do children in Turkey understand death? *Nesnedergisi*, 9(20), 221–239. https://doi.org/10.7816/nesne-09-20-01

Bluebond-Langner, M., Clemente, I. (2021). Children's views of death. In R. Hain, A. Goldman, A. Rapport, M. Mering (eds), *Oxford textbook of palliative care for children* (3rd edn). Oxford University Press.

Bonoti, F., Leondari, A., Mastora, A. (2013). Exploring children's understanding of death: Through drawings and the death concept questionnaire. *Death Studies*, 37, 47–60. https://doi.org/10.1080/07481187.2011.623216

Bridgewater, E. E., Menendez, D., Rosengren, K. S. (2021). Capturing death in animated films: Can films stimulate parent-child conversations about death? *Cognitive Development*, 59, 101063. https://doi.org/10.1016/j.cogdev.2021.101063

Chong, P. H., Walshe, C., Hughes, S. (2019). Perceptions of a good death in children with life-shortening conditions: An integrative review. *Journal of Palliative Medicine*, 22(6), 714–723. https://doi.org/10.1089/jpm.2018.0335

Clement de Clety, S., Friedel, M., Verhagen, A. E., Lantos, J., Carter, B. S. (2016). Please do whatever it takes to end our daughter's suffering! *Pediatrics*, 137(1), e20153812. https://doi.org/10.1542/peds.2015-3812

Connor, S. (ed.) (2020). *Global atlas of palliative care at the end-of-life* (2nd edn). Available at: https://thewhpca.org/resources/global-atlas-of-palliative-care-2nd-ed-2020/ (accessed 8 June 2024).

Cooke, R., Randall, D. (2021). Death and dying in childhood. In E. A. Glasper, J. Richardson, D. Randall (eds), *A textbook of children and young people's nursing*. Elsevier.

Cox, M., Garrett, E., Graham, J. A. (2005). Death in Disney films: Implications for children's understanding of death. *Journal of Death and Dying*, 50(4), 267–280. https://doi.org/10.2190/Q5VL-KLF7-060F-W69V

Currie, E. R., Christian, B. J., Hinds, P. S., Perna, S. J., Robinson, C., Day, S., Bakitas, M., Meneses, K. (2019). Life after loss: Parent bereavement and coping experiences after infant death in the neonatal intensive care unit. *Death Studies*, 43(5), 333–342. https://doi.org/10.1080/07481187.2018.1474285

Das, R. (2017). Key lessons from the role of the media in the Charlie Gard case. Available at: https://blogs.surrey.ac.uk/sociology/2017/08/08/key-lessons-from-the-role-of-the-media-in-the-charlie-gard-case/ (accessed 8 June 2024).

Deak, C., Saroglou, V. (2017). Terminating a child's life? Religious, moral, cognitive and emotional factors underlying non-acceptance of child euthanasia. *Psychologica Belgica*, 57(1), 59–76. https://doi.org/10.5334%2Fpb.341

Dempers, C., Gott, M. (2017). Which public health approach to palliative care? An integrative literature review. *Progress in Palliative Care*, 25(1), 1–10, https://doi.org/10.1080/09699260.2016.1189483

Devos, T. (ed.) (2019). *Euthanasia: Searching the full story, experiences and insights of Belgian doctors and nurses* (pp. 11–12, 49–59). Springer.

Downdey, L. (2000). Annotation: Childhood bereavement following parental death. *Journal of Child Psychology and Psychiatry*, 41 (7); 819–830.

Downing, J., Randall, D., McNamara-Goodger, K., Ellis, P., Dunlop, S., Palat, G., Ali, Z., Hunt, J., Kiman, R., Friedel, M., Neilson, S. (2024, in press). Children's Palliative Care and Public Health: Position statement. *BMC Palliative Care*.

Dunlop, S. (2008). The dying child: Should we tell the truth? *Paediatric Nursing*, 20(6), 28–31. https://doi.org/10.7748/paed2008.07.20.6.28.c6628

Ekore, R. I., Abass, B. L. (2016). African concept of death and advance care directives. *Indian Journal of Palliative Care*, 22(4), 369–372. https://doi.org/10.4103/0973-1075.191741

Farmer, P. (2020). *Fevers, feuds, and diamonds: Ebola and the ravages of history*. Farrar, Straus and Giroux.

Girgin, B. A, Gozen, D., Aktas, E., Ergun, K. (2022). Attitudes towards neonatal palliative care amongst Turkish nurses and physicians: A comparative cross- sectional study. *Journal of Hospice and Palliative Nursing*, 24(5), E185–E196 https://doi.org/10.1097/NJH.0000000000000875

Graeber, D., Wengrow, D. (2021). *The dawn of everything: A new history of humanity*. Penguin Random House.

Grinyer, A. (2012). *Palliative and end-of-life care for children and young people: Home, hospice and hospital*. Wiley-Blackwell.

Hendrickson, K., McCorkle, R. (2008). A dimensional analysis of the concept: Good death of a child with cancer. *Journal of Pediatric Oncology Nursing*, 25(3), 127–138. https://doi.org/10.1177/1043454208317237

Hexem, K., Feudtner, C. (2012). A public health framework for paediatric palliative and hospice care. In J. Cohen, L. Deliens (eds), *A public health perspective on end-of-life care* (pp. 168–172). Oxford University Press.

Higo, M. (2012). Surviving death-anxieties in liquid modern times: Examining Zygmunt Bauman's cultural theory of death and dying. *OMEGA: Journal of Death and Dying*, 65(3), 221–238. https://doi.org/10.2190/OM.65.3.e

Howell, C. (2014). *The Foundling Museum: An introduction*. The Foundling Museum.

ICPCN. (2014). ICPCN Mumbai Declaration 2014. ICPCN, 12 February 2014. Available at: https://icpcn.org/wp-content/uploads/2022/12/Mumbai-Declaration.pdf (accessed February 2024).

Jakobsson, J., Ormon, K., Axelsson, M., Berthelsen, H. (2023). Exploring workplace violence on surgical wards in Sweden: A cross-sectional study. *BMC Nursing*, 22,106. https://doi.org/10.1186/s12912-023-01275-z

Jenkins, E. J., Wang, E., Turner, L. (2014). Beyond community violence: Loss and traumatic grief in African American elementary school children. *Journal of Child and Adolescent Trauma*, 7, 27–36. https://doi.org/10.1007/s40653-014-0001-4

Kavanaugh, K., Moro, T. T., Savage, T. A. (2010). How nurses assist parents regarding life support decisions for extremely premature infants. *Journal of Obstetric, Gynecologic & Neonatal Nursing*, 39, 147–158. https://doi.org/10.1111/j.1552-6909.2010.01105.x

Kellehear, A. (2007). The end of death in late modernity: An emerging public health challenge. *Critical Public Health*, 17(1), 71–79. https://doi.org/10.1080/09581590601156365

Kendrick, A. (2023). Caring for children with infectious diseases: Children's experiences of fever hospitals and sanatoria in Scotland. *Journal of the History of Childhood and Youth*, 16(1), 9–27., https://doi.org/10.1353/hcy.2023.0006

King, J., Hayslip, B. (2002). The media's influence on college students' views of death. *Omega: Journal of Death and Dying*, 44(1), 37–56. https://doi.org/10.2190/HGXD-6WLJ-X56F-4AQL

Knecht, C., Hellmers, C., Metzing, S. (2015). The perspective of siblings of children with chronic illness: A literature review. *Journal of Pediatric Nursing*, 30, 102–116. https://dx.doi.org/10.1016/j.pedn.2014.10.010

Kübler-Ross, E. (1970). *On death and dying*. Macmillan.

Lane, I., Zhu, L., Evans, E., Wellman, H. (2016). Developing concepts of the mind, body and after life:. Exploring the roles of narrative context and culture. *Journal of Cognition and Culture*, 16; 50–82. http://dx.doi.org/10.1163/15685373-12342168

Lee, J. S., Kim, E. Y., Choi, Y., Koo, J. H. (2014). Cultural variances in composition of biological and supernatural concepts of death: Content analysis of children's literature. *Death Studies*, 38, 538–545. https://doi.org/10.1080/07481187.2014.899653

Leong Marc-Aurele, K., Nelesen, R. (2013). A five-year review of referrals for perinatal palliative care. *Journal of Palliative Medicine*, 16(10). https://doi.org/10.1089/jpm.2013.0098

Longbottom, S., Slaughter, V. (2018). Sources of children's knowledge about death and dying. *Philosophical Transactions of the Royal Society B*, 373, 20170267. https://doi.org/10.1098/rstb.2017.0267

Mancini, A., Price, J., Kerr Elliott, T. (eds) (2020). *Neonatal palliative care for nurses*. Springer Nature.

McBennett, K. A., Davis, P. B., Konstan, M. W. (2021). Increasing life expectancy in cystic fibrosis: Advances and challenges. *Pediatric Pulmonology*, 57, S5–S12. https://doi.org/10.1002/ppul.25733

McClatchey, I. S., Wimmer, J. S. (2012). Healing components of a bereavement camp: Children and adolescents give voice to their experiences. *Omega, Journal of Death and Dying*, 65(1), 11–32. https://doi.org/10.2190/om.65.1.b

McPoland, P., Grossoehme, D. H, Sheehan, D. C, Stephenson, P., Downing, J., Deshommes, T., Gassant, P. Y. H., Friebert, S. (2023). Children's understanding of dying and death: A multinational grounded theory study. *Palliative and Supportive Care*. http//doi.org/10.1017/S1478951523000287

Meleis, A. I. (2012). *Theoretical nursing development and progress* (5th edn). Lippincott Williams and Wilkins.

National Disease Registration Service. (2021). Children, teenagers and young adults UK cancer statistics report 2021. Available at: https://digital.nhs.uk/ndrs/data/data-outputs/ctya-uk-cancer-statistics-report-2021 (accessed 8 June 2024).

Neuberger, J. et al. (2013). Independent review of the Liverpool Care Pathway: More care, less pathway, a review of the Liverpool Care Pathway. Crown. Available at: https://assets.publishing.service.gov.uk/government/uploads/system/uploads/attachment_data/file/212450/Liverpool_Care_Pathway.pdf (accessed 8 June 2024).

Nguyen, S. P., Gelman, S. A. (2002). Four and 6 year olds' biological concept of death: The case of plants. *British Journal of Developmental Psychology*, 20, 495–513.

Odd, D., Stoianova, S., Williams, T., Sleap, V., Blair, P., Fleming, P., Wolfe, T. I., Luty, K. (2022). Child mortality in England during the COVID-19 pandemic. *Archives of Disease in Childhood*, 107, 14–20. https://doi.org/10.1136/archdischild-2020-320899

Okechi, O. S. (2017). Culture, perception/belief about death and their implication to the awareness and control of the socio-economic, environmental and health factors surrounding lower life expectancy in Nigeria. *Acta Psychopathologica*, 3(5), 56. https\\doi.org\10.4172/2469-6676.100128

Panagiotaki, G., Hopkins, M., Nobes, G., Ward, E., Griffiths, D. (2018). Children's and adults' understanding of death: Cognitive, parental and experiential influences, *Journal of Experimental Child Psychology*, 166, 96–115. https://doi.org/10.1016/j.jecp.2017.07.014

Panagiotaki, G., Nobes, G., Ashraf, A., Aubby, H. (2015). British and Pakistani children's understanding of death: Cultural and developmental influences. *British Journal of Developmental Psychology*, 33, 31–44. https://doi.org/10.1111/bjdp.12064

Patel, T. (2007). The mindset behind eliminating the female foetus. In T. Patel (ed.), *Sex-selective abortion in India: Gender, society and new reproductive technologies* (pp. 135–174). Sage.

Public Health and Palliative Care International. (2023). *The public health approach to palliative care*. Available at: https://www.phpci.org/public-health-approach (accessed 8 June 2024).

Randall, D. (2016a). Pragmatics and bringing dying back into children's nursing. *eHospice*, International children's edition published online 11 August 2016. Available at: https://ehospice.com/inter_childrens_posts/pragmatics-and-bringing-dying-back-into-childrens-nursing/ (accessed February 2024).

Randall, D. (2016b). *Pragmatic children's nursing: A theory for children and their childhoods.* Routledge.

Randall, D. (2021). Nursing, children and their childhoods. In E. A. Glasper, J. Richardson, D. Randall (eds), *A textbook of children and young people's nursing* (pp. 20–30). Elsevier.

Raus, K. (2016). The extension of Belgium's euthanasia law to include competent minors. *Bioethical Inquiry*, 13, 305–315. https://doi.org/10.1007/s11673-016-9705-5

Rodriguez Velásquez, S., Jacques, L., Dala, l. J., Sestitoa, P., Habibi, Z., Venkatasubramanianc, A., Nguimbis, B., Botero Mesaa, S., Chimbetete, C., Keiser, O., Impouma, B., Mboussoue, F., Sie Williame, G., Ngoye, N., Talisuna, A., Salam Gueyee, A., Barroso Hofer, C., Waogodo Caboree, J. (2022).The toll of COVID-19 on African children: A descriptive analysis on COVID-19-related morbidity and mortality among the pediatric population in Sub-Saharan Africa. *International Journal of Infectious Diseases*, 110, 457–465. https://doi.org/10.1016/j.ijid.2021.07.060

Rolls, L., Payne, S. A. (2007). Children and young people's experience of UK childhood bereavement services. *Mortality*, 12(3), 281–303. https://doi.org/10.1080/13576270701430585

Rosengren, K. S., Miller, P. J., Gutierrez, I. T., Chow, P. I., Schein, S. S., Anderson, K. N., Callanan, M. A. (2014). Children's understanding of death: Toward a contextualized and integrated account. IV. Cognitive dimensions of death in context. *Monographs of the Society for Research in Child Development*, 79(1), 62–82.

Rowse, V. (2006). Palliative care for children: A public health initiative. *Paediatric Nursing*, 18(4), 41–45.

Sharma, R. M. (2007). The ethics of birth and death: Gender infanticide in India. *Bioethical Inquiry*, 4,181–192. https://doi.org/10.1007/s11673-007-9060-7.

Spellman, W. M. (2014). *A brief history of death.* Reaktion Books.

Stroebe, M. S., Schut, H. (1999). The dual process model of coping with bereavement: Rationale and description. *Death Studies*, 23(3), 197–224. https://doi.org/10.1080/074811899201046

Stroebe, M. S., Schut, H. (2010). The dual process model of coping with bereavement: A decade on. *Journal of Death and Dying*, 61(4), 273–289. https://doi.org/10.2190/om.61.4.b

Talwar, V., Harris, P. L., Schleifer, M. (2011). *Children's understanding of death: From biological to religious conceptions.* Cambridge University Press.

Tredgold, A. (1952). *A textbook of mental deficiency* (8th edn). Balliere, Tindall and Cox.

Triggle, N. (2017). Charlie Gard: A case that changed everything? Available at: https://www.bbc.co.uk/news/health-40644896 (accessed 8 June 2024).

Vázquez-Sánchez, J. M., Fernández-Alcántara, M., García-Caro, M. P., Cabaneor Martínez, M. J., Martí-García, C., Montoya-Juarez, R. (2019). The concept of death in children aged from 9 to 11 years: Evidences through inductive and deductive analysis of drawings. *Death Studies*. https://doi.org/10.1080/07481187.2018.1480545

Verhagen, E., Sauer, P. J. J. (2005). The Groningen Protocol: Euthanasia in severely ill newborns. *The New England Journal of Medicine*, 352, 959–962. https://doi.org/10.1056/NEJMp058026

Welch, S. B. (2008). Can the death of a child be good? *Journal of Pediatric Nursing*, 23(2), 120–125. https://doi.org/10.1016/j.pedn.2007.08.015

WHO (World Health Organization). (2014). *WHA67.19. Strengthening of palliative care as a component of comprehensive care throughout the life course.* WHO.

WHO (World Health Organization). (2022). Universal health coverage. Available at: https://www.who.int/health-topics/universal-health-coverage#tab=tab_1 (accessed February 2024).

WHO and UNICEF. (2018). *Declaration of Astana.* WHO.

Wilkins, K. L., Woodgate, R. L. (2005). A review of qualitative research on the childhood cancer experience from the perspective of siblings: A need to give them a voice. *Journal of Pediatric Oncology Nursing: Official Journal of the Association of Pediatric Oncology Nurses*, 22, 305–319. http//doi.org/10.1177/1043454205278035

Wilkinson, D., Savulescu, J. (2017). Hard lessons: Learning from the Charlie Gard case. *Journal of Medical Ethics*, 44, 438–442. https://doi.org/10.1136/medethics-2017-104492

Wilkinson, D., Savulescu, J. (2018). Alfie Evans and Charlie Gard – Should the law change?, *BMJ*, 361, k1891. https://doi.org/10.1136/bmj.k1891

Winger, A., Kvarme, L., Loyland, B., Kristianses, C., Helseth, S., Ravn, I. (2020). Family experiences with palliative care for children at home: A systematic literature review. *BMC Palliative Care*, 19, 165. https://doi.org/10.1186/s12904-020-00672-4

Yang, S. C. (2013). Assessment and quantification of Taiwanese children's views of a good death. *Omega: Journal of Death and Dying*, 66(1), 17.

Yang, S. C., Park, S. (2017). A sociocultural approach to children's perceptions of death and loss. *Omega: Journal of Death and Dying*, 76(1), 53–77.

# PART II

# Core

## CHAPTER 4

# Delivery of bad or unwanted news

## Diagnosis and assessment of needs

...............................................

*Rima Saad Rassam and Stacey Power Walsh*

### INTRODUCTION

Communication presents as a core domain in palliative care for children. During the journey of living with palliative care needs many circumstances prompt attention to insightful communication as a means to alleviate suffering. In particular, the delivery of difficult news emerges as an indispensable skill recurrently used in many circumstances in the disease trajectory. Difficult news may be perceived as bad or unwanted news by patients and families. Bad news has historically been referred to as any news that is "likely to alter drastically a patient's view of her or his future" (Buckman, 1984, p. 1597). However, as Price et al. (2006) state, it can mean different things to different people. Bad news can include any information that is unwelcomed, such as news of disability, life-threatening illness or impending or actual death (Price et al., 2006). The nature in which bad news is delivered by healthcare professionals influences how a person interprets, understands and deals with it (National Council for Hospice and Specialist Palliative Care Services, 2003). Traditionally, breaking bad news was regarded as a doctor and nurse delivering a poor prognosis to a patient as a one-off event (Warnock, 2014). Breaking bad news, however, is now considered as a process and refers to the ongoing delivery of difficult or upsetting news that alters patients' perceptions of their present and their future (Warnock, 2014).

Although delivering bad or unwanted news often appears in the end-of-life context, a closer look into the patients' and families' experiences denotes a broader use. From the first day of a child's abnormal symptoms, both the parents and child receive unexpected information. Between that day and last stages of the disease, the journey is full of ups and downs with information they do not wish to hear. Regardless of how they process these stimuli, the various emotional and cognitive repercussions and responses can be challenging. After all,

DOI: 10.4324/9781003384861-7

the entire disease experience is an "unwanted" experience. As professionals, it is our duty to gain prior understanding and competence in navigating the delivery of unwanted news to help children and families process the information to the best of their capacity.

This chapter describes a range of bad or unwanted news and how children and parents perceive them. The main section addresses the different models used in disclosing information to the children and their families. The processing of information and the provider's response form the last sections before ending with two case studies (Boxes 4.1 and 4.2). We hope that this overview will help the reader develop patterns of communication when delivering bad or unwanted news, analyse the practice and approaches to address the communication needs of children and their carers, and examine children's and parents' understanding and reactions to a diagnosis of a life-limiting or life-threatening conditions.

---

**LEARNING OBJECTIVES**

The reader will be able to do the following:

1.  Develop insight into positive cultures and patterns of communication when delivering bad or unwanted news/information.
2.  Analyse the practice and approaches to identify palliative and end-of-life care needs of children and their carers.
3.  Examine children's understanding and reactions to the diagnosis of a life-limiting or life-threatening condition and dying and death in childhood.

---

## THE CONTEXT OF BAD OR UNWANTED NEWS

The spectrum of palliative care for children encompasses many categories of disease conditions (Hain et al., 2013). The prevalence of these diseases is rising in England (Fraser et al., 2021). Globally, 98% of children who die with serious health-related suffering (due to cancer and other diseases) live in low- and middle-income countries (LMICs), which accentuates the need for paediatric palliative care (PPC) in these regions (Knaul et al., 2018). The highest rates of children in need of palliative care are found in Africa (51.8%), followed by Southeast Asia (19.5%) and the Eastern Mediterranean region (12%) (Connor et al., 2020).

The palliative care needs of children cover physical, psychosocial and spiritual domains, all of which necessitate skilful communication for timely prevention, proper assessment, and effective management. Effective, compassionate, and developmentally appropriate communication is essential for quality palliative care (National Consensus Project for Quality Palliative Care, 2018). In particular, the communication of difficult news has captured professional education and research attention (Jalali et al., 2023; Neilson et al., 2021). The literature interchangeably uses the terms "bad", "difficult" and "unwanted" to denote the same negative aspect of the information, essentially on the psychological level. A closer look is needed to distinguish the entities involved in the news and where the "difficulty" resides. For a better understanding, it is important to triangulate the communication (professional, child, parent), and recognise what constitutes "difficult" news for all the entities involved.

For some parents, the delivery of "unwanted" news can occur antenatally. Congenital anomalies affect approximately 2–4% of all births worldwide (Bashir, 2019; Coleman, 2015; Health Service Executive, 2024; Lotto et al., 2017). Despite their low prevalence, congenital anomalies are a leading cause of foetal death, infant mortality and childhood morbidity (Kinsner-Ovaskainen et al., 2021). Despite international guidance of eight recommended antenatal visits (Tunçalp et al., 2017), antenatal care provided to women varies worldwide. Inequalities and socio-economic deprivation exist worldwide in relation to access and timing of antenatal screening (Budd et al., 2015; Finlayson and Downe, 2013; Maxwell et al., 2011; Smith et al., 2011). Furthermore, significant differences in antenatal care provided are evident between low- and middle-income countries compared to upper-middle and high-income countries (WHO, 2018). Boyle et al. (2018) identified that there has been little progress in the prevention of congenital anomalies in Europe over the last 30 years and associates this with the lack of implementation of public health policy in antenatal care.

Most of the identified studies examined "difficult" news from the narrow angle of end-of-life. Yet, in the context of child illness, the "difficult" news would have started long before the diagnosis. Any information that diverges the person's plans negatively is difficult and unwanted (Buckman, 1984). From the parents' and children's perspectives, any disruption of a healthy childhood is unwanted and difficult to manage and process. Even the presence of a mild symptom is not an easy information to learn, if we consider the example of flu or earache, despite their temporary nature, they can impact a child's health and family routine, so these also constitute relatively "bad news". In the context of life-limiting and life-threatening conditions, the disruption often occurs from the start of the symptoms. Therefore, even before seeking professional advice, the parents and children are already dealing with difficult news alone. In the first encounter with the patient/family, professionals deal with the disturbance and often face difficulty navigating the information that parents and children are processing. Then comes the information about procedures and often invasive, diagnostic tests. All of them are not easy news for children, their parents, or professionals.

At the diagnosis of a serious condition in children, truth-telling poses a considerable challenge for healthcare professionals and families. In many societies, such as in the Middle East, the cultural norms drive caregivers to take a protective stance and oppose disclosure to the child (Rosenberg et al., 2017). In the medical field, disclosure has transformed over the years to lately advocate for the "overall" best interest for each child individually (Gillam et al., 2022). It is essential to carefully explore the child's traits, family dynamics, concerns and cultural context to collectively reach a consensus and implement a child- and family-centred approach.

During the disease journey, children and families navigate through much news that may seem a simple part of the treatment yet creates difficulties as they arise. Within a limited resource setting, an additional layer of difficulty overacts. For example, learning about the need for transfusion during the nadir of a chemotherapy cycle is expected by professionals, sad for any parent, but devastating for parents who do not have access to blood units, particularly in countries where blood banks are limited.

## THE DELIVERY OF BAD OR UNWANTED NEWS

Perhaps the most difficult communication with a child with a serious paediatric condition and their family is the one occurring at the end of life (Ulrich et al., 2018). Many barriers challenge the effective and honest communication of poor prognosis, including doctors' concerns about the emotional impact of the information, lack of training, and lack of clarity on the goals of care (Janvier et al., 2014; Mack and Joffe, 2014). Professionals may have difficulty having such conversations since they realise their vulnerability; the treatment failure may be seen as their own failure as clinicians. Yet, redefining hope based on an open-goals-of-care discussion would help a smooth transition. For clinicians, no matter how difficult the information is, the delivery of it remains a skill to be learned and conveying it is a decision to be made. For children and their parents, it is never their choice to learn how to handle the news nor to carry it! Compassionate communication is essential.

## The importance of communication

Clear communication is of the utmost importance during the diagnosis of a life-limiting condition. Following an antenatal fatal diagnosis, parents face multiple challenges, primarily whether to continue or terminate the affected pregnancy. An integrated approach to care, inclusive of bereavement care that continues through the pregnancy, delivery, and into the postnatal period is required (Bereavement Care Standards Development Group, 2016; O'Donoghue, 2019; Royal College of Obstetricians and Gynaecologists, 2010). Healthcare professionals are required to be definitive in their knowledge and decision-making on all aspects of a congenital anomaly presentation and diagnosis. They should be knowledgeable and skilful in providing families with comprehensive and balanced counselling, where the best available information on potential outcomes is provided (Marokakis et al., 2016; O'Donoghue, 2019; Royal College of Obstetricians and Gynaecologists, 2010). Language used in antenatal counselling can be influential and so healthcare professionals providing information on congenital anomaly to parents following a diagnosis are required to be mindful of the language used. Non-medical language and repetition of information are warranted (McNamara et al., 2013). Empathetic healthcare professionals offering compassionate care should deliver honest, accurate, unbiased and non-judgemental information, taking their cues from the parents themselves (McCoyd, 2009; McNamara et al., 2013). How such information is delivered to parents has been reported to need improvement in the past (Lalor et al., 2007). More recently, Wilkinson et al. (2012) suggest that healthcare professionals' use of "fatal" and related terminology is potentially due to their discomfort with the uncertainty of death coupled with the expected quality of life, and to aid parents' decision-making around care. Wilkinson et al. (2012), however, argue that terminology may not be of importance if healthcare professionals are clear in their communication.

Regardless of whether a diagnosis is delivered antenatally or postnatally, communication of news has a central influence on decision-making, regardless of how it is processed (de Vos et al., 2015). From the parents' perspective, decisional conflicts often derive from the lack of adequate communication, ambiguity in their sense of duty and family dynamics (Morrison et al., 2015; Winter et al., 2019). From the child's perspective, especially older children and adolescents, being involved in treatment discussions enables them to convey their preferences and make decisions (Jacobs et al., 2015; Kelly et al., 2017). The American Academy of Pediatrics provides guidance on informed consent in paediatric practice, including the disclosure of information to foster decision-making and mediate a trusting relationship (Katz et al., 2016).

## What parents and children would like to know

A qualitative study in the Netherlands described what parents would like to know during the communication of bad news (Brouwer et al., 2021). Parents asked for honest revelation of uncertainty (Rajasooriyar et al., 2016), a clear plan of care including their input and contributions, explanation of medical terminology, and a timely follow-up conversation to address their questions and concerns (Brouwer et al., 2021). Parents often seek written resources such as the internet, books and pamphlets to enhance information retention (Xafis et al., 2015). In the neonatal intensive care setting, parents want doctors to know about their child and the predicted course of disease and to be given time, assurance and hope (Wege et al., 2023).

Although communication happens first with parents, conversation with children is as important. Whether the patient or the sibling, they need an open, honest and compassionate discussion of information to navigate through their, or their sibling's, plan of care. The developmental age plays a pivotal role in delineating both the content and the way of communicating.

Historically, disclosing bad news to children has constantly challenged healthcare professionals and parents (Sisk et al., 2016). Whether in truth-telling or discussing the concept of death, the initial recommendations from the 1950s supported a "protective" stance to shield loved ones from the psychological burden of the experience. In the late 1960s, the views started shifting to an "open" approach and supported the inclusion of children in such conversations. Currently, the best practice converges with an individualised approach based on the myriad of personal, developmental and cultural factors (Sisk et al., 2016). Recent evidence suggests that disclosing information to children can enhance family stability (Rost and Mihailov, 2021).

In the end-of-life context, children's understanding of the concept of death varies based on their developmental stage. Accordingly, they may exhibit different reactions while processing the information. Infants have no concept of death. For toddlers, death carries little meaning and is often associated with anxiety due to emotions in the surrounding environment. Pre-schoolers begin to formulate an understanding of death as a temporary event. At school age, children start to realise the permanent nature of death. Adolescents understand death as permanent, universal and inevitable (Irish Hospice Foundation, 2020; Murphy, 2017; The Irish Childhood Bereavement Network, 2018).

It is essential to adapt the disclosure to the child's current understanding of the situation and, at the same time, explore prior experience and support needed with processing stressful news (Murphy, 2017). Children, especially adolescents, often obtain cues about their condition even before the open disclosure (Ciobanu and Preston, 2021). Similar to the communication with adults, honest and concrete language can ease accurate understanding. It is advisable to avoid euphemism (such as "sleeping" or "gone") and use the word "died" and to name the part of the body that is not functioning such as "the heart stopped beating" (Murphy, 2017; The Irish Childhood Bereavement Network, 2018). Children's reactions to a death can be very intense but brief, they may experience strong emotions suddenly and then seem to go back to normal everyday activities very quickly, such as playing with friends. But they will revisit those strong emotions again and again (The Irish Childhood Bereavement Network, 2018).

When communicating difficult news to children and their siblings, a sensitive and compassionate conversation promotes understanding and mediates the family unity by not leaving behind any members who are affected by the information.

## FACTORS TO CONSIDER WHEN DELIVERING BAD OR UNWANTED NEWS

Formal training in communication skills, particularly in breaking bad news, is limited among healthcare professionals (Dobrozsi et al., 2019; Oliveira et al., 2020). Furthermore, advances in technology and excessive workloads have led to poorer communication between healthcare professionals and the patient (Atienza-Carrasco et al., 2018; Guerra et al., 2011). It is argued that more focus is placed on treating the illness and the patient's physical well-being rather than on their emotional and spiritual well-being (Atienza-Carrasco et al., 2018). Additionally, the personal and professional threat that breaking bad news has on the healthcare professionals may also contribute to the ineffectiveness of their method in delivering a diagnosis (Price et al., 2006). On the personal level, such threat could be attributed to the potential emotional involvement of healthcare professionals during the discussion. On the professional level, disclosing bad news may induce a perception of failure in performing the traditional curative role as expected.

Effective communication of difficult news relies on important attributes. Besides the information to convey, clinicians are urged to consider the timing and delivery while focusing on the individuality of each situation.

1. *Time*: preparing and delivering news constitutes a lengthy task. Key times in communication encompass the periods of diagnosis, new procedures, change in

health or functioning and end of life. The novelty of each period for the child and family accentuates their unique communication needs, each recipient processes the information differently. Another way to look at time is the duration and reiteration of the communication. Allocating enough time to deliver the news is crucial (Kessel et al., 2013; Wege et al., 2023). Parents indicated that the appropriate duration of communication about diagnosis is between 30 minutes and 90 minutes (Kessel et al., 2013). In the clinical setting, the complexity of medical information poses an additional layer of difficulty for the child and parent. Therefore, they understandably ask for reiteration of information either from the same person who delivered the information or from another multidisciplinary team member.

2. *Honesty and transparency*: clear, accurate and honest information is paramount. A robust body of knowledge supports use of a direct and clear vocabulary and avoidance of euphemisms (Brouwer et al., 2021; National Consensus Project for Quality Palliative Care, 2018). Ultimately, a trusting relationship with the patient and family stems from this communication and contributes to co-designing and engaging in the action plans.

3. *Cultural/religious considerations*: preferences regarding disclosure and discussion of bad news are largely shaped by cultural and religious background. In Lebanon, evoking death remains a taboo (Mouhawej et al., 2017). Some cultural groups, such as Native Americans and Asians, believe that speaking about the possibility of death can induce it (Wiener et al., 2013). As such, many families opt to withhold information about serious health conditions or possibility of death from the patient, especially in paediatric settings. Additionally, in some cultures, treatment decisions are not solely taken by the concerned patient or family. For example, Native American families engage members from the wider family in making treatment decisions, the decisions being made collectively rather than by the caregiver alone (Wiener et al., 2013). In such cultural contexts, the different stakeholders are involved in the discussion of news and decision-making processes. Cultural considerations also relate to the suppression or expression of emotion during the delivery of bad news. Suppression of emotions is common among Arab males to convey a sense of strength and control. In Saudi Arabia, mothers preferred to have close bodily contact with their babies in newborn setting when breaking bad news (Al-Abdi et al., 2011). Historically, in Muslim countries, it is common to find families opposing the disclosure of bad news or doctors making decisions on behalf of patients and families as a means to maintain hope (Qaddoumi et al., 2009). Such traits may lead to the formation of specific guidelines for breaking bad news in Muslim communities (Salem and Salem, 2013).

A correct approach to communication of bad news is tailored to the child and family needs and background. The memory of the conversation is carried for life. Regardless of the information, the way in which the news was communicated has the power to enhance trust, facilitate action and foster a new hope.

## MODELS OF DELIVERING BAD AND UNWANTED NEWS

In his landmark book, *How to Break Bad News: A Guide for Health Care Professionals*, Buckman (1992) delineated the criteria for delivering bad news. These criteria entail in-person communication, exploring the patient's understanding, delivering information in alignment with the patient's understanding, confirming understanding of the new information, developing and following through a plan. Baile et al. (2000) propose four goals for disclosing bad news:

1.  Obtain information from the patient to assess expectations and readiness to receive the news.
2.  Provide individualised information according to the patient's needs.
3.  Provide emotional support.
4.  Develop a plan of care in collaboration with the patient and family.

Several models incorporate these criteria and goals. The most widely described model in a paediatric setting is the SPIKES protocol (Baile et al., 2000). As the communication of bad news entails conversation with parents (adults), this section provides the reader with an overview of available models. Most of these models are represented by mnemonics to remind the professional of the steps to follow while delivering the news.

### The SPIKES protocol

The SPIKES protocol was initially designed for adult oncology care, specifically for difficult discussions such as relapse or introduction of hospice care (Baile et al., 2000). Modifications were suggested to be used in paediatric settings (Wolfe et al., 2014). The elements of the protocol include the following:

S = Setting up the meeting
*   Ensure a quiet and private environment where the patient and the family can comfortably discuss the condition.
*   Determine who will be present from the family and from the multi-disciplinary team. While a multi-disciplinary approach is extremely important in the care of a child with a life-limiting condition, it is important to ensure the presence of only those who are essential and have a good therapeutic relationship with the parents (Boyd, 2001).
*   Preparing ahead of time is an important step that conveys empathy and respect towards the patient and family. Do a mental rehearsal and be prepared to handle tough questions and emotions.
*   Invite both parents and the child (Novak et al., 2019).
*   Avoid outside interruptions and calls during the meeting, for example, turn pagers or phones off, and allow enough time for the meeting.
*   Sit down and avoid physical barriers.

Wolfe et al. (2014) proposed the additional measures to prepare the setting:
- If the child is not present, arrange for the child to have company during the parents' absence.
- Before the meeting, discuss the child's results with the multi-disciplinary team and agree recommendations.
- In a multi-linguistic setting, ensure the presence of an interpreter to facilitate accurate understanding.
- Introduce all team members and their roles.

**P = Perceptions**
- Assess the existing perception and comprehension of the medical situation before presenting the news. Asking open-ended questions to determine the level of knowledge (e.g. "What have you been told …?" or "What is your understanding …?" (Novak et al., 2019, p. 2)) will help tailor the information to the family's level of understanding.
- Correct any misconceptions.

**I = Invitation**
- Ask about the level and type of information that parents would like to receive. Some patients/family want all the details, others prefer a summary.
- Invite the family members present to share their concerns, questions and feelings.
- Offer to answer future questions as they arise.

**K = Knowledge**
- Warn the patient/family of the news to facilitate processing of information. For example, "I have some bad news to share."
- Share the medical facts and plan, using simple, direct and clear language, avoiding medical jargon.
- Align the information with the child's and family's level of understanding.
- Give the information in small pieces and check periodically for understanding.
- Listen and use silence (Buckman, 2005).
- Avoid statements of hopelessness such as "There is nothing more we can do."
- Highlight positive findings, when possible (Wolfe et al., 2014).
- Use age-appropriate language and visuals aids, if possible.
- Provide written material. Parents may forget what was said, so written information will help processing the news later or be shared with others (Novak et al., 2019).

**E =Emotions**
- Allow the patient/parent to express their feelings. The conversation cannot move forward unless the emotions are addressed.
- Respond to emotions empathetically by observing, naming and encouraging discussion of feelings.
- Observe the emotional reactions and expression of shock that could vary from silence to denial, crying, anger.

- Identify the emotion by naming it to help validate the feeling and connect to the patient/family. For example, "It is normal to feel sad … with this type of bad news" (Novak et al., 2019, p. 2).
- Demonstrate empathy, e.g. "I wish the news were better."
- Invite them to discuss the news and use open-ended questions to clarify thoughts/feeling:" Could you tell me what you are worried about most?" (Wolfe et al., 2014, p. 1013).
- Offer assistance to the wider family members (Wolfe et al., 2014).
- Allow compassionate silence and pause to give space for emotions.

S = Strategy and Summary

- Ask the patient/family if they are ready to move forward with the discussion.
- Reconfirm their participation in decision-making (Wolfe et al., 2014).
- Present the treatment options and collaboratively develop a plan by encouraging discussion.
- Assess patient/family understanding. Use "teach back" as needed (Wolfe et al., 2014, p. 1013).
- Emphasise the presence of hope in parallel to a realistic plan. Helpful statements include: "There are always options", "We are here to support you."
- Offer help sharing information with other family members such as siblings or grandparents (Wolfe et al., 2014).
- Provide information about support services (Wolfe et al., 2014).
- End the session with a practical plan for the patient/parents (Novak et al., 2019).
- Summarise mutual goals and timeline (Wolfe et al., 2014).

## S-P-w-ICE-S

Recently, some authors have suggested an updated version of SPIKES called "S-P-w-ICE-S" (Meitar and Karnieli-Miller, 2022). The new version shares many similarities with the traditional SPIKES, particularly emphasising the importance of creating an appropriate and comfortable setting for the conversation, assessing the patient's perception, communicating compassionately, addressing emotions, and providing support. The primary difference resides in the structure and specific steps. SPIKES follows a more linear approach with steps to follow. The elements in S-P-w-ICE-S are:

Setting
Perception
What
Invitation
Communication
Emotions
Strategy and Summary

**TABLE 4.1** Protocols for breaking bad news similar to the SPIKES steps

| Protocol names | Steps | Highlighted features |
| --- | --- | --- |
| ABCDE (Rabow and McPhee, 1999) | **A** = Advance preparation<br>**B** = Build a therapeutic environment/ relationship<br>**C** = Communicate well<br>**D** = Deal with patient and family reactions<br>**E** = Encourage and validate emotions | The protocol emphasises the importance of therapeutic relationship before and after communicating the information |
| BREAKS (Narayanan et al., 2010) | **B** = Background<br>**R** = Rapport<br>**E** = Explore<br>**A** = Announce<br>**K** = Kindling (emotions carefully)<br>**S** = Summarise | The protocol emphasises paying attention to the various aroused emotions and validating understanding |
| PEWTER (Nardi and Keefe-Cooperman, 2006) | **P** = Prepare<br>**E** = Evaluate<br>**W** = Warn<br>**T** = Tell<br>**E** = Emotional Response<br>**R** = Regroup | The protocol highlights hope in the "regrouping" element. The discussion after disclosure explores the future outlook of the patient/family to redefine goals of care. |

The introduced "What" element prompt focuses on what the patient/family already knows before proceeding with the disclosure. This helps tailor the information delivery according to the level of awareness and reduces confusion or anxiety. The "C" for "Communication" reflects the importance of effective dialogue in the disclosure (Meitar and Karnieli-Miller, 2022).

Three other models have similar steps to SPIKES, shown in Table 4.1.

## The Fine Protocol (Fine, 1991)

The Fine Protocol involves five phases:

1. *Preparation*: in this phase the clinician would prepare the appropriate location and time, revisiting the patient's needs, cultural and religious background, and goal of the discussion.
2. *Information acquisition*: during this phase the clinician explores the patient's understanding and existing information about his/her medical condition.
3. *Information sharing*: in this phase the clinician provides the news.
4. *Information reception*: the clinician assesses the information processing, clarifying any miscommunication, and addresses disagreements.
5. *Response*: this entails observing and acknowledging the patient's response to the information and closing the interview.

## IGAD (Salem and Salem, 2013)

The IGAD protocol acknowledges the specificities of Muslim countries with regards to the religious views and backgrounds, family interactions and educational structure. In Muslim communities, illness is considered a trial from God, and an opportunity for spiritual reward and removal of sins (Badawi, 2011). Disease is a family event and healthcare decisions are led by the family (Salem and Salem, 2013). Families prefer not to disclose bad news as a means to maintain hope (Qaddoumi et al., 2009). The IGAD guideline (Salem and Salem, 2013) proposes the following steps while emphasising the unique contextual characteristics:

I = *Interview:* while acknowledging the family ties, this phase entails asking the patient "in private" to identify the family members or friends he/she would like to be present during the disclosure meeting. Accordingly, the location of the meeting will be decided based on the number, while maintaining privacy.

G = *Gather background information*, including the verbal and non-verbal clues to guide the discussion. This phase helps determine the level of awareness of the patient about his/her condition and of the desire to be informed. Within this phase, the body language of the patient and family provides useful information on their readiness for the news.

A = Assess or Achieve

*Assess* the influence of patient's perception, expectations, and self-image. This phase assesses the religious influence (through costumes, reference to religious beliefs during the discussion) and family influence on the patient (for example, trying to hide the news from the patient).

*Achieve rapport with the patient* as much as possible. The information gathered from the background helps set the stage of the conversation. With patients having strong religious views, it is advisable to emphasise optimistic religious statements such as '"God is merciful". With patients preferring non-disclosure, statements like "you are in good hands" can be reassuring.

D = Decide or Disclosure or Discuss

*Decide on the level and appropriate method of disclosure.* It is often more culturally acceptable to ask the caregiver instead of the patient for the preferred level of information. This approach may pose a dilemma in some clinicians; therefore, it is essential to obtain thorough information about the patient's background. For patients preferring full disclosure, a sensitive conversation is needed. For patients preferring minimal details, "one step below" is suggested (for example, 'Bone tumour' instead of 'Osteosarcoma'). For patients preferring non-disclosure, the family will receive the information. Circumstances where non-disclosure is preferred by patients and family should be avoided.

*Disclosure of bad news*: This phase entails providing the information as clearly and sensitively as possible, taking into consideration the educational background.

*Discuss, summarise and use supportive statements.* In this phase, clinicians should encourage questions, respond compassionately, and provide supportive words according to the background information previously gathered.

## ARCHES

In the event of the parents' or families' request not to disclose difficult news to the patient, Holmes and Illing (2021) suggest the ARCHES protocol (Table 4.2). Within protectionist cultures, the protocol may be useful in paediatric contexts, particularly in adolescents. The authors' intent is to offer a six-step protocol to use in response to non-disclosure requests. If an agreement is achieved, the actual delivery of the difficult news can follow the SPIKES protocol.

In the neonatal settings, two protocols were identified: SOBPIE and NEO-SPEAK.

## SOBPIE

This mnemonic stands for:

S = situation
O = opinions or options
B = basics
P = parents' stories
I = information
E = emotions

It is developed for use in neonates, particularly in the context of withholding or withdrawing life-sustaining measures. As described by Janvier et al. (2014), the six steps reflect an individualised approach. It is commenced as the baby's situation deteriorates and encourages the initiation of the conversation of their deterioration at this time. Step two encourages an exploration of the personal biases of healthcare professionals and explores appropriate options for the baby and family. The third "basic" step alludes to basic human interactions that are required to ensure compassionate communication. These include preparing the location, arranging a suitable time, reducing interruptions, and creating an environment conducive to breaking bad news. Furthermore, it promotes the need to explore parents' understanding of the situation, their concerns and questions and readiness to hear the information. The step involving information entails communicating to the parents about withholding or withdrawing life-sustaining measures while providing a clear medical background about possible complications of these interventions. Lastly, in the emotion phase, the healthcare professional addresses emotions, social resources, and strategies for parents to cope and move forward.

**TABLE 4.2** The ARCHES steps

| ARCHES steps | Description | Example of statements in paediatric context |
|---|---|---|
| **A** = Acknowledge the request | During this step the dilemma is voiced which provides opportunity to address it | "We understand that you prefer not to tell your child about the diagnosis. We would like to further understand your perspective." |
| **R** = Build relationship | The clinician explores the caregiver's/ family's values and fears to gain a deeper understanding and promote trust | "What are your worries or fears? What are things most important to the patient?" |
| **C** = Find common ground | At this stage the clinician and caregiver identify a shared goal or view | "Your priority is not to emotionally disturb the patient and this is also our goal." |
| **H** = Honour the patient's preference; outline the harm of non-disclosure | The clinician explains the benefits of informing the patient based on his/her preference, and the potential disadvantages and burden of non-disclosure | "Many loving families ask us the same request. Most patients want to know about their condition. We need to honour these choices. When the patient understands, he/she will feel connected and able to make a choice. When we hide information, he/she will feel isolated and possibly learn about the information without receiving the needed support." |
| **E** = Provide emotional support | The clinician will reassure the caregiver that compassionate communication will be used, and the information offered and not forced | "We will be sensitive to the patient's needs for information, we will ask his/her permission before starting the conversation or sharing the information." |
| **S** = Devise a supportive solution | If the consensus is reached, the clinician and caregiver agree on who will carry out the conversation with the patient<br>In cases of a persistent non-disclosure request, the approach should be tailored to the cultural and legal context | Scenario 1: "We are glad that you see the benefit in disclosing. Our approach is to talk with the patient together with the caregiver. Let's plan the encounter."<br>Scenario 2: "It is important to know that you are still concerned about an additional emotional burden. However, if he/she shows curiosity about his/her condition, we will need to reassess the decision." |

## NEO-SPEAK

More recently, qualitative researchers have developed a framework for communicating bad news in neonatology called NEO-SPEAK (Seifart et al., 2022). The determinants of successful conversation were derived from data from interviews conducted with 17 senior neonatologists from six neonatal centres in Germany. The elements of NEO-SPEAK are:

N = neonatal prognostic uncertainty
E = encounter in partnerships triangulating parents-patients-doctors and parents-nurses-doctors
O = organisation and teamwork
S = situational stress
P = processuality, emphasising that the conversation happens over time depending on the parents' needs and development of the baby's condition
E = emotional burden
A = attention to individuality
K = knowledge and experience, including expertise in delivering difficult news.

## CONSEQUENCES AND IMPACT OF RECEIVING BAD OR UNWANTED NEWS

### Parents

A diagnosis of a fatal congenital anomaly/life-limiting condition can result in an intense grief reaction and a long-lasting effect on the overall well-being of parents and families (Boyle et al., 2015; Fleming et al., 2016; Maijala et al., 2003; Meaney et al., 2017; Nuzum et al., 2018; Statham et al., 2000). It is traumatic and emotionally distressing, shattering parents' dreams and transforming families' lives (Hurley et al., 2021). Parents' emotional distress and intensified grief are associated with the absence of appropriate follow-up care and social acknowledgement (Boyle et al., 2015; Due et al., 2018; Heazell et al., 2016; Lalor et al., 2007; Meaney et al., 2017) highlighting the need for parents to receive various levels of support at the time of their perinatal bereavement (Bereavement Care Standards Development Group, 2016; Nuzum et al., 2018). It is important to note that a child's diagnosis can also provide a sense of clarity and relief to some families where once there was an unwavering uncertainty (Demarest et al., 2022).

The emotional experience of receiving bad news can have a significant physical response of feeling dizzy and sick, with parents describing a feeling of their heart tightening (Nelson et al., 2017). Parents report being in shock, feeling numb, heavy, fearful and hopeless (Nelson et al., 2017) and experiencing a feeling of grief (Demarest et al., 2022). The emotional responses of shock, fear, sadness and devastation experienced by parents when receiving bad or unwanted news can act as a barrier to comprehension and inhibit their ability to process information being presented to them, hurling them into a haziness (Ashtiani et al., 2014; Hurley et al.,

2021). However, the impact of the delivery of bad news is a complex one. The manner in which bad news is delivered can have a lasting effect on parents, affecting not only their ability to cope and adapt but their perception, acceptance and ability to care for their child (Boyd, 2001). However, one study found parents' strong emotional reactions, including physical collapse, following delivery of bad news in an oncology setting were a consequence of the news itself and not an indicator of ineffectual delivery (Nelson et al., 2017). The news of no further active treatment for cancer, for example, can cause a complex response in parents such as a feeling of relief due to the discontinuation of treatment, especially if it was responsible for the pain experienced by their child. Yet the terminal prognosis simultaneously squashes the possibility of, and any hope they had for, successful treatment (Nelson et al., 2017). Hearing that their child is dying can leave parents feeling powerless and helpless due to their inability to protect their child (Ashtiani et al., 2014; Hurley et al., 2021; Nelson et al., 2017).

Despite this, there is a paucity of literature pertaining specifically to parental experiences of receiving the bad news of a life-limiting condition or pending death of their child. Much of the relatable literature refers to the delivery of news of a genetic or metabolic condition and developmental delay, and does not highlight if these diagnoses were life-limiting. This genre of literature reports parental dissatisfaction with suboptimal delivery of unwanted news from healthcare professionals, usually doctors (Ashtiani et al., 2014; Boyd, 2001; Das et al., 2021; Haitjema et al., 2022; Hurley et al., 2021). Ashtiani et al. (2014) described parents' frustration with a passive role, their only purpose was to listen and receive information with limited occasions to voice their queries. Ashtiani et al. (2014) presented that 61.5% of parents (n = 13) experienced the delivery of bad news (a genetic diagnosis) negatively. Healthcare professionals' attitudes, communication and language have been perceived at times as insensitive and brief with moments of inappropriateness (Das et al., 2021). Lawton et al. (2015), in a mixed-methods study on the diagnosis of spinal muscular atrophy, concurred with these studies' findings as parents described the delivery and nature of the information as suboptimal. However, parents specifically related this to the difficulties predicting clinical severity and the delay in diagnosis (Lawton et al., 2015), their appreciation of the situation resulting in reported forgiveness of healthcare professionals (Ashtiani et al., 2014). Parents need hope despite the delivery of bad news (Ashtiani et al., 2014; Boyd, 2001). Parents require acknowledgement that it will be hard and different to what they had imagined and reassured that it will be okay and that they will be supported through the diagnosis (Ashtiani et al., 2014; Boyd, 2001). Being directed to support can be beneficial, and parents often find comfort in speaking, in particular with other parents who have experienced something similar (Boyd, 2001). Boyd acknowledged that facilitating and normalising the expression of emotion, providing support and allocating time for questions were beneficial to parents.

The use of medical terminology can also prove a challenge with parents needing to look things up at home (Ashtiani et al., 2014). Clear, accurate, honest and straightforward information is essential to support understanding (Boyd, 2001; Haitjema et al., 2022). As well as identifying the need for clear, plain language, and an honest and compassionate diagnosis, establishing a rapport with the doctor who had time to address parents' needs was suggested (Demarest et al., 2022). A diagnosis that included the development of a plan for next steps and resources was also valued (Ashtiani et al., 2014; Demarest et al., 2022).

Consideration of the timing and location of delivery of bad news is essential for the delivery of bad news (Ashtiani et al., 2014). Boyd (2001) described the need for a private, comfortable and quiet environment that creates a space for expression of feelings and asking of questions. Timing is important, in particular ensuring that both parents are present to receive the news to ensure a sense of support and avoid one parent needing to deliver the devastating news of their child's condition to the other (Boyd, 2001). Furthermore, parental preparedness for receiving the information is also an essential factor to consider before disclosing bad news (Ashtiani et al., 2014). Parent preparedness can be informed by the duration of the family's journey to diagnosis (Ashtiani et al., 2014).

Parents have an overwhelming need for healthcare professionals to demonstrate empathy, caring and sensitivity when delivering bad news and normalise parents' response and expression of their multitude of feelings (Ashtiani et al., 2014; Boyd, 2001). For many parents, it is the respect and dignity shown to their child, and feeling that their medical needs were met, that lend to their parental satisfaction (Wool et al., 2016). Ultimately, the delivery of bad news needs to be individualised to ensure the needs of all family members are met (Boyd, 2001; Hurley et al., 2021). Furthermore, the evaluation of parental satisfaction is necessary to determine the healthcare organisation's quality of care (Wool et al., 2016).

Das et al. (2021) promote training of healthcare professionals in communication and usage of context-specific communication protocols and materials in order to improve the quality of care.

## Child

Delivering a life-limiting condition diagnosis to a child is one of the most daunting challenges for healthcare professionals (Stein et al., 2019). The communication is influenced by several factors, such as the relationship between child, parent and healthcare professional, with these factors evolving over time in response to the change in the child's developmental understanding and disease progression (Stein et al., 2019).

While the disclosing of a life-limiting condition to a child is still a relatively new approach to this day, a wide variation in practice, whether and how children are told about their diagnosis, still exists (Stein et al., 2019). Despite recommendations to inform children of their diagnosis, medical teams often withhold an end-of-life disclosure to children until death is imminent (Marsac et al., 2018). This can occur due to family influences and medics' own discomfort with end-of-life discussions (Marsac et al., 2018). Parents often try to protect their child and/or themselves through avoiding discussions about death (Marsac et al., 2018). Like their parents, children report a preference for honest, complete information of their prognosis to be delivered with sensitivity (Bluebond-Langner, 1978; Marsac et al., 2018). The siblings' desire to be included in these discussions is also recognised (Marsac et al., 2018). Although the majority of papers present the parents' perspective (Ciobanu and Preston, 2021), there are studies that examine the impact of a diagnosis of a life-limiting condition on the children themselves (Adduci et al., 2012; Last and van Veldhuizen, 1996; Mellins et al., 2002; Menon et al., 2007; van der Geest et al., 2015). Insight into both the child's and their parents' perspective and experience of a serious diagnosis would allow a comparison between the two groups and inform practice.

Upon receiving a diagnosis of a life-limiting condition, similar to their parents, children experience psychological indicators of distress. They can initially experience a range of emotions including shock, anger, confusion and sadness (Mellins et al., 2002). Distress indicators include anxiety and depression, being fearful, social problems and withdrawal (Adduci et al., 2012). The level of fear, anxiety, and depression can be reduced when children are communicated to about their illness, particularly when the news is delivered competently and effectively (Last and van Veldhuizen, 1996; Menon et al., 2007; van der Geest et al., 2015). Fortier et al. (2013) suggest the disclosure of a life-limiting condition can improve the quality of life through alleviating uncertainty. When communication was considered avoidant, or there was a delay in disclosure of the illness, children have described feeling angry, betrayed and a sense of being deceived (Cluver et al., 2015; Kajubi et al., 2016; Lester et al., 2002). However, there are other studies that have shown no adverse effects of disclosure, nor significant benefits, for the child or family relationship outcomes (Mellins et al., 2002).

Effective communication around end-of-life planning, within and between the family and multi-disciplinary team, is beneficial (Marsac et al., 2018). It is important to be aware of culture, traditions, ethnicity and belief systems that influence patient and family perspectives on the meaning of illness and death to ensure communication is meaningful and individualised (Stein et al., 2019).

---

**LEARNING ACTIVITY**

- If you have been involved in the disclosure of a life-limiting condition to a child and/or their family, take a moment to think: What worked well? What would you have done differently? What were the parents' reactions? What were the child's reactions?
- In your clinical experience, what differences have you noted regarding information children sought about their condition/diagnosis and how their age/development age influenced this?

---

## THE NURSE'S ROLE

While nurses themselves do not routinely deliver bad or unwanted news, they can play an essential role in supporting the family during the disclosure and influencing how it takes place (Boyd, 2001). The nurse's bedside presence, and their unique opportunity and time to develop a therapeutic relationship with a child and family, have led some authors to suggest that the nurse is best placed to deliver bad or unwanted news (Price et al., 2006). However, families expect bad news to be delivered by a doctor (Cooley, 2000). Delivering bad news is a process of providing information and assisting patients in understanding and coping with the news (Warnock, 2014). It can be undertaken by more than one professional. Buckman (1992) regards the responsibility of delivering bad news as the duty of the healthcare professional who provides continuity of care to the patient. In relation to the diagnosis of a life-limiting condition, there may be a need for the nurse to encourage parents to disclose the news to the child, if deemed in their best interest and the information sought after. Regardless of who delivers the news, as the nurse is in direct contact, it is important for them to seek assurance that the child and parent(s) have understood the diagnosis and plan of care and to address any queries and questions. In doing so, the nurse may need to act as a patient advocate (Agrawal et al., 2023). Communication needs to be clear and easily understood, and delivered using an approach and a rate that optimise child and parental understanding of what is being said.

## CASE STUDIES

Boxes 4.1 and 4.2 present two case studies.

---

**BOX 4.1 PAEDIATRIC CASE STUDY**

The following case study illustrates the use of the SPIKES protocol in disclosing difficult news. Nadia is a 6-year-old girl with neuroblastoma being treated with chemotherapy. Her family members include her parents, Susan and Joe, and older sibling Leo, who is 10 years old. Nadia's medical condition has worsened over the last couple of weeks. Recent imaging revealed a metastatic spread with incurable disease. The multi-disciplinary team treating Nadia includes the paediatric oncologist (Dr Fair), the palliative care nurse (Laila) and the social worker (Hana). The team is getting ready to disclose Nadia's situation regarding the spread of disease and prognosis to the parents.

- *Setting:* Susan and Joe are present in the hospital room. The team gathered all the background and medical information needed. Laila agreed a suitable time for the parents, and reserved the family room on the unit that was equipped with comfortable furniture. She also arranged with Nadia, her parents and the nursing staff on the unit to have a staff member stay with Nadia during the meeting. At the time of the meeting, the parents and team convened and sat down in the reserved room.
- *Perception:* After a round of introductions, Dr Fair explored the parents' understanding of Nadia's current condition, hearing from Susan and Joe. Both expressed concerns about Nadia's disease and hopes for a clear treatment plan. The parents mentioned that they were worried about Nadia's pain and wanted to know what was causing it and how to manage it.
- *Invitation:* Dr. Fair expressed empathy and acknowledged the parents' concern. She said, "I understand that you're worried about Nadia 's pain and disease status and you would like to know what's happening. We have recently done some medical tests and have results that provide more information, and I'd like to share them with you. Is now a good time for us to discuss this?" The parents agreed and Dr Fair proceeded.

- *Knowledge:* Dr Fair used clear simple terms to deliver the information, "Unfortunately, the results showed that the chemotherapy is not working as planned, the cancer has spread and will not be cured", then paused. The pause allowed parents to process the information.
- *Emotions/Empathy:* After few seconds of silence (therapeutic silence) Laila came closer to Susan as she saw she was tearful. Laila gave her a tissue and a glass of water. She acknowledged that it is a hard news to hear, saying, "I can imagine how difficult it must be for both of you to hear such news. I wish the results were different (pause). We're here to support Nadia and support you through this. Please feel free to ask any questions or share your concerns." The parents mentioned maybe they have done something wrong or missed a part of the treatment, expressing guilt. Hana added, "We understand that you experience feelings of guilt. Loving parents always experience this feeling. What worries you most? We can explore how to alleviate this feeling."
- *Strategy and Summary:* In the final phase, Dr Fair asked both parents if they would like to have further discussions or reschedule another time. After their agreement on continuing the discussion, the three team members explored the goals of care in light of the new findings. The parents wanted to optimise pain management at the hospital and continue the care at home. Dr Fair and Laila explained the pain management plan and Hana arranged to see the parents the next day to discuss the community resources needed for home care. A plan for communicating with Nadia and her brother Leo was also discussed. Before leaving, the team summarised the key points of the conversation and reiterated their readiness to answer any questions, as they arise.

The team followed the SPIKES protocol and provided compassionate and sensitive communication of bad news, while taking into consideration the family's needs and dynamics. The use of non-verbal communication helped create an empathetic environment through the use of silence and body gestures. The team supported the parents to express feelings and make decisions during and after the discussion.

---

**BOX 4.2 ANTENATAL CASE STUDY**

During the anatomy scan at 21 weeks gestation, Sarah and her partner were informed that their baby was presenting foetal abnormalities. At this time, it was explained in layman terms, that their baby was small for gestational age and displayed some heart defects and a cleft lip. Sarah was given an appointment for the Foetal Medicine Specialist (FMS) for the next day and informed that another scan would be provided, and that the doctor would explain in detail how their baby was developing. This gave Sarah and her partner a "warning shot", an opportunity to digest the news that something was "wrong" with their baby and return to the appointment with the FMS with questions they had prepared.

During this appointment, the FMS confirmed the abnormalities and explained to the couple that the sonographic findings were suggestive of Trisomy 18 (Edward Syndrome). Sarah and her partner were informed that an amniocentesis would be required to diagnose Trisomy 18. In layman terms they received a description of what was involved in this diagnostic test, the risks, and when results would be available. A description of Trisomy 18 was also provided. Sarah and her partner were given time in a quiet undisturbed environment afterwards where their questions were answered. A contact number for the Foetal Medicine Midwife Specialist was shared alongside written information on Trisomy 18. Sarah and her partner were encouraged to contact the specialist if they had any questions.

Following the amniocentesis, the couple were given the option of coming into the clinic for the results or receiving them over the phone. Encouragement was given to them to attend in person. The option for a telephone consultation is useful for those who have to travel to an FMS appointment. The FMS ensured that they allocated sufficient time to deliver a diagnosis of Trisomy 18 to the couple and provided clear, accurate and unbiased prenatal counselling. The couple were fully informed of their choice to continue with the pregnancy and receive perinatal palliative care or terminate the pregnancy. Prenatal counselling ensures parents are made aware of what both options entail and a description of perinatal palliative care provided. During this meeting, Sarah and her partner were encouraged to ask any questions they had, their individual needs at this time were identified and support offered. They were introduced to the Bereavement Midwife Specialist and their contact details provided, along with details of voluntary organisations who support parents who receive a diagnosis of Trisomy 18 and who experience pregnancy loss and perinatal death shared.

The couple's subsequent appointments were provided away from other pregnant people with minimal waiting times. These appointments were scheduled more frequently and allocated additional time to facilitate input from the Bereavement Midwife Specialist. This allowed adequate support for the parents in the incident of death of their baby in utero.

Through utilising both SOBPIE and NEO-SPEAK protocols in clinical practice, individualised patient-centred care was provided, and compassionate and non-judgemental communication promoted and delivered by a knowledgeable and skilled multi-disciplinary team. This facilitated parental understanding and met the parents' unique needs.

## SUMMARY

In children's palliative care, the skill of communicating bad or unwanted news is an intricate necessity and impactful intervention. The challenges reside in deeply understanding the child and family, respecting their uniqueness, and humanely disclosing information. Communication models and acronyms provide tangible guidance on the technique of delivering bad or unwanted news. Yet, a compassionate presence is needed before, during and, most importantly, after the disclosure. Children and parents will carry a lasting memory of the disclosure encounter for the rest of their lives, a sensitive disclosure can instil hope even in the most difficult conversations. As nurses, we have the ethical responsibility to prevent and alleviate suffering when bad or unwanted news is communicated.

## KEY POINTS

- The disclosure of difficult news should be delivered by a knowledgeable, competent healthcare professional who has a therapeutic relationship with the child and family.

- Communication must be clear, easily understood and provided at a time where the child and family can be supported, and questions answered in a quiet conducive environment.
- Communication should be delivered in a holistic and individualised approach and at a pace that facilitates the child and family's understanding of what is being said. A child- and family-centred approach is of utmost importance.

## REFERENCES

Adduci, A., Jankovic, M., Strazzer, S., Massimino, M., Clerici, C., Poggi, G. (2012). Parent-child communication and psychological adjustment in children with a brain tumor. *Pediatric Blood & Cancer, 59*(2), 290–294. https://doi.org/10.1002/pbc.24165

Agrawal, U. S., Sarin, J., Garg, R. (2023). Nursing perspective of providing palliative care to the children: A narrative review. *Journal of Health and Allied Sciences NU, 14*(02), 157–162. https://doi.org/10.1055/s-0043-1769081

Al-Abdi, S. Y., Al-Ali, E. A., Daheer, M. H., Al-Saleh, Y. M., Al-Qurashi, K. H., Al-Aamri, M. A. (2011). Saudi mothers' preferences about breaking bad news concerning newborns: A structured verbal questionnaire. *BMC Medical Ethics, 12*, 1–8. https://doi.org/10.1186/1472-6939-12-15

Ashtiani, S., Makela, N., Carrion, P., Austin, J. (2014). Parents' experiences of receiving their child's genetic diagnosis: A qualitative study to inform clinical genetics practice. *American Journal of Medical Genetics, Part A, 164*(6), 1496–1502. https://doi.org/10.1002/ajmg.a.36525

Atienza-Carrasco, J., Linares-Abad, M., Padilla-Ruiz, M., Morales-Gil, I. M. (2018). Breaking bad news to antenatal patients with strategies to lessen the pain: a qualitative study. *Reproductive Health, 15*, 1–11.https://doi.org/10.1186/s12978-018-0454-2

Badawi, G. (2011). Muslim attitudes towards end-of-life decisions. *The Journal of IMA, 43*(3), 134–139. https://doi.org/10.5915/43-3-8602

Baile, W. F., Buckman, R., Lenzi, R., Glober, G., Beale, E. A., Kudelka, A. P. (2000). SPIKES— A six-step protocol for delivering bad news: Application to the patient with cancer. *The Oncologist, 5*, 302–311. https://doi.org/10.1634/theoncologist.5-4-302

Bashir, A. (2019). Congenital malformations: Prenatal diagnosis and management. *American Journal of Biomed Science Research, 2*(1), 24–2q17. https://doi.org/10.34297/AJBSR.2019.02.000565

Bereavement Care Standards Development Group. (2016). *National standards for bereavement care following pregnancy loss and perinatal death.* Dublin: Health Service Executive. Available at: https://www.hse.ie/eng/services/list/3/maternity/bereavement-care/ (accessed 8 June 2024).

Bluebond-Langner, M. (1978). *The private worlds of dying children.* Princeton University Press.

Boyd, J. R. (2001). A process for delivering bad news: Supporting families when a child is diagnosed. *The Journal of Neuroscience Nursing: Journal of the American Association of Neuroscience Nurses, 33*(1), 14–20. https://doi.org/10.1097/01376517-200102000-00003

Boyle, B., Addor, M. C., Arriola, L., Barisic, I., Bianchi, F., Csáky-Szunyogh, M., de Walle, H. E. K., Dias, C. M., Draper, E., Gatt, M., Garne, E., Haeusler, M., Källén, K., Latos-Bielenska, A., McDonnell, B., Mullaney, C., Nelen, V., Neville, A. J., O'Mahony, M., Queisser-Wahrendorf, A., … Dolk, H. (2018). Estimating global burden of disease due to congenital anomaly: An analysis of European data. *Archives of Disease in Childhood – Fetal and Neonatal Edition, 103*(1), F22–F28. https://doi.org/10.1136/archdischild-2016-311845

Boyle, F. M., Mutch, A. J., Barber, E. A., Carroll, C., Dean, J. H. (2015). Supporting parents following pregnancy loss: A cross-sectional study of telephone peer supporters. *BMC Pregnancy and Childbirth*, *15*, 291. https://doi.org/10.1186/s12884-015-0713-y

Brouwer, M. A., Maeckelberghe, E. L. M., van der Heide, A., Hein, I. M., Verhagen, E. A. A. E. (2021). Breaking bad news: What parents would like you to know. *Archives of Disease in Childhood*, *106*(3), 276–281. https://doi.org/10.1136/archdischild-2019-318398

Buckman, R. (1984). Breaking bad news: Why is it still so difficult? *British Medical Journal (Clinical research edition)*, *288*(6430), 1597–1599. https://doi.org/10.1136/bmj.288.6430.1597

Buckman, R. (1992). *How to break bad news: A guide for health care professionals*. Johns Hopkins University Press.

Buckman, R. (2005). Breaking bad news: The S-P-I-K-E-S strategy. *Community Oncology*, *2*(2), 138–142. https://doi.org/10.1016/S1548-5315(11)70867-1

Budd, J. L., Draper, E. S., Lotto, R. R., Berry, L. E., Smith, L. K. (2015). Socioeconomic inequalities in pregnancy outcome associated with Down syndrome: A population-based study. *Archives of Disease in Childhood – Fetal and Neonatal Edition*, *100*(5), F400–F404. https://doi.org/10.1136/archdischild-2014-306985

Ciobanu, E., Preston, N. (2021). Hearing the voices of children diagnosed with a life-threatening or life-limiting illness and their parents' accounts in a palliative care setting: A qualitative study. *Palliative Medicine*, *35*(5), 886–892. https://doi.org/10.1177/02692163211000238

Cluver, L. D., Hodes, R. J., Toska, E., Kidia, K. K., Orkin, F. M., Sherr, L., Meinck, F. (2015). 'HIV is like a tsotsi. ARVs are your guns': Associations between HIV-disclosure and adherence to antiretroviral treatment among adolescents in South Africa. *AIDS*, *29* (Suppl. 1), S57–S65. https://doi.org/10.1097/QAD.0000000000000695

Coleman, P. K. (2015). Diagnosis of Fetal Anomaly and the increased maternal psychological toll associated with pregnancy termination. *Issues in Law & Medicine*, *30*(1), 3–23.

Connor, S., Morris. C., Jaramillo, E., Harding, R., Cleary, J., Haste, B., Knaul, F., de Lima, L., Krakauer, E., Bhadelia, A., Jiang, X., Arreola-Ornelas, H., Mendez Carniado, O., Brennen, F., Clark, D., Clelland, D., Centeno, C., Garralda, E., López-Fidalgo, J., Downing, J., Radbruch, L. (2020). *Global atlas for palliative care* (2nd edn). World Hospice and Palliative Care Alliance. Available at: http://www.thewhpca.org/resources/global-atlas-on-end-of-life-care (accessed 4 January 2022).

Cooley, C. (2000). Communication skills in palliative care. *Professional Nurse*, *15*(9), 603–605.

Das, M. K., Arora, N. K., Chellani, H. K., Debata, P. K., Meena, K. R., Rasaily, R., Kaur, G., Malik, P., Joshi, S., Kumari, M. (2021). Perceptions of the parents of deceased children and of healthcare providers about end-of-life communication and breaking bad news at a tertiary care public hospital in India: A qualitative exploratory study. *PloS One*, *16*(3), e0248661. https://doi.org/10.1371/journal.pone.0248661

Demarest, S., Marsh, R., Treat, L., Fisher, M. P., Dempsey, A., Junaid, M., Downs, J., Leonard, H., Benke, T., Morris, M. A. (2022). The lived experience of parents' receiving the diagnosis of CDKL5 deficiency disorder for their child. *Journal of Child Neurology*, *37*(6), 451–460. https://doi.org/10.1177/08830738221076285

de Vos, M. A., Bos, A. P., Plötz, F. B., van Heerde, M., de Graaff, B. M., Tates, K., Truog, R. D., Willems, D. L. (2015). Talking with parents about end-of-life decisions for their children. *Pediatrics*, *135*(2), e465–e476. https://doi.org/10.1542/peds.2014-1903

Dobrozsi, S., Trowbridge, A., Mack, J. W., Rosenberg, A. R. (2019). Effective communication for newly diagnosed pediatric patients with cancer: Considerations for the patients, family members, providers, and multidisciplinary team. *American Society of Clinical Oncology Educational Book. American Society of Clinical Oncology: Annual Meeting*, *39*, 573–581. https://doi.org/10.1200/EDBK_238181

Due, C., Obst, K., Riggs, D. W., Collins, C. (2018). Australian heterosexual women's experiences of healthcare provision following a pregnancy loss. *Women and Birth: Journal of the Australian College of Midwives, 31*(4), 331–338. https://doi.org/10.1016/j.wombi.2017.11.002

Fine, R. L. (1991). Personal choices: Communication among physicians and patients when confronting critical illness. *Texas Medicine, 87*(9), 76–82.

Finlayson, K., Downe, S. (2013). Why do women not use antenatal services in low- and middle-income countries? A meta-synthesis of qualitative studies. *PLoS Medicine, 10*(1), e1001373. https://doi.org/10.1371/journal.pmed.1001373

Fleming, V., Iljuschin, I., Pehlke-Milde, J., Maurer, F., Parpan, F. (2016). Dying at life's beginning: Experiences of parents and health professionals in Switzerland when an 'in utero' diagnosis incompatible with life is made. *Midwifery, 34*, 23–29. https://doi.org/10.1016/j.midw.2016.01.014

Fortier, M. A., Batista, M. L., Wahi, A., Kain, A., Strom, S., Sender, L. S. (2013). Illness uncertainty and quality of life in children with cancer. *Journal of Pediatric Hematology/Oncology, 35*(5), 366–370. https://doi.org/10.1097/MPH.0b013e318290cfdb

Fraser, L. K., Gibson-Smith, D., Jarvis, S., Norman, P., Parslow, R. C. (2021). Estimating the current and future prevalence of life-limiting conditions in children in England. *Palliative Medicine, 35*(9), 1641–1651. https://doi.org/10.1177/0269216320975308

Gillam, L., Spriggs, M., McCarthy, M., Delany, C. (2022). Telling the truth to seriously ill children: Considering children's interests when parents veto telling the truth. *Bioethics, 36*(7), 765–773. https://doi.org/10.1111/bioe.13048

Guerra, F. A. R., Mirlesse, V., Baião, A. E. R. (2011). Breaking bad news during prenatal care: A challenge to be tackled. *Ciencia & Saude Coletiva, 16*(5), 2361–2367. https://doi.org/10.1590/s1413-81232011000500002

Hain, R., Devins, M., Hastings, R., Noyes, J. (2013). Paediatric palliative care: development and pilot study of a 'Directory' of life-limiting conditions. *BMC Palliative Care, 12*(1), 43. https://doi.org/10.1186/1472-684X-12-43

Haitjema, S., Lubout, C. M. A., Zijlstra, J. H. M., Wolffenbuttel, B. H. R., van Spronsen, F. J. (2022). Communication of an abnormal metabolic new-born screening result in the Netherlands: The parental perspective. *Nutrients, 14*(19), 1–9. https://doi.org/10.3390/nu14193961

Health Service Executive. (2024). *Congenital anomaly registers in Ireland*. Available at: https://www.hse.ie/congenitalanomalyregistersireland (accessed 30 May 2024).

Heazell, A. E. P., Siassakos, D., Blencowe, H., Burden, C., Bhutta, Z. A., Cacciatore, J., Dang, N., Das, J., Flenady, V., Gold, K. J., Mensah, O. K., Millum, J., Nuzum, D., O'Donoghue, K., Redshaw, M., Rizvi, A., Roberts, T., Toyin Saraki, H. E., Storey, C., Wojcieszek, A. M., Lancet Ending Preventable Stillbirths Investigator Group. (2016). Stillbirths: Economic and psychosocial consequences. *Lancet (London, England), 387*(10018), 604–616. https://doi.org/10.1016/S0140-6736(15)00836-3

Holmes, S. N., Illing, J. (2021). Breaking bad news: Tackling cultural dilemmas. *BMJ Supportive & Palliative Care, 11*(2), 128–132. https://doi.org/10.1136/bmjspcare-2020-002700

Hurley, F., Kiernan, G., Price, J. (2021). 'Starting out in haziness': Parental experiences surrounding the diagnosis of their child's non-malignant life-limiting condition in Ireland. *Journal of Pediatric Nursing, 59*, 25–31. https://doi.org/10.1016/j.pedn.2020.12.015

Irish Hospice Foundation. (2020). Children's grief. Available at: https://hospicefoundation.ie/i-need-help/i-am-bereaved/types-of-grief/childrens-grief/ (accessed 8 June 2024).

Jacobs, S., Perez, J., Cheng, Y. I., Sill, A., Wang, J., Lyon, M. E. (2015). Adolescent end of life preferences and congruence with their parents' preferences: Results of a survey of adolescents with cancer. *Pediatric Blood & Cancer, 62*(4), 710–714. https://doi.org/10.1002/pbc.25358

Jalali, R., Jalali, A., Jalilian, M. (2023). Breaking bad news in medical services: A comprehensive systematic review. *Heliyon, 9*(4), e14734. https://doi.org/10.1016/j.heliyon.2023.e14734

Janvier, A., Barrington, K., Farlow, B. (2014). Communication with parents concerning withholding or withdrawing of life-sustaining interventions in neonatology. *Seminars in Perinatology, 38*(1), 38–46. https://doi.org/10.1053/j.semperi.2013.07.007

Kajubi, P., Whyte, S. R., Kyaddondo, D., Katahoire, A. R. (2016). Tensions in communication between children on antiretroviral therapy and their caregivers: A qualitative study in Jinja District, Uganda. *PLoS One, 11*(1), e0147119. https://doi.org/10.1371/journal.pone.0147119

Katz, A. L., Webb, S. A., Committee on Bioethics. (2016). Informed consent in decision-making in pediatric practice. *Pediatrics, 138*(2), e20161485. https://doi.org/10.1542/peds.2016-1485

Kelly, K. P., Mowbray, C., Pyke-Grimm, K., Hinds, P. S. (2017). Identifying a conceptual shift in child and adolescent-reported treatment decision making: "Having a say, as I need at this time". *Pediatric Blood & Cancer, 64*(4), 10.1002/pbc.26262. https://doi.org/10.1002/pbc.26262

Kessel, R. M., Roth, M., Moody, K., Levy, A. (2013). Day One Talk: Parent preferences when learning that their child has cancer. *Supportive Care in Cancer: Official Journal of the Multinational Association of Supportive Care in Cancer, 21*(11), 2977–2982. https://doi.org/10.1007/s00520-013-1874-8

Kinsner-Ovaskainen, A., Perraud, A., Lanzoni, M., Morris, J., Garne, E. (2021). European Monitoring of Congenital Anomalies: JRC-EUROCAT report on statistical monitoring of congenital anomalies (2009–2018). Publications Office of the European Union. Available at: https://eu-rd-platform.jrc.ec.europa.eu/system/files/public/EUROCAT-Statistical-Monitoring-Report-2021.pdf (accessed 8 June 2024).

Knaul, F. M., Farmer, P. E., Krakauer, E. L., De Lima, L., Bhadelia, A., Jiang Kwete, X., Arreola-Ornelas, H., Gómez-Dantés, O., Rodriguez, N. M., Alleyne, G., Connor, S. R., Hunter, D. J., Lohman, D., Radbruch, L., Del Rocío Sáenz Madrigal, M., Atun, R., Foley, K. M., Frenk, J., Jamison, D. T., Rajagopal, M. R., Lancet Commission on Palliative Care and Pain Relief Study Group. (2018). Alleviating the access abyss in palliative care and pain relief: An imperative of universal health coverage: The Lancet Commission report. *Lancet, 391*(10128), 1391–1454. https://doi.org/10.1016/S0140-6736(17)32513-8

Lalor, J. G., Devane, D., Begley, C. M. (2007). Unexpected diagnosis of fetal abnormality: Women's encounters with caregivers. *Birth, 34*(1), 80–88. https://doi.org/10.1111/j.1523-536X.2006.00148.x

Last, B. F., van Veldhuizen, A. M. (1996). Information about diagnosis and prognosis related to anxiety and depression in children with cancer aged 8–16 years. *European Journal of Cancer, 32A*(2), 290–294. https://doi.org/10.1016/0959-8049(95)00576-5

Lawton, S., Hickerton, C., Archibald, A. D., McClaren, B. J., Metcalfe, S. A. (2015). A mixed methods exploration of families' experiences of the diagnosis of childhood spinal muscular atrophy. *European Journal of Human Genetics, 23*(5), 575–580. https://doi.org/10.1038/ejhg.2014.147

Lester, P., Chesney, M., Cooke, M., Weiss, R., Whalley, P., Perez, B., Glidden, D., Petru, A., Dorenbaum, A., Wara, D. (2002). When the time comes to talk about HIV: Factors associated with diagnostic disclosure and emotional distress in HIV-infected children. *Journal of Acquired Immune Deficiency Syndromes, 31*(3), 309–317. https://doi.org/10.1097/00126334-200211010-00006

Lotto, R., Smith, L. K., Armstrong, N. (2017). Clinicians' perspectives of parental decision-making following diagnosis of a severe congenital anomaly: A qualitative study. *BMJ Open, 7*(5), e014716–e014716. https://doi.org/10.1136/bmjopen-2016-014716

Mack, J. W., Joffe, S. (2014). Communicating about prognosis: Ethical responsibilities of pediatricians and parents. *Pediatrics, 133*(Suppl. 1), S24–S30. https://doi.org/10.1542/peds.2013-3608E

Maijala, H., Astedt-Kurki, P., Paavilainen, E., Väisänen, L. (2003). Interaction between caregivers and families expecting a malformed child. *Journal of Advanced Nursing*, 42(1), 37–46. https://doi.org/10.1046/j.1365-2648.2003.02577.x

Marokakis, S., Kasparian, N. A., Kennedy, S. E. (2016). Prenatal counselling for congenital anomalies: A systematic review. *Prenatal Diagnosis*, 36(7), 662–671. https://doi.org/10.1002/pd.4836

Marsac, M. L., Kindler, C., Weiss, D., Ragsdale, L. (2018). Let's talk about it: Supporting family communication during end-of-life care of pediatric patients. *Journal of Palliative Medicine*, 21(6), 862–878. https://doi.org/10.1089/jpm.2017.0307

Maxwell, S., Brameld, K., Bower, C., Dickinson, J. E., Goldblatt, J., Hadlow, N., Hewitt, B., Murch, A., Murphy, A., Stock, R., O'Leary, P. (2011). Socio-demographic disparities in the uptake of prenatal screening and diagnosis in Western Australia. *The Australian and New Zealand Journal of Obstetrics and Gynaecology*, 51(1), 9–16. https://doi.org/10.1111/j.1479-828X.2010.01250.x

McCoyd, J. L. M. (2009). What do women want? Experiences and reflections of women after prenatal diagnosis and termination for anomaly. *Health Care for Women International*, 30(6), 507–535. https://doi.org/10.1080/07399330902801278

McNamara, K., O'Donoghue, K., O'Connell, O., Greene, R. A. (2013). Antenatal and intrapartum care of pregnancy complicated by lethal fetal anomaly. *The Obstetrician & Gynaecologist*, 15(3), 189–194. https://doi.org/10.1111/tog.12028

Meaney, S., Corcoran, P., O'Donoghue, K. (2017). Death of one twin during the perinatal period: An interpretative phenomenological analysis. *Journal of Palliative Medicine*, 20(3), 290–293. https://doi.org/10.1089/jpm.2016.0264

Meitar, D., Karnieli-Miller, O. (2022). Twelve tips to manage a breaking bad news process: Using S-P-w-ICE-S – A revised version of the SPIKES protocol. *Medical Teacher*, 44(10), 1087–1091. https://doi.org/10.1080/0142159X.2021.1928618

Mellins, C. A., Brackis-Cott, E., Dolezal, C., Richards, A., Nicholas, S. W., Abrams, E. J. (2002). Patterns of status disclosure to perinatally HIV-infected children and subsequent mental health outcomes. *Clinical Child Psychology and Psychiatry*, 7(1), 101–114. https://doi.org/10.1177/1359104502007001008

Menon, A., Glazebrook, C., Campain, N., Ngoma, M. (2007). Mental health and disclosure of HIV status in Zambian adolescents with HIV infection: Implications for peer-support programs. *Journal of Acquired Immune Deficiency Syndromes*, 46(3), 349–354. https://doi.org/10.1097/QAI.0b013e3181565df0

Morrison, W., Womer, J., Nathanson, P., Kersun, L., Hester, D. M., Walsh, C., Feudtner, C. (2015). Pediatricians' experience with clinical ethics consultation: A national survey. *The Journal of Pediatrics*, 167(4), 919–924.e1. https://doi.org/10.1016/j.jpeds.2015.06.047

Mouhawej, M. C., Maalouf-Haddad, N., Tohmé, A. (2017). Cultural challenges in implementing palliative services in Lebanon. *Palliative Medicine and Hospice Care*, SE(1), S15–S18. http://doi.org/10.17140/PMHCOJ-SE-1-104

Murphy, K. L. (2017). Talking with children and death and dying. In K. Kobler, R. Limbo (eds), *Conversations in perinatal, neonatal, and pediatric palliative care* (pp. 203–216). Hospice and Palliative Nurses Association.

Narayanan, V., Bista, B., Koshy, C. (2010). 'BREAKS' protocol for breaking bad news. *Indian Journal of Palliative Care*, 16(2), 61–65. https://www.ncbi.nlm.nih.gov/pmc/articles/PMC3144432/pdf/IJPC-16-61.pdf

Nardi, T. J., Keefe-Cooperman, K. (2006). Communicating bad news: A model for emergency mental health helpers. *International Journal of Emergency Mental Health*, 8(3), 203–207. https://digitalcommons.liu.edu/cgi/viewcontent.cgi?article=1004&context=post_coundfpub

National Consensus Project for Quality Palliative Care. (2018). *Clinical practice guidelines for quality palliative care* (4th edn). National Coalition for Hospice and Palliative Care. Available at: https://www.nationalcoalitionhpc.org/ncp (accessed 8 June 2024).

National Council for Hospice and Specialist Palliative Care Services. (2003). *Breaking bad news regional guidelines*. National Council for Hospice and Specialist Palliative Care Services.

Neilson, S., Randall, D., McNamara, K., Downing, J. (2021). Children's palliative care education and training: Developing an education standard framework and audit. *BMC Medical Education, 21*(1), 539. https://doi.org/10.1186/s12909-021-02982-4

Nelson, M., Kelly, D., McAndrew, R., Smith, P. (2017). 'Just gripping my heart and squeezing': Naming and explaining the emotional experience of receiving bad news in the paediatric oncology setting. *Patient Education and Counseling, 100*(9), 1751–1757. https://doi.org/10.1016/j.pec.2017.03.028

Novak, I., Morgan, C., McNamara, L., Te Velde, A. (2019). Best practice guidelines for communicating to parents the diagnosis of disability. *Early Human Development, 139*, 104841. https://doi.org/10.1016/j.earlhumdev.2019.104841

Nuzum, D., Meaney, S., O'Donoghue, K. (2018). The impact of stillbirth on bereaved parents: A qualitative study. *PloS One, 13*(1), e0191635. https://doi.org/10.1371/journal.pone.0191635

O'Donoghue, K. (2019). Pathway for management of fatal fetal anomalies and/or life limiting conditions diagnosed during pregnancy. *Perinatal Palliative Care.* Available at: https://pregnancyandinfantloss.ie/perinatal-palliative-care-pathway/ (accessed 8 June 2024).

Oliveira, F. F., Benute, G. R. G., Gibelli, M. A. B., Nascimento, N. B., Barbosa, T. V. A., Bolibio, R., Jesus, R. C. A., Gaiolla, P. V. V., Setubal, M. S. V., Gomes, A. L., Francisco, R. P., Bernardes, L. S. (2020). Breaking bad news: A study on formal training in a high-risk obstetrics setting. *Palliative Medicine Reports, 1*(1), 50–57. https://doi.org/10.1089/pmr.2020.0014

Price, J., McNeilly, P., Surgenor, M. (2006). Breaking bad news to parents: The children's nurse's role. *International Journal of Palliative Nursing, 12*(3), 115–120. https://doi.org/10.12968/ijpn.2006.12.3.20695

Qaddoumi, I., Ezam, N., Swaidan, M., Jaradat, I., Mansour, A., Abuirmeileh, N., Bouffet, E., Al-Hussaini, M. (2009). Diffuse pontine glioma in Jordan and impact of up-front prognosis disclosure with parents and families. *Journal of Child Neurology, 24*(4), 460–465. https://doi.org/10.1177/0883073808325650

Rabow, M. W., McPhee, S. J. (1999). Beyond breaking bad news: How to help patients who suffer. *The Western Journal of Medicine, 171*(4), 260–263. https://www.ncbi.nlm.nih.gov/pmc/articles/PMC1305864/

Rajasooriyar, C., Kelly, J., Sivakumar, T., Navanesan, G., Nadarasa, S., Sriskandarajah, M. H., Sabesan, S. (2016). Breaking bad news in ethnic settings: Perspectives of patients and families in northern Sri Lanka. *Journal of Global Oncology, 3*(3), 250–256. https://doi.org/10.1200/JGO.2016.005355

Rosenberg, A. R., Starks, H., Unguru, Y., Feudtner, C., Diekema, D. (2017). Truth telling in the setting of cultural differences and incurable pediatric illness: A review. *JAMA Pediatrics, 171*(11), 1113–1119. https://doi.org/10.1001/jamapediatrics.2017.2568

Rost, M., Mihailov, E. (2021). In the name of the family? Against parents' refusal to disclose prognostic information to children. *Medicine, Health Care, and Philosophy, 24*(3), 421–432. https://doi.org/10.1007/s11019-021-10017-4

Royal College of Obstetricians and Gynaecologists. (2010). Termination of pregnancy for fetal abnormality in England, Scotland and Wales report of a working party. Available at: https://www.rcog.org.uk/guidance/browse-all-guidance/other-guidelines-and-reports/termination-of-pregnancy-for-fetal-abnormality-in-england-scotland-and-wales/ (accessed 8 June 2024).

Salem, A., Salem, A. F. (2013). Breaking bad news: Current prospective and practical guideline for Muslim countries. *Journal of Cancer Education: The Official Journal of the American Association for Cancer Education, 28*(4), 790–794. https://doi.org/10.1007/s13187-013-0523-8

Seifart, C., Falch, M., Wege, M., Maier, R. F., Pedrosa Carrasco, A. J. (2022). NEO-SPEAK: A conceptual framework that underpins breaking bad news in neonatology. *Frontiers in Pediatrics, 10*, 1044210. https://doi.org/10.3389/fped.2022.1044210

Sisk, B. A., Bluebond-Langner, M., Wiener, L., Mack, J., Wolfe, J. (2016). Prognostic disclosures to children: A historical perspective. *Pediatrics, 138*(3), e20161278. https://doi.org/10.1542/peds.2016-1278

Smith, L. K., Budd, J. L., Field, D. J., Draper, E. S. (2011). Socioeconomic inequalities in outcome of pregnancy and neonatal mortality associated with congenital anomalies: Population based study. *BMJ, 343*(7818), 301. https://doi.org/10.1136/bmj.d4306

Statham, H., Solomou, W., Chitty, L. (2000). Prenatal diagnosis of fetal abnormality: Psychological effects on women in low-risk pregnancies. *Bailliere's Best Practice & Research: Clinical Obstetrics & Gynaecology, 14*(4), 731–747. https://doi.org/10.1053/beog.2000.0108

Stein, A., Dalton, L., Rapa, E., Bluebond-Langner, M., Hanington, L., Stein, K. F., Ziebland, S., Rochat, T., Harrop, E., Kelly, B., Bland, R., Communication Expert Group. (2019). Communication with children and adolescents about the diagnosis of their own life-threatening condition. *The Lancet, 393*(10176), 1150–1163. https://doi.org/10.1016/S0140-6736(18)33201-X

The Irish Childhood Bereavement Network. (2018). Children and grief by age & stage. Available at: https://www.childhoodbereavement.ie/families/

Tunçalp, Ö., Pena-Rosas, J. P., Lawrie, T., Bucagu, M., Oladapo, O. T., Portela, A., Metin Gülmezoglu, A. (2017). WHO recommendations on antenatal care for a positive pregnancy experience—going beyond survival. *BJOG: An International Journal of Obstetrics & Gynaecology, 124*(6), 860–862. https://doi.org/10.1111/1471-0528.14599

Ulrich, C. M., Mooney-Doyle, K., Grady, C. (2018). Communicating with pediatric families at end-of-life is not a fantasy. *The American Journal of Bioethics: AJOB, 18*(1), 14–16. https://doi.org/10.1080/15265161.2017.1401175

van der Geest, I. M., van den Heuvel-Eibrink, M. M., van Vliet, L. M., Pluijm, S. M., Streng, I. C., Michiels, E. M., Pieters, R., Darlington, A. S. (2015). Talking about death with children with incurable cancer: Perspectives from parents. *The Journal of Pediatrics, 167*(6), 1320–1326. https://doi.org/10.1016/j.jpeds.2015.08.066

Warnock, C. (2014). Breaking bad news: Issues relating to nursing practice. *Nursing Standard, 28*(45), 51–58. https://doi.org/10.7748/ns.28.45.51.e8935

Wege, M., von Blanckenburg, P., Maier, R. F., Knoeppel, C., Grunske, A., Seifart, C. (2023). Do parents get what they want during bad news delivery in NICU?. *Journal of Perinatal Medicine, 51*(8), 1104–1111. https://doi.org/10.1515/jpm-2023-0134

WHO (World Health Organization). (2018). *World health statistics 2018: Monitoring health for the SDGs, sustainable development goals.* Available at: https://iris.who.int/bitstream/handle/10665/272596/9789241565585-eng.pdf?sequence=1 (accessed 8 June 2024).

Wiener, L., McConnell, D. G., Latella, L., Ludi, E. (2013). Cultural and religious considerations in pediatric palliative care. *Palliative & Supportive Care, 11*(1), 47–67. https://doi.org/10.1017/S1478951511001027

Wilkinson, D. J., Thiele, P., Watkins, A., De Crespigny, L. (2012). Fatally flawed? A review and ethical analysis of lethal congenital malformations. *BJOG: An International Journal of Obstetrics and Gynaecology, 119*(11), 1302–1308. https://doi.org/10.1111/j.1471-0528.2012.03450.x

Winter, M. C., Friedman, D. N., McCabe, M. S., Voigt, L. P. (2019). Content review of pediatric ethics consultations at a cancer center. *Pediatric Blood & Cancer, 66*(5), e27617. https://doi.org/10.1002/pbc.27617

Wolfe, A. D., Frierdich, S. A., Wish, J., Kilgore-Carlin, J., Plotkin, J. A., Hoover-Regan, M. (2014). Sharing life-altering information: Development of pediatric hospital guidelines and team training. *Journal of Palliative Medicine, 17*(9), 1011–1018. https://doi.org/10.1089/jpm.2013.0620

Wool, C., Black, B. P., Woods, A. B. N. (2016). Quality indicators and parental satisfaction with perinatal palliative care in the intrapartum setting after diagnosis of a life-limiting fetal condition. *Advances in Nursing Science, 39*(4), 346–357. https://doi.org/10.1097/ANS.0000000000000147

Xafis, V., Wilkinson, D., Sullivan, J. (2015). What information do parents need when facing end-of-life decisions for their child? A meta-synthesis of parental feedback. *BMC Palliative Care, 14*, 19. https://doi.org/10.1186/s12904-015-0024-0

# Self-care for nurses and nursing teams delivering and evaluating palliative care

....................................................

*Anna Oddy, Doris Corkin and Becky Davis*

## INTRODUCTION

The presentation of the child or young person with palliative care needs, in both the hospital and community care setting, poses a unique set of stressors to clinicians and nursing teams, which can be overwhelming and significantly affect their mental health, if not managed appropriately. Supporting the family of a child who is receiving palliative and end-of-life care can be immensely rewarding, though particularly stressful and challenging for children's nurses and their students who may feel unprepared. We, the authors of this self-care chapter, acknowledge the inherent difficulties in this, identifying the challenge of striking the right balance of emotional investment without becoming too involved or overwhelmed. Caring for children receiving palliative care and their families has been the most privileged experiences we have had within our own nursing careers.

We appreciate this opportunity to inspire pre-registration and postgraduate nursing students, alongside qualified nurses, with a specific interest in children's palliative care nursing. The importance of self-care is "threaded" throughout this chapter and the need to find sustainable and nourishing ways to deliver children's palliative care highlighted.

Self-care is the process of engaging in activities that promote and maintain health and well-being: fostering nurses' resilience and reducing emotional labour (Delgado et al., 2017). For nurses delivering palliative care, self-care has become a key feature in the literature, frameworks, research, documents and textbooks (Wakefield, 2000; Goodrich et al., 2015; Gómez-Urquiza et al., 2020; RCN, 2021; Hughes and McNeilly, 2024). However, practising and sustaining self-care as well as supporting the health and well-being of patients, their families and inter-professional colleagues can be challenging. Reported current themes that contribute to work-related stress include provision of out-of-hours care, the challenge of developing and maintaining clinical skills, ambiguity of professional roles and relationships with the child

DOI: 10.4324/9781003384861-8

**LEARNING OBJECTIVES**

The reader will be able to do the following:

1.  Identify and discuss the professional roles and responsibilities within a multi-disciplinary (or inter-professional) specialist team delivering children's palliative and end-of-life care.
2.  Understand the specific challenges related to delivering children's palliative care that can lead to an increased risk of burnout and compassion fatigue.
3.  Critically gain knowledge and a deeper understanding regarding a variety of strategies for practising self-care and how you can use these to reduce the risk of burnout and compassion fatigue.

and family, a lack of resources, emotional impact and a lack of staff support (Reid, 2013a; 2013b; Samuelson et al., 2015). Therefore, improving the working experiences of children's palliative care nurses and nursing students should be a health priority with the aim of enhancing job satisfaction, fostering self-awareness, and promoting resilience and overall well-being.

Important self-care is individually directed, as well as offered, by the healthcare organisations within which we work. Healthcare organisations can and should support employee well-being. A healthy workforce will have a wide range of abilities, be resilient and effective. We need to embed a culture of "self-care" within nursing so that individuals can sustain their health and wellbeing, and consequently provide compassionate patient care. The Royal College of Nursing (RCN) campaign "Healthy Workplace, Healthy You" (RCN, 2016) sought to enhance the overall well-being of nursing professionals by addressing workplace conditions and promoting healthier practices. It emphasised the importance of staff well-being (both physical and mental), suggesting that supporting and encouraging nurses to improve their own health could, in turn, positively impact patient outcomes.

## REFLECTION ON THE NURSE'S ROLE IN TEAMS DELIVERING CHILDREN'S PALLIATIVE CARE

Children's palliative care is an ever-growing speciality that focuses on the care of babies, children and young people facing life-limiting and life-threatening conditions and their families. Palliative care often involves multi-disciplinary teams working across several organisations, including community settings, hospices and hospitals (Knapp et al., 2011). COVID-19 made its impact upon children, with healthcare staff responding to this ongoing pandemic (Figure 5.1), in innovative and appropriate ways, in order to continue to meet service demands and ensure palliative care of the highest standard (Southhall et al., 2021). New ways of working, such as remote telephone and digital healthcare consultations, were necessary to mitigate the spread of the virus. Home visits were arranged when needed and personal protective equipment (PPE) was required to protect both patients and staff.

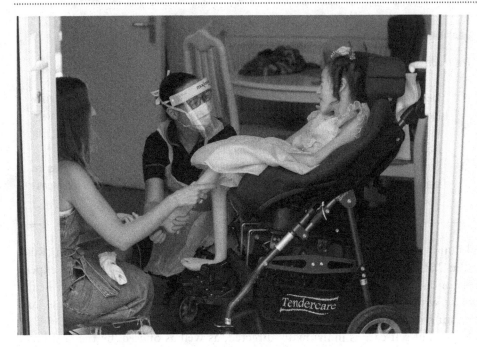

**FIGURE 5.1** CPC provision during COVID-19

Source: Reproduced with kind parental permission.

## PROFESSIONAL BOUNDARIES

It is important to note that palliative care is "often provided" to the child over many years and may include the end-of-life phase and bereavement support. For nurses and care staff providing this high level of physical, emotional, social and spiritual care, a re-negotiation of traditional professional boundaries is required to enable individualised care with the focus on quality of life for the child and their family (McCloskey and Taggart, 2010). This necessitates balancing "remaining professional" while ensuring a therapeutic relationship with the child and their family.

Navigating professional boundaries in nursing involves maintaining a therapeutic relationship with patients and families, while upholding ethical standards (NMC, 2018a). This includes maintaining confidentiality, setting appropriate physical and emotional boundaries, avoiding dual relationships, and seeking supervision or consultation when needed. On reflection, it is about striking a balance between empathy and maintaining a professional distance, to ensure the best possible care for patients. By establishing and maintaining clear boundaries between work and personal life, palliative care nurses can provide compassionate, ethical and effective care while safeguarding their own well-being and professional integrity and promoting a healthy work-life balance.

Erikson and Davies (2017) have discussed managing professional boundaries in the context of providing palliative care to children and families; maintaining integrity when integrating the competing aspects of the nursing role, behaving professionally while connecting personally. There is an art to managing this balance in tension as one seeks separation from the child and family, while the other strives for engagement with them. However, professional boundaries are not always black and white in practice and Buder and Fringer (2016) acknowledge the inherent difficulties in maintaining these. They acknowledge that some nurses identify "professional distance" with a lack of caring and that understanding and managing these boundaries cannot be taught, but must be learned from role models, experience and a sense of one's own vulnerabilities and resilience.

According to Epstein and Krasner (2013), resilience is the capacity to respond to stressors in a healthy way so that goals are achievable. Therefore, the individual must have reasonable expectations, an ability to cope with adversity and maintain a healthy engagement with difficulties at work. Building resilience is crucial for managing the emotional challenges that come with providing palliative care (Grauerholz et al., 2020). A narrative literature review of nurse-parent relationships in children's palliative care by Brimble et al. (2019) identified four main themes: (1) bonds, attachments and trust; (2) sharing the journey; (3) going the extra mile; and (4) boundaries and integrity. The very things that enhance the nurse-parent/family relationship in palliative care nursing pose the greatest challenges in emotional burden with the very real risk of compassion fatigue and occupational burnout (Gómez-Urquiza et al., 2020).

## ETHICAL DILEMMAS

Children's nurses working in acute hospital settings may face ethical dilemmas. Indeed, situations where medical interventions take priority may expose the nursing staff to further challenging and distressing situations. An example of this is 14-year-old Jack (pseudonym) for whom active treatment for a brain tumour has become futile, as the tumour continues to grow even while on active treatment. Offering palliative chemotherapy might extend Jack's life for a few more weeks or months, giving him and his family precious time. But the palliative chemotherapy brings with it a number of unpleasant side effects, which could negatively impact on Jack's quality of life. It may be better to focus on quality of life for Jack, even if this means a shorter life, by foregoing palliative chemotherapy. Jack's parents want the treatment but Jack does not. Witnessing these discussions and the emotion and distress that inevitably accompany such situations, while supporting children and families to make these difficult decisions, can be emotionally challenging for all healthcare staff involved. Indeed, nurses have reported their distress when futile treatments leave no time for the family to deal with the imminent death (Bergstrasser et al., 2017).

Parallel planning "planning for life while also planning for deterioration or death" (Widdas et al., 2013, p. 13) is a key recommendation for good palliative care and can be helpful when dealing with ethical dilemmas. Parallel planning acknowledges unexpected health and care trajectories, while planning for end-of-life care. However, parallel planning may not always be possible when decisions need to be actioned extremely quickly, especially in the neonatal or children's intensive care unit.

## INDIVIDUALISED CARE

In the UK, the Nursing and Midwifery Council (NMC, 2018a) reminds nurses that they have a responsibility to treat all patients and colleagues fairly, with dignity and respect and act in accordance with their organisation's policies. Inclusion requires recognising, valuing and engaging with others, therefore considering age, disability, race, religion, gender and sexual orientation (Equality Act, 2010). Overall, each of us collectively shapes our culture, therefore how we choose to work and interact with one another is what makes an impact.

A detailed assessment of a family's holistic needs involves ongoing gathering and recording of information, with the child and family at the heart of the process (Brown et al., 2021). This provides the opportunity to share hopes and raise concerns and explore and address faith or spiritual wishes as part of the child's palliative nursing care.

The importance of individualised care (Figure 5.2) when addressing the needs of families with dying children is recognised (Cacciatore et al., 2019). Children with palliative care needs may require input from many different professionals across multiple agencies and care settings (Carter et al., 2007). There is a clear need for integrated multi-professional working and care collaboration, but there must be role clarity. The varying numbers of health professionals who can be involved in a child's palliative care delivery can result in confusion surrounding roles and responsibilities, influencing the caregiver (Reid, 2013a).

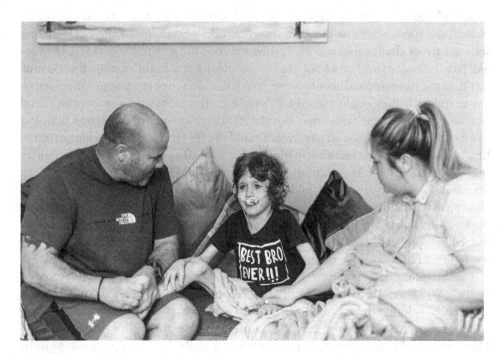

**FIGURE 5.2** Individualised family-centred care

Source: Reproduced with kind parental permission.

International policy and guidance acknowledge the vital role that children's nurses have in providing palliative care. Two primary studies (Slocum-Gori et al., 2013; Zambrano et al., 2014) highlighted the shared experiences between health professional groups that may provide palliative care and the impact that providing this level of care may have on them. Common findings included the potential for burnout, compassion fatigue and compassion satisfaction, and strategies used to manage these. There is still, however, a need for further research to improve the quality of palliative care (Dombrecht et al., 2023).

## SPECIFIC CHALLENGES

Caring for children with palliative care needs, especially at end of life, exposes professionals to emotionally demanding clinical experiences. Papadatou (2001) identified the emotional involvement needed in supporting such families, with the risk of stress, burnout and emotional exhaustion/compassion fatigue. Bergstrasser et al. (2017) also identified these experiences as challenging and stressful. Children's palliative care nursing can often lead to high levels of burnout, compassion fatigue and psychological distress. Emotional distress is an afflicting experience when providing intensive family-centred care. This distress may be a result of many factors, including giving care that it is not in the best interest of the child (Brandon et al., 2014) such as the fictitious example of Jack, discussed above. Furthermore, the quality of the child's death will influence the level of distress that the nurse may experience (Brazil et al., 2010).

A deeper understanding of personal and professional growth could help healthcare organisations implement innovative approaches that would counterbalance compassion fatigue and enhance healthcare providers' well-being (Beaune et al., 2018). Symptom management is a key area linked to stress experienced by the

---

**LEARNING ACTIVITY**

Ali (pseudonym) is a 6-year-old child with high-risk neuroblastoma stage 4 (wide spread cancer) who is receiving end-of-life care at home. He is suffering with increased pain and has shown signs of agitation over the last day. Ali is taking oral morphine for break-through pain relief and an anti-emetic medication. He is spending most of his time in bed, is restless and finding it difficult to settle. His pain has increased, he is quiet and withdrawn and no longer tolerating his oral medications. Ali's symptom management is discussed with the oncology team and the plan is to convert his medications to the subcutaneous route and start a syringe driver to deliver the medication over a 24-hour period. As the community nurse caring for Ali, this is your first time supporting a child for end-of-life care at home and you are feeling anxious and overwhelmed.

Reflect upon the following points:

- Would you feel stressed managing the medication change?
- What might help minimise or alleviate this stress, for example, training?
- What support or self-care strategies could you consider to help you if faced with this situation?

nursing workforce caring for children at the end-of-life stage (Neilson et al., 2013). This may be due to a lack of confidence, knowledge of symptom control, management of the syringe driver and administration of medications that are not frequently used (Davies et al., 2008).

## EMOTIONAL INTELLIGENCE

According to Heffernan et al. (2010), self-care is a vital part of nursing practice, which helps nurses to care for patients with emotional intelligence, compassion and resilience. Emotional intelligence is generally described as the ability to manage one's own and others' emotions to guide thoughts and actions (Mayer et al., 2008). The UK Nursing and Midwifery Council Standards of Proficiency for Registered Nurses (NMC, 2018b) states: "the registered nurse will be able to demonstrate resilience and emotional intelligence". In order to respond to the impact and demands of professional nursing practice, nurses must be resilient individuals who are able to manage their own personal health and well-being. Compassion and care are listed as being among the six fundamental values of nursing (Department of Health, 2012).

It is natural for palliative care nurses to experience emotional reactions when a child dies, given the deeply empathetic nature of their work. While it is important to maintain professionalism and provide support to the child's family during such difficult times, it is also human to feel emotions such as sadness, grief, and empathy. However, we should be mindful to manage our emotions in a way that does not overwhelm or burden the child's family. In a study by Kaplan (2000), nurses who cared for terminally ill children experienced a form of "emotional tension" in struggling to balance the intense emotional feelings of loss, with their desire to maintain their professionalism in remaining competent caregivers. When children die, nurses can feel a sense of sorrow and experience emotional stress arising from feeling powerless, the loss of the patient and the inability to alleviate the pain of bereavement. This is generally unrecognised by society.

Showing appropriate emotions can enhance the nurse-patient/family relationship, for example, demonstrating compassion and empathy while allowing the professional to grieve for their loss. Costello and Trinder-Brooke (2000) found that nurses understood and valued sharing emotions with parents even in light of the professional assumption that to do so is unprofessional. Wakefield (2000) identified difficulty with emotional responses and suggests that nurses who grieve and express their emotions are better able to manage their distress. The capacity to feel grief and to identify with the misfortune of others is the basis of our humanity. Without the recognition of suffering, there can be no compassion for children and families (Rushton and Ballard, 2004). The ability to recognise our own suffering empowers us to find ways to preserve our professional integrity. If we do not acknowledge our feelings and address feelings of grief, then we risk affecting our own mental health, which in turn will inevitably compromise our capacity for compassion (Hindmarch, 2009). Ultimately, striking a balance between empathetic expression and professional conduct is key when dealing with the death of a child.

## THE MULTI-DISCIPLINARY TEAM AND THE INTERACTION WITH SPECIALIST CARE

Members of the multi-disciplinary team who provide palliative care for children of all ages and their families in a range of settings do report positive experiences (McCloskey and Taggart, 2010; Reid, 2013a; 2013b). These experiences include developing rewarding relationships and a reduction in the child's suffering (Plante and Cyr, 2011). The work of Feudtner et al. (2007) showed the correlation between increased palliative care education and personal comfort in providing palliative care. Nurses exposed to the field of children's palliative care for many years, who had received training and education, reported increased competence and confidence in working with dying children and their families (Feudtner et al., 2007).

Child death remains a taboo subject, a rarity, making it difficult to broach, let alone discuss, openly, which can feel isolating in itself, for both professionals and families. This isolation can also be amplified by location, for example, when providing end-of-life care to children in their own homes, community children's nurses often work alone. It can be more difficult to access the peer support that might be available if working within the hospital or hospice environment, where nurses may share the experience of supporting a child at end-of-life stage. As healthcare professionals immersed in this world, we need a way to express our own emotional distress and overcome isolation by sharing with others who understand (Macpherson, 2008). These are unique experiences and talking to others similarly affected, sharing our experiences, give meaning and comfort and help us to manage professional grief (McCloskey and Taggart, 2010). This can help reduce the impact of emotional issues, resulting from our professional roles, on our personal lives (Keene et al., 2010). There are a number of ways in which we can achieve this both informally and formally, including peer support and clinical supervision.

"All in a day's work" (Figure 5.3) was captured during a home visit. A complex symptom assessment and conversations with a patient around her fears of dying were undertaken in party hats, in between games of Uno and Poo bingo. Moments of humour can help build resilience for the difficult conversations that often follow.

According to Bailey (2021), avoiding a difficult conversation is not an option for the nurse, therefore, it is important to engage in self-care steps. An integral part of our role as children's nurses is the necessity to look after ourselves, and our own needs. Children and families benefit from nursing care that is rooted in empathy for their situation. Providing individualised empathic care is immensely rewarding but can also be highly stressful. As professionals, we have to acknowledge the emotional component of our work and the associated intensity of stress that can accompany this. We need to identify ways in which we cope with this level of stress, ensuring we utilise appropriate and effective mechanisms, in order to be able to maintain and

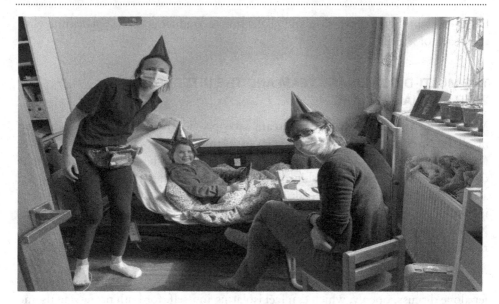

**FIGURE 5.3** All in a day's work for two children's palliative care clinical nurse specialists

Source: Reproduced with kind parental permission.

deliver compassionate care, the essence of palliative care (Larkin, 2015). Not managing our own stress can have a profoundly negative impact on the families we support, as roles can reverse, and families may find themselves supporting the healthcare professional (Black, 2011).

Costello and Trinder-Brook (2000) and Papadatou (2001) found peer support to be the most used type of support used by nurses. Four levels of support were identified by Papadatou (2001): (1) informational; (2) clinical/practical; (3) emotional; and (4) meaning making. The first two enabled nurses to provide best care, the latter two involved sharing experiences and feelings with peers. Understandably, finding meaning was attributed to being able to contribute to a "good death" (see Box 5.1).

---

**BOX 5.1 BEGUM FAMILY CARE**

The following fictitious case study (using pseudonyms) sets out an example of how a Community Children's Nurse, along with the children's hospice and palliative nurse specialist, provided nursing care, including end-of-life, emotional and informational support to a family. Providing high-quality care requires resilience and sustained compassion. This case study details how to manage self-care and support of others in these situations.

A children's community nursing team alongside a palliative care nurse specialist, hospice team and wider multi-disciplinary team provided care to the Begum family for over 12 years. The Begum family consisted of a single mother, Bhoomi, and her three children. All three children were known to healthcare services due to their complex medical needs, as all suffered with an undiagnosed degenerative condition.

The children had a joint funded package of care, to provide the mother with carer support to meet the children's individual care needs. The eldest child (Aaheli) received support until the age of 10 years, when she deteriorated over a period of time. End-of-life care was delivered in the family home. Aaheli died peacefully with her family around her, with the support of the specialist nurse and hospice teams. At the time her mother refused specialist counselling support but was informally supported through home visits and phone calls from the palliative care specialist nurse. Often during these conversations, they would talk about Aaheli and discuss memories. These conversations offered the mother a safe space to talk and discuss how she was feeling and coping with her grief. The team around Aaheli recognised that the wishes of the family in the Advance Care Plan had been achieved. This enabled them to view the death of Aaheli in a positive manner.

Less than two years later, the middle child (Vikat) suffered with an acute illness which led to a sudden decline. Vikat needed in-patient admission to paediatric intensive care, but died before transfer to the family home could be arranged, as detailed in his Advance Care Plan. Bhoomi was present at his time of death, but it was not the peaceful death that she had envisaged. Overall, the team were disappointed that they had not been able to deliver gold standard care as they previously had delivered to Aaheli.

The team compared the deaths of Aaheli and Vikat and felt that they failed in their duty of care. They voiced their disappointment at not achieving the family's preferred place of care at death for Vikat. Perceiving that their involvement 'had been reduced' and that they had provided limited support to the family while they were in intensive care, they questioned how they would continue to provide care to the third sibling (Shayna), knowing that she would also require end-of-life care in the future. The team feared for Bhoomi's future health and well-being following her loss; the deaths of her children, loss of identity as a mother, loss of financial support, and loss of the therapeutic relationship she had had with the team of healthcare professionals over many years.

Bhoomi talked about her suffering being indescribable, and questioned how she would continue to live after the death of her children and the loss of everyone who supported her throughout the difficult journey. Recognising the uniqueness of this family, and how Bhoomi may grieve differently, was essential in order to address her individual needs. The team could see the impact of her children's deaths on Bhoomi, and the anticipatory grief for her remaining child, and this visible and verbalised impact prompted the team to revisit the possibility of a counselling referral with Bhoomi.

The nurses involved had to balance their professional boundaries over a significant period of time, starting with the referral into the service when Aaheli was acknowledged to have a life-limiting illness and required nursing support, which then extended into bereavement support. The nurses knew this support would inevitably have to come to an end at some point and Bhoomi would need to be signposted to other services for ongoing support.

When children's nurses and nursing students are caring for a child and/or young person (CYP) at the end of life, this opportunity is a privilege, but also a responsibility. The nurse needs to ensure the very best individualised and meaningful care is provided to the child and family, as there are no second chances to get it right. Therefore, focus must be on prioritising and adapting to individual needs and working in partnership with appropriate and timely services (NMC, 2018a).

## SELF-CARE STRATEGIES

There are numerous strategies for building resilience, including improving work-life balance by undertaking regular clinical supervision and critically reflecting on practice experiences.

### Debriefing/group supervision

According to Keene et al. (2010), professional distress can relate to sharing long-term relationships with the child and family alongside witnessing parental pain following the death of their child. Strategies such as team debriefing and clinical supervision provide opportunities for healthcare professionals to reflect upon the care given in a safe environment without fear of judgement, particularly if there are feelings of failure or inadequacy to address. Debriefing provides a supportive environment in which staff can reflect on events, providing opportunities to identify what went well, what did not, and ways in which practice may need to be changed, in order to address those issues in the future. Nurses who used reflective practice are more able to make sense of their feelings, thereby helping them to cope with difficult emotions and experiences (Wakefield, 2000).

### Clinical supervision

Overall, clinical supervision provides a more formal line of support. It is supportive (enabling you to monitor your own well-being, a safety net for identifying and exploring feelings and reactions, both positive and negative) and educational (integrating theory and practice, identifying learning, developing further insight). Self-management can help to balance and maintain professional boundaries (Hindmarch, 2009).

### Schwartz Rounds

Schwartz Rounds are designed to provide healthcare professionals with a non-judgemental space to discuss and reflect on personal emotions, experiences and work challenges. In palliative care settings, Schwartz Rounds can be particularly valuable for staff members to process the emotional impact of caring for patients and families facing end-of-life situations. These sessions offer opportunities for all members of the multi-disciplinary team to share their perspectives, learn from one another, and develop strategies for coping with the complex emotions associated with providing palliative care (Robert et al., 2017). Schwartz Rounds aim to promote empathy, resilience and well-being among healthcare professionals, fostering a culture of compassion and collaboration, which can enhance the quality of care provided to patients and families (Maben et al., 2018). For further information, access: www.Pointofcarefoundation.org.uk. Taylor et al. (2018) carried out a review of studies in relation to Schwartz Rounds. Despite the weak evidence base for Schwartz Rounds and other interventions, the authors do acknowledge that, given the high rates of work-related stress, it is not acceptable for employers not to act.

By practising self-care, healthcare professionals can sustain their energy, compassion and empathy, enabling delivery of high-quality compassionate care to the children and families within their care, while preserving their own well-being and job satisfaction (McConnell et al., 2016). Prioritising self-care can sustain health and well-being, prevent burnout, and allow the continuation of providing compassionate, fundamental and effective care. Therefore, creating a self-care plan may be a useful tool (Box 5.2).

---

**BOX 5.2 CREATING A SELF-CARE PLAN: A USEFUL TOOL**

1.  Physical self-care

    - *Regular exercise*: engage in physical activities, even if it is just a short walk or stretching exercises. Exercise helps in reducing stress and improving overall well-being.
    - *Practise stress-reduction*: techniques such as mindfulness, meditation, deep breathing exercises, or yoga can help to manage work-related stress.
    - *Healthy diet*: ensure you are eating nutritious meals. Avoid excessive caffeine and sugar, as they can affect your energy levels. Stay hydrated.
    - *Adequate rest*: try and ensure you get enough sleep and rest to recharge your energy levels.
    - *Health check-ups*: schedule regular health check-up/screenings to monitor your own health.

2.  Emotional self-care

    - *Professional counselling*: do not hesitate to seek counselling if you find it challenging to cope with the emotional burden of your work. Consider talking to a therapist or counsellor who specialises in trauma and healthcare-related stress.
    - *Mindfulness and relaxation*: practise mindfulness, meditation or yoga to manage stress and stay emotionally grounded.
    - *Creative outlets*: engage in creative activities like painting, writing or music to express your emotions.
    - *Journaling*: write about your experiences, thoughts and emotions in a journal. It can be a therapeutic way to process your feelings.
    - *Humour*: this can be a powerful coping mechanism. Finding moments of humour, even in challenging and sad situations, can provide relief.

3.  Social self-care

    - *Maintain personal relationships*: nurture your relationships with family and friends who understand the challenges you face. Make time for them.
    - *Socialise*: spend time with people who uplift you. This can be colleagues, friends, or people outside of the healthcare profession.

4. Professional self-care

- *Self-reflection*: take time to reflect on experiences, emotions, and reactions to work situations to gain insight and promote self-awareness.
- *Supervision:* regular clinical supervision with suitable trained staff, such as a clinical psychologist, and timely multi-disciplinary structured debriefing sessions with colleagues, can provide an outlet for discussing challenging cases and emotions. These can help to bring closure, particularly after the death of a child.
- *Debriefing*: always attend debriefs following the death of a child.
- *Networking and peer support groups*: connect with other professionals in your field. These provide a safe space for sharing experiences, and coping strategies. They can help put things in perspective and can be incredibly validating and helpful.
- *Education*: stay updated with the latest developments in palliative care. Attend workshops and conferences, if available. Engage in professional development opportunities to enhance knowledge and skills, which can increase confidence and job satisfaction.
- *Training*: consider additional training in areas such as communication skills, stress management or conflict resolution.
- *Delegate/share responsibilities*: ask for help, and share complex or difficult patients/ families, to help prevent feeling overwhelmed and avoid burnout.
- *Boundaries*: set and maintain appropriate professional boundaries with children and families – seek support from more experienced colleagues if you need help with this.
- *Break times*: ensure you take regular breaks during your shifts. Short breaks can significantly improve your resilience throughout the day.
- *Teamwork*: remember the importance of working as a team. Open communication within teams fosters a supportive working environment.
- *Celebrate success*: acknowledge your achievements and milestones. Focus on the positive aspects of your work. Celebrate the positive impact you make on the lives of the children and families you care for.
- *Work-life balance*: maintain a healthy balance between your work life and your personal life. Understand your limits at work and do not be afraid to say no. It is okay to decline additional responsibilities if you feel overwhelmed. Overworking can lead to burnout.
- *Separate work from home life*: Develop a routine to mentally transition from work to home. This could involve a specific activity or ritual that signifies the end of your workday.

5. Spiritual self-care

- *Reflection and gratitude*: find a quiet place for self-reflection.
- *Gratitude*: practise this by focusing on positive aspects of your work and life. Keep a gratitude diary.
- *Religious or spiritual practices*: engage in activities that align with your beliefs, whether it is prayer, meditation, attending religious services, or simply spending time in nature.

6.  Personal self-care

    *   *Hobbies and interests*: engage in creative activities and interests outside of work, that bring joy and fulfilment into your life, whether it's gardening, reading, cooking, music, sports, or spending time with loved ones.
    *   *Holidays and time off*: plan regular vacations and take your allotted time off. Use this time to relax and rejuvenate.
    *   *Self-compassion*: be kind and compassionate to yourself. Acknowledge that it is okay to feel a range of emotions and seek support when needed. Use positive affirmations to reinforce your self-worth and capabilities.

Finally, it can be helpful to perform a going home checklist at the end of your day, in which you check in with yourself, acknowledge any difficulties and recognise what has gone well. An example might look like the going home checklist in Box 5.3.

---

**BOX 5.3 GOING HOME CHECKLIST**

✓ Take a moment to think about today.
✓ Acknowledge *one* thing that was difficult during your shift: let it go.
✓ Be proud of the care you gave today.
✓ Consider *three* things that went well.
✓ Check on your colleagues before you leave: are they OK?
✓ Are you OK? Your senior team and colleagues are there to listen and support you. Talk to them.
✓ Now switch your attention to home. *Rest and recharge!*

---

Remember, building resilience is a gradual process. It involves self-reflection, self-compassion, self-care and a willingness to seek help when needed. Regularly assess your self-care strategies and adjust them according to your needs. Also regularly assess how you are feeling. If you notice signs of burnout, compassion fatigue, or emotional exhaustion, do not hesitate to seek professional help. Your well-being is crucial not just for you, but also for the special children and families you support.

## SUMMARY

Supporting a family at the end of a child's life can be very stressful and challenging for those closely involved. It is important that the palliative care team members reflect upon their own self-care, to prevent compassion fatigue and occupational burnout (Gómez-Urquiza et al., 2020).

Repeated exposure to emotional labour and grief highlights the importance of managing professional boundaries and integrity with families in long-term professional relationships (NMC, 2018a; RCN, 2021). The transition, when palliative care ends, also needs to be sensitive and appropriately managed for both nursing staff and families. Ensuring that families have clear information about available support, how long this will continue for/when it will eventually end, allows nurses to set boundaries which are crucial to the well-being of all involved (Buder and Fringer, 2016). Navigating these endings carefully with healthcare staff is important, as they may also be grieving and feel the loss professionally, particularly if they have supported the family for a long time.

In summary, self-care refers to the proactive and deliberate actions taken to maintain and enhance physical, mental and emotional well-being. It involves engaging in practices and activities that help manage stress, prevent burnout and compassion fatigue, and promote overall health and resilience. Self-care for children's palliative care nurses and nursing students is crucial for maintaining emotional resilience and providing the highest quality of patient care. This includes setting boundaries between work and personal life and seeking support from colleagues and supervisors. Practising stress management techniques, such as mindfulness or relaxation exercises, engaging in regular physical activity, maintaining hobbies and interests outside of work, attending counselling or therapy if needed and recognising when to take breaks or time off to recharge.

## KEY POINTS

- Palliative care nursing teams need access to debrief and regular clinical supervision across the workplace to help them cope with patient death and family grief.
- The palliative nursing community should identify and invest in effective strategies to help manage work-related stress associated with children's palliative care, such as promoting a healthy work life balance, regular exercise and access to counselling.
- Debriefing provides a supportive environment in which staff can reflect on events – establishing emotional support and helping to manage grief.

## Points for reflection

- Consider which elements of Equality, Diversity and Inclusion need addressing in the care of children and young people with palliative care needs.
- Critically appraise how you manage professional boundaries within your practice.
- Critically reflect upon the cultures within your nursing team and consider any improvements to enhance self-care practice for staff.
- Acknowledge the need for support and self-care within the work environment.
- Critically reflect on your own experiences of self-care and sustaining compassion. What strategies might you find most helpful?

## USEFUL LINKS AND RESOURCES

- The Professional Quality of Life Scale (The Centre for Victims of Torture, 2021) can be useful for assessing the impact of caring. The tool measures compassion fatigue, work satisfaction and burnout in helping professionals. The quality is what one feels in relation to one's work as a carer. Both the positive and negative aspects of a job influence one's professional quality of life. The overall tool is particularly useful for professionals to self-monitor their satisfaction and as a prompt for self-care. In addition, service managers seeking to facilitate staff well-being can use the scale to track professional quality of life over time to help inform workload and support decision-making. This tool measures three aspects of professional quality of life:
  - Compassion satisfaction (pleasure you derive from being able to do your work well).
  - Burnout (exhaustion, frustration, anger and depression related to work).
  - Secondary traumatic stress (feeling fear in relation to work-related primary or secondary trauma).
- Home Creative Tool: https://www.creativetoolkit.online/is an evidence-based well-being intervention to combat burnout in healthcare workers. The website provides a digital version of the Creative Toolkit, a suite of resources that employ creativity to support mental health and well-being.
- Self-care matters: https://palliativecare.org.au/resources/self-care-matters is a Palliative Care Australia resource aimed at supporting you, whatever your role in palliative care, to prevent burnout and build resilience. It includes a range of planning tools to help prioritise and practise self-care.
- Resources for improving resilience and well-being can be found at https://www.salt-box.co.uk/resources.
- The Royal College of Nursing, "Stress and You: A Guide for Nursing Staff" can be accessed at: https://www.rcn.org.uk/-/media/Royal-College-Of-Nursing/Documents/Publications/2015/September/004967.pdf.
- Professional quality of life self-care tools can be found at https://proqol.org/self-care-tools-1.
- Useful resources for how to be healthy at work and how to manage stress, such as using a mind wellness action plan for the workplace, can be found at www.mind.org.uk.
- WHO 5 Well-being Index, available at: https://www.psykiatri-regionh.dk/who-5/Documents/WHO-5%20questionaire%20-%20English.pdf.
- See also Topp et al. (2015).

## REFERENCES

Bailey, S. (2021). Seven steps for having difficult conversations. *American Nurse Journal*, 16(4), 14–17.

Beaune, L., Muskat, B., Anthony, S. J. (2018). The emergence of personal growth amongst healthcare professionals who care for dying children. *Palliative & Supportive Care, 16*(3). 298–307. https://doi.org/10.1017/S1478951517000396

Bergstrasser, E., Cignacco, E., Luck, P. (2017). Health care professionals experiences and needs when delivering end-of-life care to children: A qualitative study. *Palliative Care: Research and Treatment, 10*, 1–10. https://doi.org/10.1177/1178224217724770

Black, R. (2011). *Living with dying children: The suffering of parents*. University of Kent.

Brandon, D., Ryan, D., Sloane, R., Docherty, S. L. (2014). Impact of a pediatric quality of life program on providers' moral distress. *MCN: The American Journal of Maternal/Child Nursing, 39*(3), 189–197. https://doi.org/10.1097/NMC.0000000000000025

Brazil, K., Kassalainen, S., Ploeg, J., Marshall, D. (2010). Moral distress experienced by health care professionals who provide home-based palliative care. *Social Science & Medicine, 71*(9), 1687–1691. https://doi.org/10.1016/j.socscimed.2010.07.032

Brimble, M. J., Anstey, S., Davies, J. (2019). Long-term nurse–parent relationships in paediatric palliative care: A narrative literature review. *International Journal of Palliative Nursing, 25*(11), 542–550. https://doi.org/10.12968/ijpn.2019.25.11.542

Brown, E., Muckaden, M., Mndende, N. (2021). Culture, spirituality, religion and ritual. In R. Hain, A. Goldman (eds), *Oxford textbook of palliative care for children* (3rd edn; pp. 44–58). Oxford University Press.

Buder, R., Fringer, A. (2016). Paediatric palliative nursing: The tension between closeness and professional distance. *European Journal of Palliative Care, 23*(6), 278–280.

Cacciatore, J., Thieleman, K., Lieber, A. S., Blood, C., Goldman, R. (2019). The long road to farewell: The needs of families with dying children. *OMEGA: Journal of Death and Dying, 78*(4), 404–420. https://doi.org/10.1177/0030222817697418

Carter, B., Cummings, J., Cooper, L. (2007). An exploration of best practice in multi-agency working and the experiences of families of children with complex health needs. What works well and what needs to be done to improve practice for the future? *Journal of Clinical Nursing, 16*(3), 527–539. https://doi.org/10.1111/j.1365-2702.2006.01554.x

Costello, J., Trinder-Brooke, A. (2000). Children's nurses' experiences of caring for dying children in hospital. *Paediatric Nursing, 12*(6), 28–32. http://doi.org/10.7748/paed2000.07.12.6.28.c674.

Davies, B., Sehring, S., Partridge, C., Cooper, B., Hughes, A., Philp, J., Amidi-Nouri, A., Kramer, R. (2008). Barriers to palliative care for children: Perceptions of paediatric health care providers. *Paediatrics, 121*(2), 282–288. https://doi.org/10.1542/peds.2006-3153

Delgado, C., Upton, D., Ranse, K., Furness, T., Foster, K. (2017). Nurses' resilience and the emotional labour of nursing work: An integrative review of empirical literature. *International Journal of Nursing Studies, 70*, 71–88. https://doi.org/10.1016/j.ijnurstu.2017.02.008

Department of Health. (2012). Compassion in Practice: Nursing, Midwifery and Care Staff – Our vision and strategy. Available at: https://www.england.nhs.uk/wp-content/uploads/2012/12/compassion-in-practice.pdf (accessed 7 June 2024).

Dombrecht, L., Lacerda, A., Wolfe, J., Snaman, J. (2023). A call to improve paediatric palliative care quality through research. *BMC Palliative Care, 22*(1), 141. https://doi.org/10.1186/s12904-023-01262-w

Epstein, R. M., Krasner, M. S. (2013). Physician resilience: What it means, why it matters, and how to promote it. *Academic Medicine, 88*(3), 301–303. https://doi.org/10.1097/ACM.0b013e318280cff0

Equality Act. (2010). c.1. Available at: www.gov.uk/guidance/equality-act-2010-guidance

Erikson, A., Davies, B. (2017). Maintaining integrity: How nurses navigate boundaries in pediatric palliative care. *Journal of Pediatric Nursing, 35*, 42–49. https://doi.org/10.1016/j.pedn.2017.02.031

Feudtner, C., Santucci, G., Feinstein, J. A., Snyder, C. R., Rourke, M. T., Kang, T. I. (2007). Hopeful thinking and level of comfort regarding providing pediatric palliative care: A survey of hospital nurses. *Pediatrics, 119*(1), e186–e192. https://doi.org/10.1542/peds.2006-1048

Gómez-Urquiza, J. L., Albendín-García, L., Velando-Soriano, A., Ortega-Campos, E., Ramírez-Baena, L., Membrive-Jiménez, M. J., Suleiman-Martos, N. (2020). Burnout in palliative care nurses, prevalence and risk factors: A systematic review with meta-analysis. *International Journal of Environmental Research and Public Health, 17*(20), 7672. https://doi.org/10.3390/ijerph17207672

Goodrich. J., Harrison, T., Cornwell, J., Richardson, H. (2015). Resilience: A framework supporting hospice staff to flourish in stressful times. Available at: https://hospiceuk-files-prod.s3.eu-west-2.amazonaws.com/s3fs-public/2022-04/Resilience%20-%20A%20framework%20supporting%20hospice%20staff%20to%20flourish%20in%20stressful%20times.pdf (accessed 30 May 2024).

Grauerholz, K., Fredenburg, M., Jones, P., Jenkins, K. (2020) Fostering vicarious resilience for perinatal palliative care professionals. *Frontiers in Pediatrics, 8*, 1–15. https://doi.org/10.3389/fped.2020.572933

Heffernan, M., Quinn Griffin, M. T., McNulty, S. R., Fitzpatrick, J. J. (2010). Self-compassion and emotional intelligence in nurses. *International Journal of Nursing Practice, 16*(4), 366–373. https://doi.org/10.1111/j.1440-172X.2010.01853.x

Hindmarch, C. (2009). *On the death of a child* (3rd edn). Routledge.

Hughes, U., McNeilly, P. (2024) Bereavement support. In S. Clarke, D. Corkin (co-eds), *Care planning in children and young people's nursing* (2nd edn; pp. 323–329). Wiley Blackwell.

Kaplan, L. J. (2000). Toward a model of caregiver grief: Nurses' experiences of treating dying children. *OMEGA: Journal of Death and Dying, 41*(3), 187–206. https://doi.org/10.2190/NGG6-YPAH-40AB-CNX0

Keene, E. A., Hutton, N., Hall, B., Rushton, C. (2010). Bereavement debriefing sessions: An intervention to support health care professionals in managing their grief after the death of a patient. *Pediatric Nursing, 36*(4), 185–190. Available at: https://patchsa.org/wp-content/uploads/2019/10/Bereavement-Debriefing-Sessions-Research-Keene-2012.pdf (accessed 7 June 2024).

Knapp, C., Woodworth, L., Wright, M., Downing, J., Drake, R., Fowler-Kerry, S., Hain, R., Marston, J. (2011). Pediatric palliative care provision around the world: A systematic review. *Pediatric Blood & Cancer, 57*(3), 361–368. https://doi.org/10.1002/pbc.23100

Larkin, P. J. (2015). Compassion: A conceptual reading for palliative and end-of-life care. In P.J. Larkin, *Compassion: The essence of palliative and end-of-life care* (pp. 1–10). Oxford University Press.

Maben, J., Taylor, C., Dawson, J., Leamy, M., McCarthy, I., Reynolds, E., Ross, S., Shuldham, C., Bennett, L., Foot, C. (2018). A realist informed mixed-methods evaluation of Schwartz Center Rounds® in England. *Health Services and Delivery Research, 6*(37). https://doi.org/10.3310/hsdr06370

Macpherson, C. F. (2008). Peer-supported storytelling for grieving pediatric oncology nurses. *Journal of Pediatric Oncology Nursing, 25*(3), 148–163. https://doi.org/10.1177/1043454208317236

Mayer, J. D., Salovey, P., Caruso, D. R. (2008). Emotional intelligence: New ability or eclectic traits? *American Psychologist, 63*(6), 503. https://doi.org/10.1037/0003-066X.63.6.503

McCloskey, S., Taggart, L. (2010). How much compassion have I left? An exploration of occupational stress among children's palliative care nurses. *International Journal of Palliative Nursing, 16*(5), 233–240. https://doi.org/10.12968/ijpn.2010.16.5.48144

McConnell, T., Scott, D., Porter, S. (2016). Healthcare staff's experience in providing end-of-life care to children: A mixed-method review. *Palliative Medicine, 30*(10), 905–919. https://doi.org/10.1177/0269216316647611

Neilson, S. J., Kai, J., McArthur, C., Greenfield, S. (2013). Using social worlds theory to explore influences on community nurses' experiences of providing out of hours paediatric palliative care. *Journal of Research in Nursing, 18*(5), 443–456. https://doi.org/10.1177/1744987113491759

NMC (Nursing and Midwifery Council). (2018a). *The Code: Professional standards of practice and behaviour for nurses, midwives and nursing associates.* Available at: https://www.nmc.org.uk/standards/code/ (accessed 30 May 2024).

NMC (Nursing and Midwifery Council). (2018b). *Standards of proficiency for registered nurses.* Available at: https://www.nmc.org.uk/standards/standards-for-nurses/standards-of-proficiency-for-registered-nurses/ (accessed 30 May 2024).

Papadatou, D. (2001). The grieving healthcare provider: Variables affecting the professional response to a child's death. *Bereavement Care, 20*(2), 26–29. https://doi.org/10.1080/02682620108657520

Plante, J., Cyr, C. (2011). Health care professionals' grief after the death of a child. *Paediatrics & Child Health, 16*(4), 213–216. https://doi.org/10.1093/pch/16.4.213

RCN (Royal College of Nursing). (2021). Nursing workforce standards. Available at: https://www.rcn.org.uk/Professional-Development/publications/rcn-workforce-standards-uk-pub-009681 (accessed 30 May 2024).

RCN (Royal College of Nursing). (2016) Healthy workplace, healthy you. Available at: https://www.rcn.org.uk/-/media/royal-college-of-nursing/documents/publications/2016/january/005450.pdf (accessed 30 May 2024).

Reid, F. C. (2013a). Lived experiences of adult community nurses delivering palliative care to children and young people in rural areas. *International Journal of Palliative Nursing, 19*(11), 541–547. https://doi.org/10.12968/ijpn.2013.19.11.541

Reid, F. C. (2013b). Grief and the experiences of nurses providing palliative care to children and young people at home. *Nursing Children and Young People, 25*(9), 31–36. https://doi.org/10.7748/ncyp2013.11.25.9.31.e366

Robert, G., Philippou, J., Leamy, M., Reynolds, E., Ross, S., Bennett, L., Taylor, C., Shuldham, C., Maben, J. (2017). Exploring the adoption of Schwartz Center Rounds as an organisational innovation to improve staff well-being in England, 2009–2015. *BMJ Open, 7*(1), e014326. https://doi.org/10.1136/bmjopen-2016-014326

Rushton, C. H., Ballard, M. K. (2004). The other side of caring: Caregiver suffering. In B. S. Carter, M. Leveton, S. F. Friebert (eds), *Palliative care for infants, children and adolescents* (pp. 220–243). Johns Hopkins University Press.

Samuelson, S., Willén, C., Bratt, E. L. (2015). New kid on the block? Community nurses' experiences of caring for sick children at home. *Journal of Clinical Nursing, 24*(17–18), 2448–2457. https://doi.org/10.1111/jocn.2015.24.issue-17pt18

Slocum-Gori, S., Hemsworth, D., Chan, W. W., Carson, A.,Kazanjian, A. (2013). Understanding compassion satisfaction, compassion fatigue and burnout: A survey of the hospice palliative care workforce. *Palliative Medicine, 27*(2), 172–178. https://doi.org/10.1177/0269216311431311

Southall, S., Taske, N., Power, E., Desai, M., Baillie, N. (2021). Spotlight on COVID-19 rapid guidance: NICE's experience of producing rapid guidelines during the pandemic. *Journal of Public Health, 43*(1), e103–e106. https://doi.org/10.1093/pubmed/fdaa184

Taylor, C., Xyrichis, A., Leamy, M. C., Reynolds, E., Maben, J. (2018). Can Schwartz Center Rounds support healthcare staff with emotional challenges at work, and how do they compare with other interventions aimed at providing similar support? A systematic review and scoping reviews. *BMJ Open, 8*(10), e024254. https://doi.org/10.1136/bmjopen-2018-024254

The Centre for Victims of Torture. (2021). Professional Quality of Life Measure (ProQOL 5.0). Available at: https://proqol.org/proqol-measure (accessed 30 May 2024).

Topp, C. W., Østergaard, S. D., Søndergaard, S., Bech, P. (2015). The WHO-5 Well-Being Index: A systematic review of the literature. *Psychotherapy and Psychosomatics, 84,* 167–176. https://doi.org/10.1159/000376585

Wakefield, A. (2000). Nurses' responses to death and dying: A need for relentless self-care. *International Journal of Palliative Nursing, 6*(5), 245–251. https://doi.org/10.12968/ijpn.2000.6.5.8926

Widdas, D., McNamara, K., Edwards, F. (2013). A core care pathway for children with life-limiting and life-threatening conditions. Available at: http://www.togetherforshortlives.org.uk/assets/0000/4121/TfSL_A_Core_Care_Pathway__ONLINE_.pdf (accessed 30 May 2024).

Zambrano, S. C., Chur-Hansen, A., Crawford, G. B. (2014). The experiences, coping mechanisms, and impact of death and dying on palliative medicine specialists. *Palliative & Supportive Care, 12*(4), 309–316.

# CHAPTER 6

# Play, education and children and carers coping, living with palliative care needs

......................................................

*Maraliza de Haan, Angela Rackstraw and Duncan Randall*

## INTRODUCTION

Play is often associated with fun and is something children especially love to do every day. Play may also be a social activity and provide occupation, but it remains joyous.

Play is frequently used by professionals in the field of psychology and social work, but using play in the field of medical care is perhaps not as common. The value of play is sometimes questioned, and it can be perceived by health professionals as an additional, nice, added extra which is time-consuming and which they may feel they are not skilled in providing. However, for children, play can help them to feel more in control of their circumstances, it can be a distraction during painful medical procedures, or a tool for communicating with others and building trustful relationships.

Play can also be used as a therapeutic intervention to help children to resolve or adapt to challenges in their lives. However, here we are thinking about play as a normative experience rather than as play therapy, thinking more of play as part of the social environment of children and their childhoods.

Childhood, irrespective of whether it is lived with palliative care needs or not, is both being and becoming. Children live a childhood; a period which ends with the transition into adulthood and one which is constructed in cultural, historical and political ways (James et al., 1998; Corsaro, 2012). While childhoods vary in and between communities within cultures and between cultural alignments, they also typically have comparable features, such as the need to play and learn.

Children are children – they play and learn. The question we seek to answer, or at least explore in more depth in this chapter is, how do we as nurses help and support children to be children, who will one day hopefully grow into adults? Of course, some of the children we see with palliative care needs will not become adults.

DOI: 10.4324/9781003384861-9

However, they are still children, living a childhood, which means they are both being a child and enacting becoming an adult. So, irrespective of prognosis, we need to understand how nurses and nursing can help, or hinder, children in both being children and in their becoming young people.

This process of a childhood, as alluded to above, occurs in social and cultural relationships, be that with parents, grandparents, siblings or other carers. Much of nursing is reliant upon the work, practices and understandings of informal carers – those who accept the responsibility for caring for children are living lives in which the child's palliative care needs are a part. So, understanding how nurses and nursing can facilitate the coping mechanisms of carers is vital to providing safe and effective care for both children and their carers.

The beauty and complexity of childhood are depicted in children playing, learning and living in their family. Simplistic naturalism can, however, blind us as nurses to the importance of play and learning – "it is just children doing what they do". But we know that people, lives and cultures are formed through children's play.

---

**LEARNING OBJECTIVES**

The reader will be able to do the following:

1. Identify coping strategies and practices for children and their carers who are living with palliative care needs.
2. Explore creatively, using play in daily nursing activities and using play as a tool in approaching children and reaching care objectives in children's palliative care.
3. Discuss nurses' and nursing's contribution to the design, delivery and evaluation of play for children living with palliative care needs.
4. Critically discuss the intersections of education and healthcare in children's palliative care, and the contribution of nursing and nurses in facilitating children living with palliative care needs to participate in their education.
5. Demonstrate evaluation and analysis of the nurses' role in the promotion, restoration and the stabilising of positive coping patterns.

---

## CHILDREN AND CARERS LIVING WITH PALLIATIVE CARE NEEDS

Receiving a diagnosis of a life-limiting or life-threatening condition is a life-altering event. This is true whether the diagnosis is for oneself or for a loved one. Facing the possibility of a child dying is perhaps even more devastating. We think not just of the loss of life but of a childhood, and of the futures of the child and adult they would have become. This affects children, those who care for children and other family members. In a sense, there is a loss of the child as a child whom one assumes will grow into an adult. The loss of a potential adult and adult life means a loss of possible future children and grandchildren.

Such loss used to be characterised in terms of a Kübler-Ross (1970) staged reaction of denial and isolation, anger, bargaining, depression and acceptance. We now recognise the dual processing model, proposed by Stroebe and Schut (1999; 2010), in which loss is processed at the same time as people function in their social roles and community contexts. It is recognised that children and their carers process the loss of their future, not in a staged way with a definite beginning and end, but in a continual process in which they have to integrate coping mechanisms into their overall functioning and relationships. Rather than a piece of "work", with stages and the possibility of completion, it is a continuum; an adaptation to a new reality of living with the diagnosis or bereavement which does not have a conclusion.

This concept of coping, as both dealing with living with palliative care needs and attempting to perform "normality", can be seen in work on parental coping strategies. Darlington et al. (2020), in their work on parental coping strategies, proposed that avoidance or denial should not necessarily be seen as a negative coping mechanism, as it traditionally has been. Rather that avoidance and approach are equally useful coping styles, depending on the context, and that over-reliance on any singular coping strategy may present problems. Their model suggests that avoidance and approach can be mapped on a quadrant with a focus on the self and on the family (Figure 6.1).

While Darlington et al. (2020) did not evaluate outcomes, they suggest that nurses should consider the quadrants and the features of parental coping when managing information and planning care. As they point out, parents can feel overwhelmed and

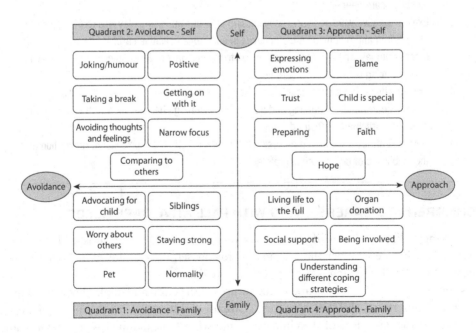

**FIGURE 6.1** Overview of parental coping strategies

Source: Darlington et al. (2020), p. 676, reproduced with permission.

may use avoidance self-strategies, such as going on a walk. These strategies can help parents to reach a point where they are ready to hear new information and feel less overwhelmed. As such, this might be a useful strategy but, as parents themselves pointed out, this can be seen as denial or avoidance and not taking responsibility, and they can feel that nurses are judging this behaviour. A more constructive approach might be to validate avoidance strategies and manage the timing of information-giving and support. Waiting until parents are ready to hear the message allows them to take time to address their self-care needs. Interestingly Darlington et al. (2020) also acknowledge the widely held belief that support from formal and informal carers (nurses and friends) can be derived from presence, without specific action or intervention. Just by being there!

This presence can be likened to "witnessing" something. We cannot always make children feel better, but we can be present, as mentioned above. Learmonth (1994) talks about "active inactivity" or "attentive silence" as being vital if one is to be present. He also says that a "precondition of witness is presence". While being present may not seem good enough, for a child's distress to be seen and acknowledged, this will help them feel less alone or isolated. Winnicott (1971), an eminent paediatrician and child psychoanalyst, who had a lot to say about the importance of play for children, wrote about the need for (the doctor to be) "a sympathetic witness to the child's distress", saying that the "unanxious recognition" of a child's situation and/or pain, is an intervention in itself. Of course, this applies to nurses, parents and other carers too. It is not easy to have to watch children suffering without being able to make them feel better, so nurses and parents need to be supported in this.

## PLAY AND EDUCATION: A CHILD BEING A CHILD

### Play

Occupational therapists agree that, for children, play is a central and vital occupation of their childhoods (Moore and Lynch, 2017). The central role of play has also been recognised in the nursing care of children (Fairclough and Bennet, 2021) and for children living with palliative care needs (Boucher et al., 2014). Play has been recognised as a human right for children which would extend to children living with palliative care needs. The United Nations (2013) offers a definition of play:

Children's play is any behaviour, activity or process initiated, controlled and structured by children themselves; it takes place whenever and wherever opportunities arise. Caregivers may contribute to the creation of environments in which play takes place, but play itself is non-compulsory, driven by intrinsic motivation and undertaken for its own sake, rather than as a means to an end. Play involves the exercise of autonomy, physical, mental or emotional activity, and has the potential to take infinite forms, either in groups or alone. These forms will change and be adapted throughout the course of childhood. The key characteristics of play are fun, uncertainty, challenge, flexibility and non-productivity. Together, these factors contribute to the enjoyment it produces and the consequent incentive to continue to play. While play is often considered non-essential, the Committee reaffirms that it is a fundamental and vital dimension of the pleasure of childhood, as well as an essential component of physical, social, cognitive, emotional and spiritual development.

Jasem et al. (2020) identified in their scoping review that play for children with palliative needs is an under-researched area, with only three studies identified that focused on play. What the literature did indicate is that play for these children is conditional on their health status and on the availability of play opportunities. Play for children is seen by children and their parents as integral to "normal everyday lives" and that accessing this "normality" helps them feel happiness (Jasem et al., 2020). Children adapt their play to their health status, so we see children with oncology diagnoses who are restricted in their movements, either by intravenous infusions or infection control measures (barrier nursing to protect children with compromised immune systems), adapt their play to within their bed space, often using computers or electronic devices to access play (Lima and Santos, 2015; Jasem et al., 2022a). Play opportunities were found to be restricted by access to play equipment and play spaces. However, children would often find opportunities to play with others, their playmates (Jasem et al., 2020). What emerges from the literature is that, despite structural challenges, children will play, and that this play is essential to their being and their connection to their community and families. As we know from other work, connection to one's family and community is essential in self-esteem and self-efficacy, which, in turn, are central to children's mental well-being (Strauman and Goetz, 2012, Chang et al., 2018). Play, then, for children with palliative care needs is a way to combat the isolation of living with their condition (Jasem et al., 2020).

Jasem et al. (2020) developed their work based on their literature review and undertook studies across two cultural contexts in the UK and in Kuwait, examining play in hospital and hospice settings. Using both observation and Q methodology, Jasem and her colleagues were able to explore not just what children and others did in these settings, but also what children and their carers thought and felt about play. Twenty-seven children aged 5–11, all with a life-limiting or life-threatening condition, took part in the Q methodology (Jasem et al., 2021). The factors that emerged were equally represented by all the participants, which shows that the inferences may be applicable across cultural and care settings. The first factor found was the social experience of play. For these children, playing with someone else was most important. This might be a child, an adult or a pet (or other animals). While children seemed to prefer to play with others, those they had relationships with already, they would also play with anyone whom they perceived as available for play. The second factor was the conditions of play. For these children, the conditions of play, for example, the type and location of play, availability of gender- and age-specific toys as well as space and opportunity to play in the care setting, were important. It was not that they did not want to play with others but for them the conditions were also an important factor. It is interesting to note that

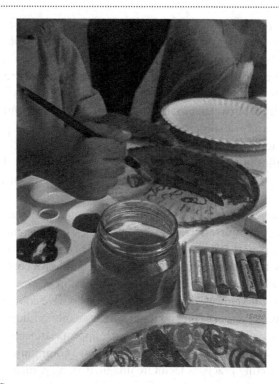

**FIGURE 6.2** Painting

while electronic-based play was important, arts and crafts play (Figure 6.2) and reading were equally important to these children, including some perhaps more traditional childhood play activities such as building or construction toys (Lego) and dressing up. These factors presented in Jasem et al. (2021) were also found in other studies, often focused on oncology conditions but with strikingly similar themes (Aldiss et al., 2009; Nabors et al., 2019).

The observational aspect of Jasem et al.'s (2022a) studies added the marginal participant observation of 31 children across the settings, amounting to over 60 hours of observation. The identified themes were the influence of the child's condition on their play, patterns of play and children's interactions during play. Findings identified that, despite the importance children associated with play, it was restricted by their physical and cognitive abilities which decline as their health status alters.

While immunosuppressed children may require nursing in isolation, thus impeding their ability to play with others, children with palliative needs may find their physical and cognitive abilities impact on their play. Needing assistance to play can often be frustrating for children (Jasem et al., 2022a). Jasem et al. (2022a) observed people assisting children with impaired cognitive abilities, which might involve movement for the child to passively engage in play, or play in front of the child. It is perhaps questionable whether this is participation in play or rather "doing" play *for* children, even imposing play *on* children. Jasem et al. found that new technologies can facilitate children's participation in play and children with palliative care needs, with variable degrees of physical and cognitive abilities, used a range of electronic devices and accessed the internet to play both on their own and with others. Interestingly Jasem et al. point to the Kuwait Hospice where play with electronic devices was less obvious but play specialist staff provided a daily range of arts-based play.

What is perhaps disappointing is that the observation found very little interaction in play activities between nurses and children. Opportunities to play were often not taken up and, in some settings, there was more often play *done to* children rather than facilitation of children playing *with* others. Although this may be a feature of the children receiving care who have less physical and cognitive ability to play, as well as the construction of children's nursing as an activity allied to medicine.

Jasem et al. give an example of an 8-year-old girl engaged in imaginative play (2022a, p. 6) which is ignored by nurses. This does flag the lack of understanding of imaginative play. Obviously play that exists in our head in our thoughts is difficult to observe. However, we know that nurses often misunderstand children's cognition and confuse verbal expression with cognitive language comprehension (Carter et al., 2016). The term "non-verbal" is often misused to mean children who have communication difficulties, i.e. have poor or no verbal expression, but we know these children may well understand language and be able to communicate with appropriate support (Carter et al., 2016). They are thus not "non-verbal" but actually have communication difficulties. It may be that some nursing practices facilitate imaginative play, such as the use of snoozariums, multi-sensory rooms, reading of stories, singing of songs and music-making (Jasem et al., 2021). How effective these are in promoting imaginative play, and if they are effective with children with cognitive impairment and communication difficulties, are undetermined. In contrast, Box 6.1 presents the story of engaging in play.

---

**BOX 6.1 ENGAGING IN PLAY**

We might contrast the view of nurses seen in Jasem et al. (2022a) with the work of a nurse-therapist (Angela Rackstraw) from Cape Town, South Africa. The nurse-therapist allows children to direct her in play or drawing when they are well enough to begin engaging with her. Until then, she just quietly sits alongside them. Sometimes she will colour in or draw, hoping they may like to try this themselves, and in this way drawing them into gentle interaction, waiting for their story to unfold. Simple art materials are used, simple objects/toys too, such as finger puppets, paper bag puppets, dolls, a small bed and bedding, or a small car. She uses the narrative too, encouraging them to tell stories about their play, asking the children if she can write them down, so that she doesn't forget what it is they are saying. This invites children to be directive, because they enjoy it when an adult tells them they are getting old or forgetful!

Interestingly, many children have asked her to make dolls, and subsequently some of these very simple dolls (Figure 6.3), always made according to colour specifications and specific instructions, have even accompanied children to theatre, or to procedure rooms, etc. Not only have these dolls been a source of comfort, but they can then retell the story on behalf of the patient, and so become a voice for these child patients too. Other simple toys are labels with messages (Figure 6.4).

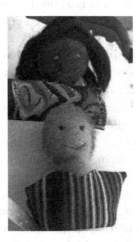

**FIGURE 6.3** Simple dolls

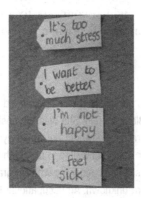

**FIGURE 6.4** Labels

As discussed above, a central theme to children's play is playing with someone, preferably a family member. Therefore, we also need to understand how care givers and playmates understand children's play. Jasem et al. (2022b) also undertook Q sorts with children's care givers. Thirty-nine carers (mostly parents) from the UK and Kuwait who cared for the children aged between 5 and 11, who accessed both hospital and hospice services, participated. Similar factors to those which featured in the children's Q sorts (Jasem et al., 2021) were found. Being with others and the social aspects of play were the most important. This reflects the similar aspects of play such as reading and arts-based activities. Humour and joking were also highlighted by carers and related directly to coping with painful and upsetting medical procedures. "He [the child] loves joking too much. He will not feel the injection if you were joking with him" (Jasem et al., 2022b, p. 6). Carers also understood that social aspects of play may be conditional on the child's health status and, in particular, their immunosuppression.

The second most important factor was again the conditions of play and children's abilities. Often this was an important factor for carers of children accessing hospices and who had physical and cognitive impairment. Predominantly these children were deemed to be in the Amber category, as set out by Shaw et al. (2015), where prognosis of death is likely in months. For these carers, it was important to have play which could be facilitated for their child and was appropriate for their child's abilities.

What we can see then is that there is alignment between various studies and the views of children and carers. Children value playing with someone, anyone, as an important social interaction within the social relationships that connect children and their carers to childhoods in communities. Play is vital to reducing the social isolation felt by children living with palliative care needs. It can also help children deal with painful, embarrassing and distressing procedures. What is less clear is the nurse's role in play and how play is integrated into the theories and practices of nursing. While how nurses participate in easily observable play, such as physical play, games and play with objects, is clear, it is less obvious how nurses engage with internal play, such as imaginative play, pretence and role playing. Yet these may be the very types of play which connects to a child's affective domain and could inform nurses of how children feel when receiving palliative care (Box 6.2).

---

**BOX 6.2 UNWANTED**

A young girl of 14 years who had a name that meant "Unwanted" in South Sotho was admitted to Sunflower Children's Hospice in Bloemfontein. She was HIV positive and had advanced disease, with severe malnutrition and depression. She did not make eye contact with the staff and sat outside on her own just gazing into space, unwilling to play with other children.

Her family history showed that she had been living with her grandmother after her mother died, and her father's whereabouts were unknown. An occupational therapy student spent time with her trying to get her interested in games and activities, without success at first. Another girl of her age tried to interact with her, but without success. The psychologist reported that the 14-year-old suffered from a very poor self-image and felt worthless; and said she was just waiting to die.

The occupational therapist then brought along two dolls, dressed alike, and the child became interested in these dolls, enjoying dressing them in different clothing and playing with their hair. Eventually she started to make up a story, telling the therapist that the one doll was called by her own name and identifying why she felt depressed, sad and lonely, and that she had never felt loved and wanted. The other doll she spoke of as the child she would like to be: happy, loved and with a dream for a future as a nurse.

Over the course of two weeks, she gradually spent more time with the "happy" doll (Figure 6.5) and eventually gave the other doll to another child. Her attitude changed to match that of the doll she played with – she responded to hugs and would sit on a staff member's lap; she smiled and laughed with the other children; and she made friends with another young girl in the hospice. At the end she was very frail and could not keep any food down. Despite this, even on the day she died, she would insist on being among the other children in the garden, trying to eat whatever they ate, and she held her special doll in her hand, even when she lay dying.

Needless to say, the doll was buried with her.

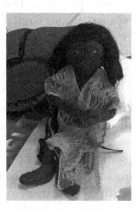

**FIGURE 6.5** An example of a "happy" doll

Source: reproduced with permission from Angela Rackstraw.

This story was shared by Joan Marston, founder of Sunflower Children's Hospice (with permission).

## Education

It is believed that humans have such an unusually long childhood because they are born with very few abilities to survive as members of their social group (Bogin, 2006), whereas other animals are normally born able to survive almost from the moment of birth. A long childhood is required in humans to learn all the social skills and linguistics to survive as an adult. We start this learning, of course, in play with songs and stories and games that help us to learn language, social norms, and cultural understandings. There is also a direct link between (pre-)school or formal education and early play experience and activities, such as pre-writing skills.

Every child has a legal right to an education. The Universal Declaration of Human Rights, passed by the United Nations in 1948, declared the "inherent dignity and inalienable rights of all members of the human family", and stated that everyone has the right to a free, compulsory education. The Convention on the Rights of the Child, adopted in 1989, reaffirmed these rights in Article 23, which states that children with disabilities should not only receive an education, but should also have effective access to education (United Nations, 1989).

The International Children's Palliative Care Network: Charter of Rights for Life-Limited and Life-Threatened Children (ICPCN, 2008) also asserts that every child or young person shall have access to education and, wherever possible, be provided with opportunities to play, access leisure opportunities, interact with siblings and friends and participate in normal childhood activities.

Besides being the right of every child, going to school is a normal part of a child's life. School can provide the routines that are so important to children, a reason to get out of bed each morning, a reason to motivate oneself, to interact with others and to acknowledge their own progress. This motivation, interaction and achievement can provide valuable distractions from the worries, trials and pains of illness (Boucher, 2021). Children have a strong desire to be like other children and to do what other children do. Parents too have a need to see their child participate in the normal routines of life. When a parent sees their child going to school and participating in the normal activities of childhood, even in a limited way, the day-to-day coping with their child's illness may seem a little more purposeful, and they may be able to celebrate each milestone, however large or small, in their child's life journey.

Children near the end of life sometimes have a particularly strong desire to be a part of school, as if they are trying to compress all their learning into their last days, or cling to the small threads that still connect them to the world of school, to that of their peers (see Box 6.3). They may wish to attend school to do maths but settle for listening to a story when their energy and attention will not allow them to carry out their desires. Right up to the end of life, children seek to be connected to the world, and for most children participation in schooling represents normality. Although life is never the same for young people and their families after a diagnosis of life-limiting illness, "normality" is an aspiration that should be encouraged. By normalising life, schools prolong life rather than postpone dying (Brown, 2009).

---

**BOX 6.3 EDUCATION TALES OF EXCELLENCE AND NEGLECT**

Anecdotally, we have talked to educators and young people who report both extraordinary efforts to facilitate children's education and the neglect of children's education.

A hospital school educator told us how she organised for a young man to take his English Language examinations for a basic qualification. She met a great deal of resistance with people telling her there was no point. He did not need the qualification as he would never work. The young man was aware of this possibility. He just wanted to be like everyone else in his cohort of friends and take the examination. We reflected that this was also something he could control. His disease and what was happening to his body he could not control, but studying for and taking the exam were things he could do to be "normal". The educator helped him sit his exam in the hospital school, obtaining special licence from the exam board – he passed. He died shortly afterwards but he had his certificate!

We also talked to young people who were not so fortunate. One young man with a complex medical condition and severe disability was left at the age of 26 years with no qualification and no prospect of finding employment. He commented, "People just kept expecting me to die, since I was six, so they didn't bother." He had been in special education but had never been expected to live and be required to find himself an occupation. He was finally training to be a computer games designer and attending Further Education college but also had to take the basic qualifications which he had missed out on.

---

Schools are expected to offer opportunities for developing friendships and being part of a caring community. School is a place where children can explore, discover, learn, and create. By participating in activities at which they can be successful, children are able to further develop their abilities, and are more likely to develop positive self-esteem. Close friendships and peer relationships have a special role in a child's life which cannot be filled by adults, and help children to feel that they are connected to their world (Boucher, 2021).

It is challenging to estimate the school population of children with palliative care needs. Connor et al. (2017) estimated that in 2010, conservatively, there were more than 21 million children in need of palliative care worldwide, with more than 8 million requiring some degree of specialist care. With an estimated world population of children aged 5–14 years of 2.1 billion in 2023 (United Nations Population Fund, 2024), the school population with palliative care needs is likely to be small. In a Greek national survey, it was estimated that 19% of teachers had a child in their classes with "a serious disease" during their career (Papadatou et al., 2002). The conditions discussed included chronic illness as well as life-threatening or life-limiting conditions, so this may be an over-estimation of palliative care needs in schools.

School populations are likely to be highly variable by country and regions. Child populations vary across the world, and it is estimated in 2024 that just under 2 billion children live in low-/middle-income countries (https://www.humanium.org/en/children-world/, see United Nations Population Fund, 2024). In addition, the palliative care needs of school-aged children vary a great deal across the world, with increased needs in Africa and South Asia (Worldwide Palliative Care Alliance, 2020). These regions also have lower national incomes, higher child population and a lower ratio of child population to working population. Thus, the areas of the world with the highest need in schools often have the least in terms of education provision. Some countries and states within these regions also have gender-based policies which limit the access to education for girls (UNICEF, 2023). Therefore, the picture in different countries around the world may well be very different, not just due to need or awareness of need but also due to provision and funding.

In the few studies we have on children's palliative care needs in school, we can see that even where need is identified, it is often unmet. For example, in Aruda et al.'s (2011) study in the USA of 21 children with "special health care needs", seven parents felt their child would benefit from palliative care but only two children were receiving palliative care. These children received complex medical care (averaging over 10 hours per month on medical appointments with an average 4.4 specialists involved in their care), yet their parents felt the communication between medical staff and the school was often poor, and that they acted as care co-ordinators relaying information between the medical team and the school.

It is interesting to note in more recent work, arising from cancer survivorship and the educational impact of treatments for central nervous system oncology conditions (dominated by brain tumours), researchers looked at how parents' skills and behaviours in advocating for their child can be supported and developed. Northman et al. (2018) report on the success of a "School Liaison Programme" which, rather than facilitating healthcare teams' communication with educators, focused more on parents' education, late treatment effects and advocacy. While this work was developed in cancer and, in particular brain tumour care, it may well have implications for children with a number of cognitive impairment conditions, some of whom may require palliative care (Northman et al., 2018). This does not challenge the communication cultures in which parents are often expected to fulfil the role of care co-ordinator.

There seems to be a perpetuation of the role of parents as care co-ordinators and advocates rather than a clear articulation of the nurse's role in co-ordination across the boundaries of the education system and the healthcare system. This work focuses on living with palliative care needs and the effects of treatment on educational attainment. There is little systematic investigation of children's dying and deaths during school and further education years.

There is, however, some work being done in the public health education sector relating to grief and bereavement work. Horn and Govender (2019), for example, describe a programme of "Train the trainers" to deliver group therapy for bereaved children in schools in South Africa. The programmes were in response to the high number of children orphaned by HIV- and AIDS-related disease in the region, whereby children were often left with no close adult relative to help them negotiate their grief. It is of note that Horn and Govender do not frame this work within nursing but relate it to educational psychology.

## PRAGMATICS AND NEGOTIATION OF CARE, PROMOTION, RESTORATION, AND THE STABILISING OF POSITIVE COPING PATTERNS

One of the challenges for nurses is to understand what their role is in play and education. Nurses work with and alongside parents, siblings for children to play with, life specialists or play therapists and teachers in schools, all of whom have a more defined role. So, nurses can struggle to find their own space and role within the education setting.

We might flip the question to ask: What is the role of play and education in the work of nurses? Randall (2016; 2021) contends that the work of children's nurses is to facilitate children having as much as is possible, a childhood which resembles that of their peers in their community. Following this argument, to help children to play and to access education is absolutely the role of the children's nurse, as these activities enable children to be children. In Figure 6.6, we have set out how nurses might use Randall's pragmatic approach to focus on play and education. The approach advocates two stages: the first, in which nurses enable and facilitate an internal and external environment such that children have the health status to play and the space, time and place to play (or learn). Once these environments have been established, we might think of these as the conditions for play and learning, and then the second phase of negotiation of care can be entered. Below we give some more practical ways to enact these strategies for play and learning.

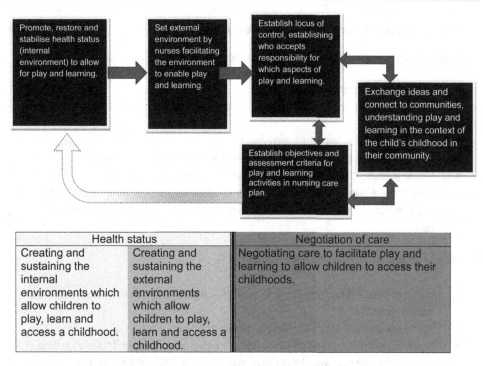

| Health status | | Negotiation of care |
|---|---|---|
| Creating and sustaining the internal environments which allow children to play, learn and access a childhood. | Creating and sustaining the external environments which allow children to play, learn and access a childhood. | Negotiating care to facilitate play and learning to allow children to access their childhoods. |

**FIGURE 6.6** Pragmatic approach to children's nursing: play and education

Source: adapted from Randall (2021).

Randall (2016) points out that children's nursing is a gendered, cultural and political act, and this would apply to nurses playing too. Randall suggests that we can understand who accepts or rejects responsibilities in nursing in light of feminist understanding (based upon the work of Walker (2007)). Thus, the negotiation of play and learning in nursing occurs in a gendered context where there is different social expectation upon men and women. For nurses, there are also professional and employment roles which have to be negotiated alongside their role in play. Other healthcare workers and managers have to accept and facilitate nurses playing as part of their work. This is most noticeable when new nurses come to a hospice and need reassurance that playing is part of "what we do at the hospice, it is OK to play".

The negotiation of play/learning is then complicated for nurses. Their own role, what they do and how much time they can invest are contingent on their other clinical and administrative roles. Other factors include how others see their participation in play/learning, or often how nurses think they may be perceived.

This balancing has to be attempted alongside facilitating the participation of children. Nurses allow, but sometimes encourage or focus, the child's play, while understanding and supporting carers and formal carers, such as play therapists or life specialists. All of this needs to be constructed within therapeutic relationships and the overall nursing care (Box 6.4).

---

**BOX 6.4 A NURSE'S TOOL KIT FOR PLAY/EDUCATION**

We could develop personal "tool kits" for play and learning in practice:

- Learn some songs or poems off by heart.
- Learn a small magic trick that you can perform with simple materials – card tricks are great!
- Paper and pens/crayons with a clipboard.
- Colouring-in books, or photocopies of simple images that can be coloured in.
- Simple puppets, made out of fabric, toilet rolls, socks or paper bags.
- Look at some widely used curricula books for ideas on activities for a child's particular interests that you could adapt (try https://www.khanacademy.org/ or https://unacademy.com/).

We could develop ward or department "tool kits":

- Start a children's song choir where all workers and parents can learn children's songs, or popular songs.
- Start a ward/service library of children's books.
- Reach out to local volunteer groups to find a musician or story tellers. This is often done in hospices, so they may well already have volunteers. For older children, you could collate a directory of local teachers who are willing to give one-to-one tuition.*

*If you have a children's hospice in your location, they may well have a volunteer programme. If you don't, you should consider that volunteers, including teachers, will require support to undertake work with children living with palliative care needs. Safeguarding practices and policies will also need to be considered and monitored.

---

It is just as well that play occurs naturally. If nurses choose to do nothing, children will find a way to play as this is what they do, a part of who they are as children. However, for nurses to harness the power of play and learning and to help children to be children, the complexities set out above have to be used to help children to live with palliative care needs.

Moment-by-moment judgements need to be considered then by nurses:

- Does the child have the health status to undertake this play/learning activity?
- Will the activity adversely affect their health status or clinical care?
- Will carer's (parental/grandparent/siblings, etc.) participation enhance the child's relationships or diminish them?
- Do the carers (parents) have the capacity to participate? (This might be energy, time, cognitive ability or just head space.)
- Will formal carers' (professional) involvement enhance or diminish children's relationships or informal carers' capacity and relationships?

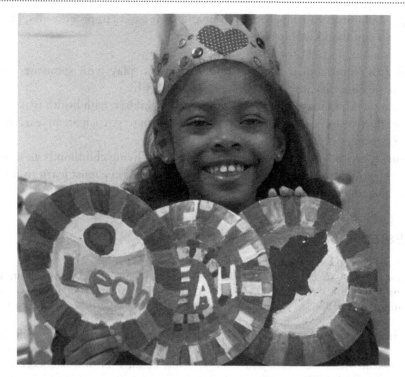

**FIGURE 6.7** Child with painted plates

Finally, we should consider how this work of playing and learning is accounted for and recorded by nurses. If we are harnessing the power of play, then we should be assessing and evaluating the effect it is having in reaching therapeutic goals. Without such assessment and evaluation being recorded, there is a danger that the work of play that nurses do is not valued and, as we have seen, it can be obscured, neglected and abandoned.

## SUMMARY

Children everywhere have a right to play and to learn. This is also true for children living with palliative care needs. It must then be a part of the role of the nurse to facilitate this play and learning. These statements are, perhaps, easier to say than to do! However, naïve simplicity of play/learning may obscure the complexities and lead us to underestimate the time, education, space and people required to guarantee children's rights. We must therefore strive to be available to play and learn and to create the cultures and environments that celebrate playing (Figure 6.7).

## KEY POINTS

- Coping with a life-limiting or life-threatening condition diagnosis is a process in which people use avoidance and approaching strategies. Both may help people to cope, and nurses can support children and their carers to process loss, grief and living a childhood with palliative care needs.

- Play is a human right for all children.
- Play is learning and is social. Children want to play with someone, anyone, above all else, they just want someone to play with.
- Education is a human right for all children and children with health issues should have effective access to education that allows them to participate in learning with their peers.
- If nurses are to facilitate children being children, living childhoods as similar as possible to that of their peers in their communities, they must learn to integrate play and education into their work and assess and evaluate the effects.

## SUGGESTED READING

International Play Association. Available at: https://ipaworld.org/
International Play Association. (2023). Article 31/general comment #17. Available at: https://ipaworld.org/childs-right-to-play/article-31/general-comment-17/#:~:text=General%20comment%20No.,31)*&text=age%20of%20the%20child%20and,cultural%20life%20and%20the%20arts.%E2%80%9D
McKendrick, J. H., Loebach, J., Casey, T. (2018). Realizing Article 31 through General Comment No. 17: Overcoming challenges and the quest for an optimum play environment. *Children, Youth and Environments*, 28(2), 1–11. https://doi.org/10.7721/chilyoutenvi.28.2.0001
Rainbow Trust. (2020). Pandemic pressures: The struggles and resilience of families caring for a seriously ill child. Available at: https://www.rainbowtrust.org.uk/uploads/other/pdfs/Pandemic_Pressures_Rainbow-Trust-Childrens-Charity.pdf

## Journals

*Children, Youth and Environments*
*International Journal of Play*
*International Journal of Play Therapy*

## REFERENCES

Aldiss, S., Horstman, M., O'Leary, C, Richardson, A., Gibson, F. (2009). What is important to young children who have cancer while in hospital? *Children & Society*, 23, 85–98. https://doi.org/10.1111/j.1099-0860.2008.00162.x
Aruda, M. M., Kelly, M., Newinsky, K. (2011). Unmet needs of children with special health care needs in a specialized day school setting. *The Journal of School Nursing*, 27(3), 209–218. https://doi.org/10.1177/1059840510391670
Bogin, B. (2006). Modern human life history: The evolution of human childhood and fertility. In K. Hawkes, R. R. Paine (eds), *The evolution of human life history*. School of American Research Press.
Boucher, S. (2021). Education and school. In R. Hain, A. Goldman, A. Rapoport, M. Meiring (eds), *Oxford textbook of palliative care for children* (3rd edn). Oxford University Press.
Boucher, S., Downing, J., Shemilt, R. (2014). The role of play in children's palliative care. *Children*, 1(3), 302–317. https://doi.org/10.3390/children1030302

Brown, E. (2009). Helping bereaved children and young people. *British Journal of School Nursing*, 4(2), 69–73. https://doi.org/10.12968/bjsn.2009.4.2.40655

Carter, B., Simons, J., Bray, L., Arnott, J. (2016). Navigating uncertainty: Health professionals' knowledge, skill, and confidence in assessing and managing pain in children with profound cognitive impairment. *Pain Research and Management*. https://doi.org/10.1155/2016/8617182

Chang, C. W., Yuan, R., Chen, J. K. (2018). Social support and depression among Chinese adolescents: The mediating roles of self-esteem and self-efficacy. *Children and Youth Services Review*, 88, 128–134 https://doi.org/10.1016/j.childyouth.2018.03.001

Connor, S. R., Downing, J., Marston, J. (2017). Estimating the global need for palliative care for children: A cross-sectional analysis. *Journal of Pain and Symptom Management*, 53(2). 10.1016/j.jpainsymman.2016.08.020

Corsaro, W. A. (2012). *The sociology of childhood* (3rd edn). Sage.

Darlington, A-S., Randall, D., Leppard, L., Koh, M. (2020). Palliative and end of life care for a child: Understanding parents' coping strategies. *Acta Paediatrica*. https://doi.org/10.1111/apa.15429

Fairclough, S., Bennet, V. (2021). Play for children and young people in hospital and healthcare settings: In E. A. Glasper, J. Richardson, D. Randall (eds), *A textbook of children and young people's nursing*. Elsevier.

Horn, J., Govender, S. (2019). Evaluating a grief programme offered in primary schools: An appreciative inquiry. *South African Journal of Childhood Education*, 9(1), a726. https://doi.org/10.4102/sajce.v9i1.726

ICPCN (International Children's Palliative Care Network). (2008). *The ICPCN Charter of Rights for Life Limited and Life Threatened Children*. Available at: https://icpcn.org/wp-content/uploads/2022/11/ICPCN-CHARTER-ENG-1.png (accessed 27 February 2024).

James, A., Jenk, C., Prout, A. (1998). *Theorizing childhood*. Polity Press.

Jasem, Z. A. M. H. M., Darlington, A-S., Grisbrooke, J., Lambrick, D., Randall, D. (2020). Play in children with life-threatening/limiting conditions: A scoping review. *The American Journal of Occupational Therapy (AJOT)*, 74(1). https://doi.org/10.5014%2Fajot.2020.033456

Jasem, Z. A. M. H. M., Darlington, A-S., Lambrick, D., Randall, D. (2022a). "Eat, sleep, internet and talk": An exploratory study of play profile for children living with palliative care needs. *Palliative Care and Social Practice*. https://doi.org/10.1177/26323524221105100

Jasem, Z. A. M. H. M., Lambrick, D., Randall, D., Darlington, A-S. (2021). The social and physical environmental factors associated with the play of children living with life threatening/limiting conditions: A Q methodology study. *Child: Care, Health & Development*. https://doi.org/10.1111/cch.12933

Jasem Z. A. M. H. M., Randall, D., Darlington, A-S., Lambrick, D. (2022b). Caregivers' perspectives on the social and physical environmental factors associated with the play of their children with palliative care needs: A Q methodology study. *Journal of Child Health Care*. https://doi.org/10.1177/13674935211044875

Kübler-Ross, E. (1970). *On death and dying*. Macmillan.

Learmonth, M. (1994). Witness and witnessing in art therapy. *Inscape*, 1, 19–22.

Lima, K., Santos, V. (2015). Play as a care strategy for children with cancer. *Revista Gaúcha de Enfermagem*, 36(2), 76–81. https://doi.org/10.1590/1983-1447.2015.02.51514

Moore, A., Lynch, H. (2017). Understanding a child's conceptualisation of well-being through an exploration of happiness: The centrality of play, people and place. *Journal of Occupational Science*, 25(1), 124–141. https://doi.org/10.1080/14427591.2017.1377105

Nabors, L., Liddle, M., Graves, M. L., Kamphaus, A, Elkins, J-L. (2019). A family affair: Supporting children with chronic illnesses. *Child: Care, Health and Development*, 45, 227–233. https://doi.org/10.1111/cch.12635

Northman, L., Morris, M., Loucas, C., Ross, S., Muriel, A. C., Guo, D., London, W. B., Manley, P., Ullrich, N. J. (2018). The effectiveness of a hospital-based school liaison program: A comparative study of parental perception of school supports for children with pediatric cancer and Neurofibromatosis Type 1. *Journal of Pediatric Oncology Nursing*, 35(4), 276–286. https://doi.org/10.1177/1043454218765140

Papadatou, D., Metallinou, O., Hatzichistou, C., Pavlidi, L. (2002). Children with a chronic and life limiting condition: Teachers' perceptions and experiences regarding students' school integration. *Illness, Crisis and Loss*, 10(2), 108–124.

Randall, D. (2016). *Pragmatic children's nursing: A theory for children and their childhoods*. Routledge.

Randall, D. (2021). Nursing, children and their childhoods. In E. A. Glasper, J. Richardson, D. Randall (eds), *A textbook of children and young people's nursing*. Elsevier.

Shaw, K. L., Brook, L., Mpundu-Kaambwa, C., Harris, N., Lapwood, S., Randall, D. (2015). The spectrum of children's palliative care needs: A classification framework for children with life-limiting or life-threatening conditions. *BMJ Support and Palliative Care*, 5(3), 249–258. https://doi.org/doi:10.1136/bmjspcare-2012-000407

Strauman, T. J., Goetz, E. L. (2012). Self regulation failure and health: Pathways to mental and physical illness. In M. R. Leary, J. P. Tangney (eds), *Handbook of self and identity* (2nd edn). The Guildford Press.

Stroebe, M., Schut, H. (1999). The dual process model of coping with bereavement: Rationale and description. *Death Studies*, 23(3), 197–224. https://doi.org/10.1080/074811899201046

Stroebe, M., Schut, H. (2010). The dual process model of coping with bereavement: A decade on. *Journal of Death and Dying*, 61(4), 273–289. https://doi.org/10.2190/om.61.4.b

UNICEF. (2023). Goal Area 2: Every child, including adolescents learns and acquires skills for the future: Global annual results report 2022. Available at: https://www.unicef.org/media/142921/file/Global%20annual%20results%20report%202022:%20Goal%20area%202.pdf (accessed 27 February 2024).

United Nations. (1989). Convention on the Rights of the Child. Resolution 44/25. General Assembly of the United Nations. Available at: https://www.unicef.org.uk/wp-content/uploads/2016/08/unicef-convention-rights-child-uncrc.pdf (accessed 27 February 2024).

United Nations. (2013). General comment No. 17 (2013) on the right of the child to rest, leisure, play, recreational activities, cultural life and the arts (art. 31), section IV legal analysis of Article 31, paragraph c. Available at: https://docstore.ohchr.org/SelfServices/FilesHandler.ashx?enc=6QkG1d%2fPPRiCAqhKb7yhsqIkirKQZLK2M58RF%2f5F0vFw58qKy0Nsttps://docstore.ohchr.org/SelfServices/FilesTuVUIOzAukKtwGqGgFkAgArTuTdZZUuSZObAaHCoPsdppxu9L6un29TyD4Jyrk0F22kRyLCMeCVm (accessed 27 February 2024).

United Nations Population Fund. (2024). World population dashboard. Available at: https://www.unfpa.org/data/world-population-dashboard (accessed 27 February 2024).

Walker, M. U. (2007). *Moral understandings: A feminist study in ethics*. Oxford University Press.

Winnicott, D. W. (1971). *Playing and reality*. Tavistock Publications.

Worldwide Hospice and Palliative Care Alliance. (2020). *Global atlas of palliative care at the end of life* (2nd edn). Available at: http://www.thewhpca.org/resources/global-atlas-on-end-of-life-care (accessed 27 February 2024).

# CHAPTER 7

# Symptom management

..........................................

*Sara Fleming, Helen Queen and Susan Neilson*

## INTRODUCTION

Over recent decades there has been a remarkable development in the progress of palliative care and pain services with the dedication of specialist experts and professionals, and a wider unified approach. Collaboration, engagement, understanding and research have led to a broader level of understanding and experiential, often anecdotal knowledge and education, yet the need for services far outweighs provision, particularly in low-resource settings (Sisk et al., 2020). Unfortunately, this has not been the experience internationally, and indeed nationally, due to barriers and hindrances preventing a global unified approach (Twamley et al., 2014; Benini et al., 2016). This has led to greater recognition of children's suffering and the concept of holistic suffering (Sisk et al., 2020).

The WHO defines palliative care as "the prevention and relief of physical, psychological, social, and spiritual suffering of adult and paediatric patients and their families due to life-threatening illnesses" (Sepúlveda et al., 2002). It widely recognises the principles of palliative care with early intervention, a parallel care plan approach and active involvement of the wider multi-professional team. As nurses, we must consider the family's transition into palliative care and on to bereavement. A focus must remain on the family, following the death of their child, provided by a multi-professional team delivering an integrated holistic approach (WHO, 2018a). Children with life-limiting or life-threatening conditions have unique palliative care needs which are different from those of adults (Marston et al., 2013). To provide holistic, unique care for the child and their families, physical, psychological, social and spiritual, care must be aimed at the individual child and the family around them, regardless of their age or diagnosis.

Symptom management in children's palliative care is a clinically advanced, complex and dynamic challenge requiring a multi-disciplinary approach. At the core of

DOI: 10.4324/9781003384861-10

this are nurses who are often the bridge between the family and the healthcare team. They are the crucial contact points, who observe closely and notice the suffering and distress, and take the necessary steps to achieve relief and keep striving through educated decision-making and compassion practicalities to make a difference. When suffering continues, the nurse remains present, offering support and compassion. There is great satisfaction in providing salve to a painful symptom and helping a family feel better. We cannot hope to cover all aspects of management for all palliative care symptoms in one chapter, even an extended one such as this. We can only address the most common symptoms we see across conditions, such as fatigue, gastrointestinal symptoms, respiratory symptoms, those experienced by children and young people with neurological impairment, and, finally, pain. We can guide the reader to the many excellent sources that already exist on assessment and management of symptoms. Finally, we can try to set out principles that underpin our nursing assessments and management and show how these relate to the multi-disciplinary team, including nurses, that surrounds each child and their carers.

We will focus on the aspects of children's pharmacology and pharmacodynamics that specifically relate to dying and end-of-life care. It may help to revise some basics of pharmacology and we will suggest some resources to help you. We will discuss non-pharmacological interventions, but again this will only scratch the surface of the possibilities and, in each location of care, what is available and appropriate may vary enormously. You may want to go back to Chapter 6 on coping, play and education to see some more examples of non-pharmacological interventions, particularly when considering distraction as an intervention.

Nurses are often the key assessors working in large teams, particularly in palliative care and the multi-model/multi-disciplinary team is vital in tackling symptoms. Nurses can be seen as weavers who search out and grasp various strands, i.e. people from other specialities, fellow professionals and informal carers, and weave them together to provide the child and family with the team that offers them the best clinical capability in support of their goals of care, and in response to the realities of their palliative care needs.

---

**LEARNING OBJECTIVES**

Readers will be able to do the following:

1. Critically discuss the assessment and management of common symptoms encountered by children living with palliative care needs.
2. Identify and discuss the complexities of symptom assessment and management in delivering care to children at the end of their lives.
3. Critically discuss the non-pharmacological and pharmacological interventions in children's palliative care and relate these to nursing theories and practices.
4. Evaluate the evidence base for symptom assessment and management of common symptoms encountered by children living with palliative care needs.

## IDENTIFYING CHILDREN WHO NEED PALLIATIVE CARE

Palliative care should begin at the point of diagnosis of a life-limiting condition. Identifying children and young people who require palliative care is important to ensure that appropriate and timely assessments of their needs are undertaken. Tools such as the Spectrum of Children's Palliative Care Needs (Shaw et al., 2015), the Paediatric Palliative Screening Scale (Bergstraesser et al., 2013, Bergstraesser et al., 2014) and the Assessment Form for Complex Clinical Needs in Pediatrics (Lazzarin et al., 2021) can aid the identification of these children. The Paediatric Palliative Screening Scale (PaPaS Scale) was designed to help identify children (over the age of 12 months) with palliative care needs, with the aim of ensuring appropriate, well-timed referrals (Bergstraesser et al., 2013; Bergstraesser et al., 2014). The scale comprises five scored domains: (1) disease trajectory/impact; (2) treatment outcomes; (3) burden of symptoms/problems; (4) patient/parent needs/preferences; and (5) anticipated life expectancy. The Assessment Form for Complex Clinical Needs in Paediatrics evaluates the clinical need of children with life-limiting conditions and is a useful tool for identifying palliative care eligibility (Lazzarin et al., 2021). A neonatal and perinatal pathway covering the trajectory from point of diagnosis to bereavement also exists (Akyempon and Aladangady, 2021). The need and the associated challenges of validating these types of tools are recognised by all the authors.

Palliative care assessment encompasses the physical, psychological, social and spiritual needs of children and the psychological, social and spiritual assessment of their families (WHO, 2018a). The WHO have identified a minimum palliative care and symptom management package that should be accessible to all children in all settings. The Essential Package of Paediatric Palliative Care and Symptom Relief consists of medicines, equipment and support systems to both prevent and relieve physical, psychological, social and spiritual suffering (WHO, 2018a). While it is difficult to predict when a child with a life-limiting condition might die, there are signs and symptoms that can help inform the timeframe in terms of hours or days, such as irregular breathing, increased pain, altered level of consciousness and family concerns.

Assessment challenges include the heterogeneity of diseases, the physiological development of the child (perinatal to adolescent) and assessing children with cognitive impairment. Recognised nursing challenges arise in part from the rarity, when compared to adult palliative assessments, and nurses' abilities to develop and maintain the required knowledge, skills and competencies. The workforce and training challenge is particularly important today as globally an estimated 95% of children requiring palliative care do not have access to any (International Children's Palliative Care Network, 2022). It is useful to add here that not all children with a palliative care need require a paediatric palliative care specialist; the majority of care can be delivered by generalist clinicians with basic/intermediate palliative care training (WHO, 2018a).

## COMMON PALLIATIVE AND END-OF-LIFE SYMPTOMS

While the range and severity of symptoms experienced by children receiving palliative care vary, recognised common symptoms include pain, lack of energy, irritability, drowsiness and shortness of breath (Feudtner et al., 2021). A range of symptom assessment tools exist (Greenfield et al., 2020; Papa et al., 2023). In this chapter fatigue, gastro-intestinal symptoms, respiratory symptoms, neurological impairment and pain are explored, along with some of the principles of end-of-life symptom management.

## FATIGUE

One of the most prevalent symptoms in patients living with palliative care needs is fatigue (WHO, 2018a), and this is one of the three most commonly reported symptoms in end-of-life care in children. There is growing evidence that the treatment of some of the causes of fatigue can relieve suffering (Wolfe et al., 2000). Children who die of a treatment-related complication are reported to have suffered from more symptoms than those who died of progressive disease (Sourkes, 2018). It is critical and crucial that the assessment of fatigue forms part of the holistic assessment of our patients and their families. Fatigue is a subjective symptom in children which compounds the difficulty and challenges in accurately identifying it and treating it. This makes it difficult for clinicians to accurately recognise and interpret the intensity of the problem and identify and develop an instrument which is multifaceted and validated to determine and quantify the fatigue experienced, including cause, frequency and intensity. In children's palliative care, both malignant and non-malignant conditions have a trajectory and a disease process which are both challenging and prevalent and will have a direct effect on the child's quality of life (WHO, 2018a). It can be a direct or indirect symptom with significant and substantial adverse physical, psychosocial, and economic consequences for both patients and caregivers. It is therefore multifaceted and can prohibit accurate and effective symptom control, management, and prevention. Understanding its impact and the child's and family's perspective is an essential component in its management and in alleviating the impact on each physical, emotional, social, psychological, and spiritual care need. Fatigue can be triggered by inflammation or the start of a therapeutic regimen, among other factors. Due to the inherent subjectivity of the symptom, quantification and assessment of fatigue are even more challenging in the paediatric population (Hockenberry-Eaton et al., 1999).

The WHO (2023) states that children's palliative care involves the active care of their body, mind and spirit and supporting their family. This needs to be expressed through their words and personal experience and perceptions and must be inclusive of the wider family and siblings who are equally sharing and living with, through and beyond the children's palliative care experience, albeit in a different way. Although psychological symptoms are often inextricable from the physical, they may also present independently as part of the overall illness experience. In our failure to address fatigue as part of the holistic care needs and assessment of our patients, if left untreated, it will adversely affect the child's and young person's quality of life and prohibit the opportunity to address and manage distress, significantly affecting quality of life and a positive life experience. Children who grow up with a chronic disease often face several challenges. One of the most prevalent challenges is fatigue, which can cause major disruptions in the child's development and social participation. As part of a nursing assessment, we need to explore the possible and potential factors that contribute to fatigue as well as factors that potentially may alleviate it.

Fatigue may be physiological and/or pathological with physical and cognitive components. It is not responsive to rest or proportional activity and affects multiple domains of life, preventing achievement of a good quality of life and becoming a significant source of distress to both the child and parent. It also prevents participation in the things that provide pleasure and meaning in life. Fatigue further compounds the feelings associated with stress, distress, anxiety and depression and manifests itself as a decline in cognition with reduced attention and concentration, and can impair emotional function, for example, depressed mood or decreased concentration (Wolfe et al., 2000). The physical, mental and emotional components may be characterised by a lack of energy, decreased physical ability and feelings of tiredness. These are subjective and multi-dimensional and may occur acutely, episodically, or chronically with multifactorial aetiology (Nap-van der Vlist et al., 2021). According to the biopsychosocial model, described by Nap-van der Vlist et al. (2021), several potentially modifiable generic biological/lifestyle, psychological and/or social factors can be associated with, and can perpetuate, fatigue in these patients. Therefore, understanding fatigue in children with chronic disease, as well as the factors that can cause or perpetuate this fatigue, may require a multi-professional diagnostic approach.

## Primary fatigue

Primary fatigue is thought to be related to the disease and disease process itself. The disease/condition produces chemicals and hormones that make the patient feel tired. This is accompanied by emotional or mental withdrawal, and mood changes, such as irritability and decreased co-operation. Alongside this, there could be a physical desire to rest or lie down and withdraw from family activities, as well as a loss of energy.

## Secondary fatigue

Secondary fatigue is influenced by multiple factors, including disease, and manifests itself as emotional distress with symptoms such as insomnia, weight loss, poor nutrition, dehydration, infection, anaemia, electrolyte imbalance, side effects of medication and co-morbidities.

## Contributory causes and factors for consideration

- Environmental influences, including care settings, such as hospital, noise, sleep disturbances.
- Personal and behavioural influences, such as anxiety or boredom.
- Cultural and family expectations and related activities.
- Treatment-related, such as medications.

- Difficulties in play or social interaction.
- Inability to concentrate and, negative emotions (Sourkes, 2018), depression and fatigue can present with similar characteristics.

Box 7.1 presents the implications for practice that fatigue presents.

---

**BOX 7.1 IMPLICATIONS FOR PRACTICE**

Consideration of fatigue in end-of-life care provision for children needs to include individually negotiated and tailored practical and emotional support for parents to establish and fulfil their parental role through death and beyond.

Policy and guidance should acknowledge the importance of parents being able to assess, advocate and parent their child at the end-of-life stage.

There is little available literature that considers fatigue for end-of-life care in different settings, and a lack of understanding of the impact of fatigue on different personal and family circumstances or on parents' ability to fulfil their preferred role (Ullrich and Mayer, 2007).

---

### Assessment

The causes of fatigue in children with cancer are multifactorial and include the natural progression of the disease, of which pain, poor appetite and nutritional status, depression, dyspnoea, and anaemia are the most reported problems. Although there may be no effective therapy for some of these factors, there is growing evidence that the treatment of some of the causes of fatigue can relieve suffering. Data suggests that there may be a lack of awareness among physicians that the suffering caused by certain symptoms typically experienced at the end-of-life may be amenable to palliation (Sourkes, 2018). Psychological symptoms are often not as predictable and will be very personal to the individual. Considerations in addressing these specific needs will require a full understanding of the child's disease or life-limiting condition and their experience, to date, of their disease trajectory and management, as well as the related trauma impact and psychological burden of the treatment and their perception of care. Separation anxiety will also be prevalent, and a full understanding of the journey will need to be performed to manage their symptoms of fatigue effectively and proactively. This broadens the concept and context of the "whole" family, and time will be required to understand this and to be effective in advocating and managing, and also considering any religious, spiritual, and social care of the child and their family while simultaneously ensuring that culturally competent care is provided. Assessment of fatigue requires consideration of disparate symptoms (Table 7.1).

The reliance is on the caregivers to give a full and well-rounded explanation of how the child is feeling. Parents often cannot describe exactly how the child is feeling due to

**TABLE 7.1** Frequently described symptoms of fatigue

| | |
|---|---|
| Physical | Pain |
| | Nausea |
| | Vomiting |
| | Fatigue: Increased and profound tiredness |
| | Weakness |
| | Heaviness |
| | Seizures |
| | Hair loss |
| | Increasing pain and need for analgesia |
| | Altered level of awareness |
| | Intractable seizures |
| Cognitive | Poor concentration |
| | Irritability |
| | Impaired memory |
| Sleep | Insomnia |
| | Hypersomnia |
| | Poor sleep |
| | Nonrestorative sleep |
| | Somnolence |
| Emotional | Depression |
| | Anxiety |
| | Avoidance in play and in family/social activities |
| | Withdrawal from family/social life |
| | Irritability |
| | Avoidance of school |
| | Apathy |
| | Decreased motivation |

many different reasons, including fear, lack of understanding and self-perception of the disease and management plan. Many parents state that decision-making adds to the burden of care for the child, but that it is an essential role of parenting (Hockenberry-Eaton et al., 1999). In addition, complicated family dynamics or familial struggles, sleeplessness, financial or other stress, and pre-existing needs, such as poverty, may complicate care and decision-making. As nurses, we must be aware of the physical and emotional fatigue of the parents and their ability to make a full, comprehensive and rational assessment of their child's care needs and associated fatigue. The responsibility and ownership of such skills and reporting of events and consequences are reliant upon a clinical evaluation which is informed, compassionate and holistic. The medical caregiving role is in addition to, and sometimes at odds with, the typical parental caregiving for the child because medical caregiving asks the parent to subject their child to difficult, and sometimes painful procedures and experiences, while the typical parental role is to protect the child from pain and discomfort.

## Management

The impact of fatigue can also inhibit care delivery, such as adequate pain management and the use of opioid administration, thereby preventing optimal pain relief (Wolfe et al., 2000; Nap-van der Vlist et al., 2021). These problems associated with life-threatening illnesses include the physical, psychological, social, and spiritual suffering of patients, and psychological, social and spiritual suffering of family members (Sourkes, 2018). As nurses, we must consider the development stages of every child as the impact of fatigue and emotional, psychological and spiritual fatigue and distress will be unique to their development stage. The holistic assessment is vital in providing tailored unique and individualised care. Developmental differences must be part of the care and management of children. This will include adaptions, regular assessments and evaluation of their fatigue. All associated symptoms and developmental changes must also be evaluated (Bowden and Greenberg, 2014). Sensitive, honest and open communication with the child and their family is paramount in addressing these needs. Regular assessment is also required to ensure timely and appropriate care planning and delivery.

This information is important because severe symptoms, if not bothersome and without morbidity, may not be addressed, with no consideration or attention paid to them. Consequently, less severe symptoms that are more easily experienced and described, due to being more easily reportable as they are perhaps more troublesome, will be prioritised. Understanding and making a holistic assessment with the child form an essential component of delivering expert and appropriate care, with a deeper understanding and exploration of the child's lived experience of fatigue. This understanding should not be limited by age. With a child with an ability to understand and communicate, every effort should be made to engage with them, with support from their parents/carers in understanding how their ability to live well is impacted by fatigue and associated symptoms. A greater understanding of fatigue experienced by children will assist in improving care and subsequent improvement in health-related quality of life. Box 7.2 presents some considerations for the management of fatigue.

---

**BOX 7.2 CONSIDERATIONS FOR THE MANAGEMENT OF FATIGUE**

- Patient-reported factors, which will include symptoms and underlying disease, treatment.
- Child factors, their age and developmental and cognition.
- Clinical factors, treatment regimes, previous treatments, and side effects of treatments.

Consideration and assessment of the above will contribute to fatigue and fatigue distress. Interpreting and understanding these factors will inform the development of effective interventions to mitigate fatigue. Understanding the prevalence and factors associated with fatigue will support care planning and create a better framework in anticipatory planning and future management.

---

Going beyond the disease-specific biological factors of a child's and young person's condition will help us to assess and understand the psychological, physical, biological and social factors which are being experienced. This will enable a broader understanding of the factors which are contributing to fatigue. These have been referred to as transdiagnostic where generic factors can be addressed, such as pain, sleep and physical activity, which are all potentially modifiable biological or lifestyle factors. Symptoms may include anxiety, sleep disturbances, mood changes and depression and may alter and have an effect on the family dynamic. All these symptoms have been associated with fatigue, therefore encouraging engagement in social participation and maintaining social function will help in supporting them in achieving psychosocial milestones. Modifiable factors, such as depression and/or anxiety, both of which are associated with fatigue and can be addressed within a psychological domain, were also identified in other studies regarding chronic disease (Nap-van der Vlist et al., 2021). These factors are suitable targets for treatment, for example, with cognitive behavioural therapy. Another example is dyspnoea and fatigue.

## GASTROINTESTINAL SYMPTOMS

Gastrointestinal (GI) symptoms are common in children's palliative care either as a manifestation of the primary diagnosis or as a side effect of therapy. These symptoms are often a source of utter misery and have a daily impact on quality of life. There is common complexity in management of these symptoms as one therapy interacts with another, such as analgesia and nausea.

Nutrition and hydration are emotional and cultural symbols of "good parenting" and require an exquisitely sensitive approach. The rise of augmented feeding via a variety of devices brings relief to provision of nutrition but a caution in net benefit-especially in end-of-life-care.

In this section, we will take a "top-down" anatomical order (1) oral health care; (2) dysphagia; (3) gastro-oesophageal reflux disease; (4) gastro-intestinal bleed; (5) nausea and vomiting; (6) constipation; (7) diarrhoea; (8) bowel obstruction; and (9) anorexia and cachexia, to review the gastrointestinal symptoms, explore the guidelines to identify cause and match this to management strategies.

We will also refer to the clinical story of Max (Boxes 7.3–7.6).

---

**BOX 7.3 MAX'S STORY 1**

Max is the 4-year-old firstborn child of Stella and Jerome. They also have a 9-month-old baby Claire, who is well. Max was diagnosed at 6 months of age with Infantile Tay-Sachs disease after he stopped crawling and had a seizure. Tay-Sachs is an autosomal recessive, genetically inherited lysosomal disease where there is a deficiency in the hexosaminidase-A enzyme and resulting accumulation of gangliosides in the brain and nerve cells. It is a progressive, lethal disease where the most common Infantile form (type 1) has a life expectancy of 5 years. He had significant issues with gastro-oesophageal reflux, poor swallowing and choking and has had a percutaneous endoscopic gastrostomy (PEG) device inserted with anti-reflux surgery at the same time. He appears to have no positive responsive interaction with his environment.

## 1. Oral health care

The mouth is the origin of the smile, of the opportunity to vocalise and a gateway to oral intake. It is an important symbol of happiness and expression, and it is mighty uncomfortable if unhealthy!

Causes of poor oral health are:

- Poor intake (dry); related to nausea and vomiting, dysphagia, pain, oral phobia.
- Chemotherapy and other medication side effects; mucositis including ulceration.
- Infection (candidiasis, herpes).
- Neurological (chewing, biting).
- Poor oral hygiene.

### Assessment

The *1988 Oral Assessment Guide* is a tool still used globally to evaluate oral cavity functions. It follows several areas of assessment: swallow, lips, tongue, saliva, mucous membranes, gums, teeth, and voice (Eilers et al., 1988; Eilers et al., 2014).

### Management

- *Treat underlying cause*, e.g. Nystatin drops for candida, manage nausea, encourage hydration, consider dental assessment. If the child is on oxygen therapy, try humidifying the flow.
- *Mouth care*: the simplest accessible mouth care solution is lightly salted water as a saline mouthwash or gentle swab four times per day. The key to what the child will tolerate may be finding tastier mouthwashes and pineapple juice is also good (but not if ulcers are present!). Use a gentle soft toothbrush, or teeth cleaning gels can be substituted if the brush is not welcome. Look after lips with a favourite flavour lip balm applied regularly; lanolin/paraffin also works well. It is easy to forget mouthcare in the daily routine and so keeping a note of that in a diary is often a way to ensure it happens regularly.
- *Ensure comfort* with use of analgesia and care with oral intake texture and temperature. Some children may require supplemental feeding while the mouth recovers.

### Evaluation

Children who have mucositis, especially those on chemotherapy, will benefit from evaluation using a formal oral assessment guide. General noting of the ability to use the mouth to eat, smile and communicate is also a key goal to measure (Eilers et al., 1988; Eilers et al., 2014).

## 2. Dysphagia

Difficulty swallowing is caused by nerve or muscle issues and is seen in children's palliative care in children with neurological or neuromuscular conditions, cancer, and HIV/AIDS (Amery, 2016; Hain et al., 2021; Paediatric Palliative Care Australia and New Zealand, 2023). Commonly children with this kind of dysmotility either avoid or stop oral intake, or they persist with recurrent choking and episodes of known or hidden aspiration with resulting respiratory issues. The neuromuscular elements of this condition mean that it is often linked with gastro-oesophageal reflux (see below).

### Assessment

Watch feeding and note that spluttering on clear fluids may be an early sign. Also enquire about history of feeding and episodes of choking, restlessness, food refusal, look for persistent drooling, be wary of increasing respiratory frailty. Specialist assessment by a speech therapy team and engagement of dietitians are good if possible (Krasaelap, 2023). Infection, in particular candidiasis, can also exacerbate dysphagia.

### Management

- *Review goals of care*, if early in trajectory of disease, this may be the time for consideration of feeding tubes. If this is at end-of-life care, it may signal a natural process of dying and so "eating" needs reframing to feeding-for-pleasure with consideration of supplementation if the child is hungry. Stomach acid suppression can alleviate symptoms of discomfort and candida should be treated.
- *Safety*: if the family wishes to persist with oral intake, then minimise the risk of aspiration with supported careful positioning, safe thickness, texture and temperature of food and fluids, and first aid training in management of choking. If available, a suction unit may be useful.

## 3. Gastro-oesophageal reflux disease (GORD)

This is common in paediatrics, especially in children with a neurodisability. The gastric contents move back up into the oesophagus with or without vomiting, regurgitation and pain. Sometimes this condition is exacerbated by commencement of tube feeding.

### Assessment

Look for a history of irritability, crying and distress with and after feeds, chronic regurgitation with spills, gagging, vomiting and foul breath, stridor, wheeze, chronic chest infections, feeding refusal, signs of pain including back arching and abnormal movements, sleep disturbance, reports of retrosternal or epigastric pain. Review medications for those which cause reflux.

## Management

- *Feeding*: thicken feeds, try smaller more frequent volumes, always elevate head of bed/cot and position carefully during, and for 30 minutes after, feeds.
- *Medication*: proton pump inhibitors such as Omeprazole relieve symptoms and prevent acid reflux damage. H2 receptor inhibitors reduce gastric acidity but do not impact frequency of GORD. Prokinetic agents can promote gastric emptying.
- *Surgery*: increasingly rarely, surgical fundoplication may be considered although the risks of the anaesthetic, wound healing complications and the procedure being unsuccessful often favour a non-surgical approach. Insertion of a tube into the jejunum/transpyloric may also be considered, which requires more onerous care but bypasses gastric issues.

---

**BOX 7.4 MAX'S STORY 2**

Max is restless and irritable, especially worse towards the end of his feeds and for about an hour after. Stella and Jerome place him flat in his bed as he isn't particularly soothed in their arms, but this doesn't help. He seems to be retching more with back arching and choking more on secretions. He was on Omeprazole prior to PEG (percutaneous endoscopic gastrostomy) and fundoplication but hasn't required any since. You agree with the family that a possible cause is gastro-oesophageal reflux. They don't want to disturb him with tests and imaging and so a trial of Omeprazole is prescribed. They will elevate the head of his bed 25 degrees and try to position him a little on his side so that secretions don't pool as easily. His parents will review his feeding with the dietitian (whom you will ask to call them).

---

## 4. Gastro-intestinal bleed

Bleeding from the mouth is distressing and gastro-intestinal haemorrhage is very rare. A large bleed is a palliative emergency (New Zealand Child Youth Clinical Networks 2022a; 2022b) and families should be prepared if a child has a high risk, such as a low platelet count, severe gastritis, or tumour erosion of the GI tract.

## Assessment

- Do not panic; exude calm!
- Where appropriate, identify the history of the blood: is it frank red (oesophageal cause); or more brown coffee grounds ± melena (gastric ulceration). Observe for small staining, and check bleeding/trauma, for example from the mouth or nose.
- Is there associated pain? Is there a clotting disorder possibility? Has there been increased nose blowing/mechanical suction?

## Management

- Calm reassurance.
- Position child to minimise risk of choking and aspiration.

- Get family to assemble dark-coloured towels, disposable cloths, vomit bowls.
- Treat oral/nasal source of bleeding with gentle mouth/nose care. Consider tranexamic acid application or topical adrenaline.
- If this is an acute end-of-life care catastrophic haemorrhage, use a sedative such as Midazolam to manage distress.
- In cases where there is an identified high risk of a bleed, think about having a "Messy Kit" in the home to grab easily to help cope with this – dark towels, disposable wipes, gloves, sedative.

## 5. Nausea and vomiting

Children vomit relatively easily, and emotional and cognitive factors can also affect the intensity of the experience. Nausea and vomiting are common symptoms which have many origins such as medication side effects, raised intercranial pressure, metabolic imbalance, constipation, upper GI inflammation, infection, liver failure, tumour pressure and psychological origins. There is a matrix of both assessment of the cause of the nausea and vomiting and choosing an agent best suited to manage this and a step-wise approach (Amery, 2016; Hain et al., 2021; Jassal, 2022; Paediatric Palliative Care Australia and New Zealand, 2023).

### Assessment

Where is the origin of the problem? Take a good history, looking at possible causes, get a sense of when the symptom is experienced, what it may be related to (food, movement, medication timing), review drug list for causative medications, review bowel actions, understand psychological and emotional state, identify any neurological features, look for signs of infection, including family history of illness.

### Management

- *Attend to basic nursing comforts*: reassurance, safe positioning to avoid aspiration, fresh air (a fan's cool breeze or open window can be very comforting), get rid of as many triggering smells as possible, provide mouth care, promote a relaxed and secure environment with distractions as appropriate.
- *Ensure that practicalities are managed*, such as the provision of vomit bowls, linen supply, cleaning up supplies.
- *Address anxiety issues and stress* associated with the meaning of this symptom. Work with therapist available and use the child's ability to express or be distracted via play, art, music, etc.
- *Treat the underlying cause as identified*, e.g. infection, raised intracranial pressure. Modify medication causes, if possible, with rotation to another drug, dose adjustment. There are multiple layers of medication which work best for different causes on different receptor sites in the body. For example, ondansetron for chemoreceptor trigger zone (Paediatric Palliative Care Australia and

New Zealand, 2023). Therapy may start simply with one medication, but in complex cases may require multiple receptor site approaches. Consider the best route of administration, given that the child may not tolerate an oral medication initially in this instance (Hain et al., 2021; Jassal, 2022; Paediatric Palliative Care Australia and New Zealand, 2023).

- *Nutrition*: the clue here is small, simple and frequent: offer ice chips, small sips of water, flat soft drink, change feeds to a slower rate and consider using an electrolyte solution, try high fluid food, such as clear soup, watermelon or jelly.

### Evaluation

This is a symptom where the family will need clear communication about how quickly you expect the management plan to work and a short review time for efficacy. Be ready to initiate "Plan B" in symptom management for times where the nausea and vomiting are frequent and distressing. Consider using a diary with the family to record nausea and vomiting and oral intake to help with clarity about this symptom.

## 6. Constipation

This symptom is common in the general population and there are many factors in children's palliative care which increase the occurrence. It often has multiple triggers, and the key here is *prediction and prevention*, or at least early detection and management. Constipation can trigger seizures and dystonia, cause pain, nausea and vomiting, inability to void, and increased anxiety (Amery, 2016; Hain et al., 2021; Jassal, 2022; Paediatric Palliative Care Australia and New Zealand, 2023).

### Assessment

Describing frequency and appearance of bowel actions can be surprisingly difficult and unreliable, unless approached with a diary and chart. Ask the family to keep a record of bowel actions, the Bristol Stool Chart (Lewis and Heaton, 1997) remains one of the best visuals and the paediatric-friendly version is well received. Also note any history of pain or strain on passing stools, abdominal cramping, soiling, bloating.

Assess for causative factors:

- Medication, e.g. opioid, anti-emetic, anti-epileptic.
- Physical abnormalities: postural curvature, gut issues, pain.
- Daily living changes: immobility, dietary changes, poor fluid intake.
- Diagnosis-related: neurological condition, gut dysmotility, autonomic failure, electrolyte disturbance, weakness.
- Local factors: anal fissures/infection, haemorrhoids.

- History-taking may give enough information, but gentle abdominal palpation can also help detect faecal loading. Occasionally a plain abdominal x-ray may help identify the extent of the problem. Rectal examination is rarely necessary.
- Watch for signs of bowel obstruction; see below.

## Management

Prevention: family education, regular assessment, identification of patients at risk, diet management, lifestyle changes.

1. Physical
   - Gentle abdominal massage can be taught to the family, as well as postural work such as "bicycling" legs, and increasing activity if possible. Preece (2002) provides a clear description of the abdominal massage technique for both small and large intestine massage.
   - Take care with ensuring optimal positioning for comfort and use of gravity, and the right defecation angle is helpful such as ensuring pain relief, holding a cushion to hunch over on the toilet, feet up on a box or stool on the toilet to raise knees to hip height, especially for little people. Ensure that privacy and support are balanced to the child's needs.
   - Care of the perianal area is vital with good hygiene and monitoring for any tears, haemorrhoids or excoriation. Use of barrier cream is often helpful, and a local anaesthetic haemorrhoid-type gel can be soothing for painful anal areas.
   - Intake: consider adding fibre to feeds (this must include increasing water volume), use of pear/prune juice and generally more water.
2. Medication
   - Stop, change or reduce unnecessary or flexible medications which are contributing to the constipation.
   - Laxative therapy: this will often depend on patient preference (what you can get into them), the degree of the problem and stage of illness. There are three drug groups within the laxative range: stool softener (e.g. docusate sodium), stimulant (e.g. senna, bisacodyl) and an osmotic agent (e.g. lactulose). Be aware that the stimulant laxatives can cause cramps and so it may be best to try the use of other drug groups first (Ahmedzai and Boland, 2010).
   - Many families and clinicians are reluctant to use enemas and suppositories and they are to be avoided in neutropenic patients; however, neonates and young children tolerate this well in small volume enemas. At end-of-life care, small volume enemas may be required to alleviate rectal discomfort (Amery, 2016; Paediatric Palliative Care Australia and New Zealand, 2023).

Impaction resistant to laxative measures may require manual removal in very rare cases, by an experienced clinician, and here it is important to ensure that the child is prepared, sedated (e.g. midazolam), and the area is well set up (lubricant, gloves, towels/pads, ventilation, privacy, support, distraction) (Amery, 2016; Jassal, 2022).

---

**BOX 7.5 MAX'S STORY 3**

Max's GORD symptoms settled well with Omeprazole but, about two months later, Max's mother calls to say that he has been increasingly unsettled in the last week. She notes, on further questioning and with reference to her in-home diary and Bristol Chart, that he has only had some small liquid poo in the last few days. He seems "squirmy" with feeds, and she has stopped them early most times because he was retching. Anti-convulsant and dystonia medications (essential), combined with immobility and likely disease progression, are working causes for what is a likely constipation. You agree that Stella will start some lactulose syrup twice a day via the PEG and if, there is no result or more straining tomorrow morning, she will give the 5 ml micro-enema which you have taught her to use. Stella will also reduce the formula feeds but supplement them with water. She does remember "tummy rubs" and legs bicycling, but you will show her abdominal massage again on a home visit tomorrow.

---

## 7. Diarrhoea

This may be caused by infection, medication, malabsorption/food intolerance, bowel dysmotility related to disease. It is also a possible flag to constipation as it can be a liquid overflow around impaction.

### Assessment

History: here again a bowel chart can be very useful to document frequency and stools.
   Assess for causative factors:

- The history of any illness in family/community
- Fluid intake
- Medication
- Disease progression
- Stool offensiveness
- Evidence of blood or pus
- Presence of fever
- Abdominal pain/cramping

The culture of stool samples may help to establish infective cause, especially over more days than expected.

### Management

Treatment of cause, e.g. adjust medication if possible, treat impaction:

- Advise family on the management of fluid intake, oral rehydration solutions, practicalities of toileting, infection control. Maintain good perianal hygiene with gentle cleaning and application of barrier cream.

- Persistent infective conditions may require antibiotics or anti-amoeba therapy, also consider treating for clostridium difficile.
- For chronic disease-related, or unavoidable medication side effects, try loperamide.

## 8. Bowel obstruction

This is a rare symptom, especially in children. It is marked by severe abdominal colicky pain, distension, nausea and vomiting and constipation. The cause is usually related to abdominal or pelvic tumours; it is a palliative emergency requiring rapid and advanced clinical management by a specialist team (New Zealand Child Youth Clinical Networks, 2022a; 2022c).

## 9. Anorexia and cachexia

Anorexia has been described as having no appetite or feeling of wanting to eat whereas cachexia is a metabolic syndrome where muscle, but not always fat, is lost (Mahant et al., 2021). The two conditions combine to a syndrome which is a malnutrition which leads to death if the underlying causes cannot be treated. This is generally seen in end-of-life care and caused by the disease itself and multiple factors such as pain, medication, anxiety, inflammation, and nausea (Mahant et al., 2021).

Providing nutrition to children is a practicality which is often paired with the emotional burden of being defined as a good parent, dependent on the success of this. There are cultural symbols surrounding this area including the reality of feeding being a source of identity, comfort and pleasure.

Many children in the western world who have life-limiting diagnoses receive part or all their nutrition via an inserted artificial nutrition device; nasogastric (NGT), nasojejunal, percutaneous gastrostomy (PEG), or percutaneous jejunostomy (PEJ). In some cases, children also receive total parenteral nutrition (TPN) via central venous or percutaneous lines (Amery, 2016; Hain et al., 2021; Paediatric Palliative Care Australia and New Zealand, 2023). For many families this relieves the burden and risks in oral feeding for many years and is a positive enhancement in their child's life. When a child is showing signs of oral feeding issues, the discussion about artificial feeding devices needs to happen early with full exploration of goals of care, the cost/benefit and expectations (Mahant et al., 2018; Anderson et al., 2021;.Paediatric Palliative Care Australia and New Zealand, 2023).

As the disease progresses, some children develop intolerance to artificial nutrition with symptoms of bloating, vomiting, reflux, irritability and pain which can be very distressing. At this time, many of these children will not experience hunger or thirst and it is a signal for a net benefit analysis of what is being achieved for the child. Visceral hypersensitivity or gastrointestinal dystonia (Hain et al., 2021; Paediatric Palliative Care Australia and New Zealand, 2023) is a severe form of this where there is an altered threshold to pain from a gut stimulus. It is seen in children with neurological impairment and generally follows a pattern of pain, anxiety and dystonia. The resulting burden of the symptoms results in poor quality of life and malnutrition. Changes to feeding regime, volume and composition may help but often this requires medication such as gabapentinoids and tricyclic antidepressants under specialist medical management (APPM, 2023a). Optimal management of GORD and constipation if present is essential. Venting the gastrostomy tube or intermittent tube aspiration can ease abdominal distention. These sensitised children benefit from high-level calming and comfort measures within a low stimulus environment and their families need additional support.

Sometimes children approaching the end of life develop feeding intolerance at a level where they "suffer to be fed" and continuing does not align with goals of care. Withdrawing artificial nutrition and hydration at this time is ethically and legally permissible but does not always feel comfortable for all involved (Anderson et al., 2021; Paediatric Palliative Care Australia and New Zealand, 2023). Sensitive and honest discussions with families at this time require sharing of the reasons to change and assurance of comfort and meeting the goals of care. Reminding the family of what other ways they are providing love and care for their child is important. Children can live for a long time without optimal, or any, nutrition and good nursing care, including mouth and skin care, positioning comfort, and sensitive clothing. It is very important that parents are well supported through this time, and that the clinical team also have an opportunity to explore any questions or doubts.

### Assessment

There needs to be sensitivity to the usefulness of multiple weight measurements – it may be helpful but, at the same time, may also be distressing if the cause is irreversible. General observation of fat coverage, muscle tone, energy and size are important facts as well as a good history of intake and tolerance of that.

There are reversible causes which should be considered, such as cancer therapies, dehydration, oral and gastrointestinal dysfunction, infection, pain. Management of these causes is addressed in other sections of this text.

### Management

Irreversible anorexia and cachexia can be gently managed with the "small, simple and frequent" approach and a feeding-as-tolerated ethos. Family discussions around this need to be inclusive of emotional, spiritual and cultural aspects, and shared decision-making about the best approaches.

Sensitivity regarding how this weight loss looks may include care with how the child is dressed, use of colour and patterns for visual distraction. Good pressure area care needs to start early with attention to regular skin checks and use of pressure area management proactively (Jassal, 2022; Paediatric Palliative Care Australia and New Zealand, 2023).

> **BOX 7.6 MAX'S STORY 4**
>
> Max has become very quiet and still in the last few days. He has had another respiratory illness and has very shallow breathing. His feeds continue as normal but today Stella notes that his breathing seems more laboured as she gives the feed, and he has been groaning a little during that time. His secretions are increasingly difficult to manage with times of choking, and anticholinergic medication just makes them too thick for him to manage. He seems to groan with nappy changes which feels to Stella like he just wants to be left alone. Stella and Jerome express that they feel their brave boy has had enough and that it is time to look at simpler end-of-life care. After two gentle but clear shared-decision-style conversations, it is agreed that artificial nutrition is no longer of net benefit to Max, and that he seems uncomfortable with it. As he has not demonstrated signs of hunger for years, he may have better secretion control if he is dryer and will require fewer nappy changes. Stella would like to give occasional water and electrolyte feeds just to "keep something in his tummy" and assuage the unbearable thought of doing nothing. She has a good pressure area mattress for Max, and positioning padding, and you have provided more mouth swabs and gentle mouthcare solution. They are prepared for Max's death with an understanding of the likely signs of this, knowledge of the 24-hour supports available, some night nursing respite and daily visits from the community nursing team. You have had an online telehealth meeting with the clinical and therapy team to discuss these changes and explore responses to them.

## RESPIRATORY SYMPTOMS

Breathing requires an organised function between healthy lungs, conducting airways, a central nervous system controlling and some good working muscles. It's not surprising then that children with life-limiting conditions are likely to experience respiratory symptoms. This causes fear and distress for the child and family and a threat to quality living; if you can't breathe well, you can't talk, or laugh or cry. Breathing is both autonomic and conscious and so it takes careful assessment and consideration to identify what the cause of the difficulty is, how it is experienced by the child and what we can and should do to relieve that.

There has been little research on dyspnoea and children with chronic illness (Pieper et al., 2018) even though in children's palliative care this is ranked in the top 10 symptoms in most studies regarding symptom prevalence (Pieper et al., 2018; Hain et al., 2021; Wolfe and Sourkes, 2022). As technology has evolved, we now have many ways to extend life and alleviate breathing difficulties from the very simple act of fresh air breezing the face to tracheostomy and long-term ventilation.

As there is an emotional and environmental component to this symptom, we are again called to be calm and use a raft of non-pharmacological measures. We as nurses can also be frightened looking at this and Amery (2016) gives us some great advice (Box 7.7).

---

**BOX 7.7 KEEP CALM**

Calm is catching, as is panic. Panic helps nobody, so try and stay calm. Momentarily drop your gaze. Breathe in, then all the way out. Imagine a quiet, protected place in your head or heart and put your feelings inside there. Drop your shoulders and unclench your jaw. Breathe in again, slowly all the way out, and then look up.

If you still feel like panicking, make an excuse to go outside for a bit (a mock phone call is always useful, or rummage around in your bag, or fetch something from the car) until you calm down.

Source: Amery (2016).

---

In this section we will explore: (1) dyspnoea; (2) cough; (3) secretions; (4) pulmonary haemorrhage; (5) weak respiratory muscles, along with ethics and advance care planning.

## 1. Dyspnoea

Simply defined, this means "breathlessness or shortness of breath" (Paediatric Palliative Care Australia and New Zealand, 2023). It is an often frightening experience of breathing discomfort characterised by increased work of breathing, a sensation of chest tightness and air hunger (Amery, 2016; Hain et al., 2021). It affects the psychological well-being and functional status of not only the child but often the whole family. The literature (Amery, 2016; Pieper et al., 2018; Hain et al., 2021; New Zealand Child Youth Clinical Networks, 2022d; Wolfe and Sourkes, 2022; Paediatric Palliative Care Australia and New Zealand, 2023) identifies many causes for this:

- Muscle weakness
- Chest wall deformity
- Airway obstruction
- Lung tissue anomaly, interstitial lung disease
- Pleural effusion, pneumothorax
- Asthma
- Blood gas abnormality, acidosis
- Mucus plugging
- Heart failure, heart disease
- CNS dysregulation, raised ICP
- Anaemia
- Infection
- Pain
- Anxiety, fear
- Reflux, dysphagia

## Assessment

What you will see is any or many of these signs; increased respiratory rate, pursed lips, gasping, use of accessory muscles, intercostal retraction/tracheal tug, laboured breathing on exertion, fever, wheeze, cyanosis (Amery, 2016; Pieper et al., 2018; Hain et al., 2021; New Zealand Child Youth Clinical Networks, 2022d; Wolfe and Sourkes, 2022; Paediatric Palliative Care Australia and New Zealand, 2023). Take caution with oximetry as the child may well be working too hard to maintain those saturations!

There are subjective self-assessment tools such as the Dalhousie dyspnoea scale which measures effort, chest tightness and throat closing sensation – these are restricted to those children with cognitive and developmental capacity (Pieper et al., 2018). General gentle questions about how a child feels works well, as does the comparative observation reporting of the parent.

Our goal is to try and differentiate what the cause is, to delineate the easily reversible such as infection, anxiety and pain and act on those, and to make sure that we are mindful of the possibility of significant disease progression and the need for shared decision-making and clinical prudence.

## Management

First steps in acute urgent management of dyspnoea (Amery, 2016; Pieper et al., 2018; Hain et al., 2021; New Zealand Child Youth Clinical Networks, 2022d; Wolfe and Sourkes, 2022; Paediatric Palliative Care Australia and New Zealand, 2023) are as follows.

Calm, rapid, assertive management:

- Identify the reversible.
- Sit patient up.
- Identify goals of care.
- Manage secretions.
- Apply oxygen, if available and tolerated.
- Then consider opioids and sedatives.

Opioids for breathlessness are front-line management and given using a 25–50% dosing to that of analgesia. They can be effective orally, parenterally, or transmucosally – there is no evidence that atomised dosing is an advantage and it can be more distressing to the child. Benzodiazepines can add effect, particularly if anxiety is a factor, but are not preferred over opioids.

Recommended therapy (Amery, 2016; Pieper et al., 2018; Hain et al., 2021; New Zealand Child Youth Clinical Networks, 2022d; Wolfe and Sourkes, 2022; Paediatric Palliative Care Australia and New Zealand, 2023) also includes:

- Treat underlying cause: antibiotics, analgesia, therapy for anxiety.
- A hand-held fan over the face, direct air flow.

- Breathing exercises, blowing bubbles, self-hypnosis.
- Bronchodilators and steroids for bronchospasm, asthma.
- Creative visualisation and active distraction.
- Upright, well-supported positioning for all locations: think about propping cushions and foam wedges, using soft toys and novelty cushions.
- Balance exercise and adventure with energy conservation support, such as walking aids.
- Oxygen/medical air, as tolerated.
- Bilevel positive airway pressure (BiPAP), continuous positive airway pressure (CPAP)
- Tracheostomy and ventilation.

The management of a child on oxygen requires attention to the safety elements and education for home, attention to which system is most comfortable, nose and mouth care, consideration of the need for humidification, and sensitivity to the portability and delivery of the equipment.

The BTF (Breathing, Thinking, Functioning) model (Table 7.2) (Spathis et al., 2017) gives us an illustration of the cognitive behavioural interactions of breathlessness and addresses the impact of negative thoughts and feelings, and deconditioning. The work of Spathis et al. (2017) describes how we can be mindful of the "vicious cycle of breathing" and find opportunities to work within this, when appropriate.

**TABLE 7.2** The BTF (Breathing, Thinking, Functioning) model (adapted from Spathis et al., 2017)

| BTF element | Domain features | Management approach |
| --- | --- | --- |
| Breathing | Dysfunctional breathing, apical breathing, sighs, yawns, increased RR, use of upper chest and respiratory muscles | • Breathing techniques<br>• Hand-held fan<br>• Airway clearance<br>• Inspiratory muscle training<br>• Chest wall vibration<br>• Non-invasive ventilation |
| Thinking | Anxiety<br>Fear<br>Panic | • Cognitive behavioural therapy<br>• Relaxation techniques<br>• Mindfulness<br>• Acupuncture |
| Functioning | Reduced activity<br>Muscle atrophy<br>Sensitivity to exertion | • Pulmonary rehabilitation<br>• Activity promotion<br>• Walking aids<br>• Pacing<br>• Neuromuscular stimulation |

## 2. Cough

Cough is a relatively common and very irritating symptom! It can be caused by aspiration, infection, tumour, fluid overload, inflammation/irritation, medication side effects and is common in HIV/AIDS. It deeply affects sleeping, eating and socialisation, and can cause sequential vomiting, fatigue, and abdominal and chest pain. Generally, cough is a body's defence mechanism to expel particles from the airway, but may be an unhelpful irritant. At end of life, this symptom is best suppressed as the fatigued and lower conscious child is unable to respond to other more physical remedies, and use of opioids will often be the best symptom control (Amery, 2016; Pieper et al., 2018; Hain et al., 2021; New Zealand Child Youth Clinical Networks, 2022d; Wolfe and Sourkes, 2022; Paediatric Palliative Care Australia and New Zealand, 2023).

### Assessment

We need to ask some questions and observe the nature of the cough to help define the cause and delineate between an ineffective mechanism, an airway irritation or inflammation or a more mechanical source. Think about the sound of the cough: is it wet or dry? Has stridor? Wheeze? Is it productive? Sputum type? Any whooping? How long does it take to recover from the episode?

### Management

- The definition of the cough, and timing within goals of care, will point to whether it needs help to expel particles, protection from irritant or outright suppression.
- Treat: infection, gastro-oesophageal reflux, secretion aspiration, pulmonary oedema.
- Avoid irritant(s): think about pollen, smoking, environmental factors.
- Antihistamine and/or anticholinergic.
- Soothing linctus, such as glycerin and honey.
- Opioids at 25–50% of analgesic dose.
- Nebulised saline and/or salbutamol for bronchospasm.
- Chest physiotherapy and positioning.
- Mechanical cough-assist machine (for neuromuscular weakness, requires child compliance).

## 3. Secretions

Excessive secretions are a terrible noisy, choking, gagging symptom with risk of aspiration, vomiting, and increasing the cycle of dyspnoea. There can be a fine line between managing copious thin stringy secretions and thickening secretions, to the level of causing mucus plugging and inability to cough these up. Ongoing monitoring and follow-up of management changes are therefore important (Amery, 2016; Pieper et al., 2018; Hain et al., 2021; New Zealand Child Youth Clinical Networks, 2022d; Wolfe and Sourkes, 2022; Paediatric Palliative Care Australia and New Zealand, 2023).

At the end of life, this symptom can increase with loss of consciousness, causing distressing noise and potential restlessness. At this time, it should be managed more aggressively to eliminate secretions and the need for suction, with drying agents and accompanying mouth care.

### Assessment

Get a good picture of the consistency, volume, and timing of secretions, for example, when are secretions mostly a problem? Are they discoloured? What discomfort are they causing the child?

### Management

- *Practicalities*: postural drainage, positioning care with child lying on their side to facilitate drainage and prevent gurgling at back of throat, use of bibs and disposable pads on pillows if on bed rest. Judicious use of suction with home unit if available; ensure that this does not become high frequency as it could be a stimulant for more secretions itself and put the child at risk of secondary trauma from repeated procedure.
- *Anticholinergics* such as glycopyrronium bromate can be carefully titrated to reduce volume; watch for mucus plugging, urinary retention and constipation as side effects of this medication.
- *Infection*, if suspected, could benefit from use of antibiotics.
- *Mouth care*, including good lip barrier cream and skin protection.
- *Botulinum Toxin A* may be offered as a local measure injected into the salivary glands with 4–6 months of relief (Wolfe and Sourkes, 2022).

### 4. Pulmonary haemorrhage

This symptom can range from blood-tinged sputum to, on rare occasions, a life-threatening catastrophic haemoptysis (a palliative care emergency). The causes of this are advanced lung disease, infection, liver disease and local cancer. It is one of those symptoms best prepared for, if it is possible it could occur, with a management kit containing dark-coloured towels, gloves, fluid absorbency products, instant acting opioids and sedation, family preparation, clear management plan and 24-hour contact support (New Zealand Child Youth Clinical Networks, 2022b). A calm but focused response is required here.

### Assessment

It is important to evaluate the volume and colour of the blood carefully as, on many occasions, the bleeding is from the upper respiratory tract and will be minimal volume and bright red. Brown or coffee grounds bleeding signals other potential causes.

## Management

- Identify patients at risk and ensure preparation to manage bleeding, minimise bleeding risk with platelet transfusions, vitamin K (liver failure), as possible.
- Treat bleeding issues with transfusions and antifibrinolytics.
- Treat infection.
- Manage tumours with radiotherapy or chemotherapy.
- Ensure that airway suction, and possible sources of upper airway irritation, are managed gently and used minimally.

## 5. Weak respiratory muscles

The most common diagnoses which cause this are Spinal Muscular Atrophy and Duchenne Muscular Dystrophy. These genetically inherited diseases are accompanied by not only profound respiratory muscle weakness but also skeletal, nutrition and multisystem challenges. They both have new medications available to extend life and many children live much longer now, but they are still life-limiting.

In these diagnoses, and others similar, we see a progression in muscle weakness with the medical capacity to meet the resultant breathing difficulties with assisted technology (Amery, 2016; Pieper et al., 2018; Hain et al., 2021; New Zealand Child Youth Clinical Networks, 2022d; Wolfe and Sourkes, 2022; Paediatric Palliative Care Australia and New Zealand, 2023).

Non-invasive ventilation:

- Oxygen: via nasal prongs, face mask, intranasal cannula.
- CPAP (continuous positive airway pressure).
- BiPAP (bilevel positive airway pressure): oral or nasal mask sealing to airway and connected to dual pressure ventilator.
- HFNC (high flow nasal cannula): a mix of air and oxygen via tubing sitting firmly inside nostrils.

The institution of these measures requires complex assessment and management and will be led by a Respiratory team. The partnership with palliative care specialists may support reflection on goals of care – balancing improvements in breathing with quality of life as interventions escalate. The next level of intervention of full invasive tracheostomy and ventilation requires considerable tender, skilled conversations and collaborative shared decision-making across the family and specialty teams.

Nursing considerations for care of children using non-invasive breathing support (Box 7.8) include:

- Assessment and support of optimum device fit
- Eye, nose, and mouth care
- Preparation of environment for equipment or power failure
- Home safety

- Mobility considerations
- Anxiety management as the child adjusts to new levels of support
- Parental education and respite support

---

**BOX 7.8 TRUDY'S STORY**

Trudy is a 3-year-old with infantile Spinal Muscular Atrophy. She did well initially with therapy for this, but has had a series of difficult respiratory infections which took weeks to months to recover from and hypervigilance in her home care. She is unsettled at night and has intermittent breathlessness and secretion issues during the day. They have recently seen the Respiratory team and, after sleep studies, have been advised that she needs BiPAP support. Her parents have managed home oxygen well and are proficient in use of home suction and managing her PEG feeds. Margo, her mother, raises concerns with the palliative care team about "when this gets worse", and a shared case conference was arranged with the Respiratory and Neurology teams to discuss goals of care and explore with the family what their options and wishes are. For this family, it is important to be at home, and to base decisions around what they can manage there. They are clear that they do not want to progress to invasive ventilation but wish to include BiPAP, cough assist, artificial nutrition, suction, and multi-disciplinary support for as long as they feel that Trudy has a net benefit from these.

---

## 6. Ethics and advance care planning

It is important that progressive respiratory conditions are addressed across several discussions, where escalating support may be appropriate but may also increase suffering for the child. The "weighing-up" of quality of life and disease progression for each situation may have increased difficulty, with prognostic uncertainty, but is best addressed early and continuously as interventions are considered.

## NEUROLOGICAL IMPAIRMENT

Children with severe neurological impairment form a high percentage of children's palliative care referrals (Amery, 2016; Hain et al., 2021; Paediatric Palliative Care Australia and New Zealand, 2023). The trajectory of neurological conditions (Hain et al., 2021) includes:

1. Static neurological injury, e.g. cerebral palsy, severe hypoxic ischaemic encephalopathy (HIE).
2. Progressive conditions, e.g. muscular dystrophy, Tay-Sachs disease.
3. Amenable to therapy diagnoses, e.g. mucopolysaccharidoses, lysosomal storage disease.

Impairment of the central nervous system also includes brain tumours and brain injured children. Duc et al. (2017, p.1114) identify the unique needs of children with life-limiting conditions and intellectual disability through literature synthesis, commentary and a best practice guide (Box 7.9).

---

**BOX 7.9 SYMPTOM ASSESSMENT AND MANAGEMENT**

- Consider use of validated scales to help assess pain/other symptoms. Consider involving parent or key carer(s) to help assess a child's pain/distress.
- Be mindful that symptoms may be multifactorial – there may be more than one cause for a child's symptom.
- Diagnostic overshadowing may affect decisions regarding palliative care. This is the phenomenon of attributing symptoms to the disability, rather than looking for an underlying physical or mental health problem (Hallyburton, 2022).
- Some children with disability may have pain insensitivity or indifference, which may further complicate diagnosing an acute episode or deterioration in an existing condition.

---

We know that children with severe neurological impairment exhibit neurological symptoms in response to stimuli such as pain, infection, and constipation. They will also often have psychosocial and existential aspects, and that these signs can also be caused by medication side effects (Duc et al., 2017; Namisango et al., 2019; Hain et al., 2021; Paediatric Palliative Care Australia and New Zealand, 2023). We also recognise that for families with children who experience these symptoms, there is often a distressing and exhausting burden of care resulting from the need for care, constant observation, sleep deprivation and the existential suffering as a child loses capacity and quality in living. The role of support, reassurance and respite cannot be overstated here.

Across all these symptoms are the non-pharmacological methods of soothing, providing distraction and modifying the environment to reduce stimulation as it applies to each child. In this section we will explore: (1) tone/movement disorders; (2) agitation and irritability; and (3) seizures.

## 1. Tone/movement disorders

Zinner and Mink (2010) and Mink and Zinner (2010) describe movement disorders as "Movement disorders involve impairment of appropriate targeting and velocity of voluntary movements, dysfunction of posture, the presence of abnormal involuntary movements, or the performance of normal-appearing movements at inappropriate or unintended times."

- *Dystonia* is a syndrome of involuntary sustained muscle contractions, frequently causing twisting and repetitive movements or abnormal postures. (Sanger et al., 2003; Mink and Zinner, 2010; Hain et al., 2021).
- *Chorea* is characterised by frequent, brief, unpredictable, purposeless movements that tend to flow from body part to body part chaotically and unpredictably. The movements are less sustained than those of dystonia but are more sustained and less "shock-like" than myoclonus (Zinner and Mink, 2010; Hain et al., 2021).

- *Myoclonus* is characterised by brief, abrupt, involuntary, non-suppressible, jerky contractions involving a single muscle or muscle group (Zinner and Mink, 2010; Hain et al., 2021).
- *Spasticity* is velocity-dependent increased resistance to stretch and results from increased tone which isn't necessarily painful, but results in associated inflammation and spasms which can be painful and hard to manage (Sanger et al., 2003; Hain et al., 2021).

## Assessment

Our goal of management for these symptoms will include assessment for definition of the movement and impact, and what might be reversible, but often an acceptance in our management that this is not reversible and a plan to decrease the frequency, duration, and severity of the experience (Amery, 2016; Hain et al., 2021). Using the definitions above, and by careful observation and history-taking, can lead to the best ability to articulate, define and then evaluate the interventions for these symptoms. Impact on comfort, tasks of daily living and distress are important assessments for children and their family.

## Management

- Manage what may be exacerbating symptoms, such as constipation, pain, stimulus. Provide support to therapy such as stretching, low intensity exercise, massage, bathing, hydrotherapy.
- Ensure optimal positioning and supports for optimal tone, e.g. seating, night supports, splinting. Take care that, as conditions progress sometimes, there becomes a place to move from corrective very structured positioning to something gentler and "cushy".
- Address functional issues with mobility, feeding and bathing aids and assistance. Pharmacological measures are usually needed and require persistent re-assessment, often a slow introduction of dosing due to side effects, and a plan for "as required" concurrent to baseline medication. There can be a requirement for several medications and care should be taken to avoid unnecessary poly pharmacy by identifying what is no longer working.
- Physical therapies such as botulinum toxin injection into dystonic muscles, insertion of intrathecal baclofen pump, surgical management, bracing and splinting may be very effective, especially earlier in the disease trajectory, in consultation with rehabilitation specialists and with ongoing review in line with family goals of care.

## 2. Agitation and irritability

Distress, which manifests as an abnormal or extended response to stimuli and restlessness with movements, is frequently seen in children with severe neurological impairment (Hain et al., 2021; APPM, 2023a; Paediatric Palliative Care Australia and New

Zealand, 2023). These symptoms can be difficult to separate from pain behaviours and movement disorders and, in essence, they can go together. Families are generally very exhausted and distressed through trying to manage these symptoms and require ongoing support and encouragement. There can also be emotional and situational triggers for these symptoms. At the end-of-life stage, this symptom may present as terminal restlessness/agitation due to the impact of hypoxia and existential changes.

A more extreme description of these symptoms is autonomic dysfunction/autonomic storming/paroxysmal hyperactivity. This is characterised by dysregulation of temperature and pulse, pallor, sweating, flushing, redness, retching, vomiting, bowel irregularities, urinary retention, hypersalivation, posturing and agitation.

### Assessment

Look for treatable causes, e.g. pain, gastro-oesophageal reflux diseases, constipation, urinary tract infection, infection, pruritus, medication side effects. Help the family to share their language set for how they describe these symptoms and how they see their child when they are resolved. Look for fear, anxiety, depression or existential elements.

### Management

- Treat identified causes: pain, infection, elimination, feeding, psychological distress.
- Recognise triggers and implement means to decrease/avoid these.
- Look for ways to calm the child and their environment and to lower stimulation and increase comfort.
- Ensure respite for families with trained carers who know soothing techniques.
- Redirect the child's senses with those which are intact; for example, massage, music.
- Medication: a combination of baseline management and good "break the cycle" medication will generally be needed. Benzodiazepines are first-line management for agitation (APPM, 2023a), gabapentin and clonidine are highly effective for cerebral irritation (Palliative Care Australia and New Zealand, 2023) and well tolerated. A benzodiazepine for breakthrough distress is usually prescribed (APPM, 2023a; Palliative Care Australia and New Zealand, 2023). Regular reassessment and slow adjustment up in dose will require vigilance and clear, reassuring communication.

## 3. Seizures

"Seizure" (also known as fit or convulsion) is the physical effect or change in behaviour that happens during and after abnormal electrical activity in the brain. Specific symptoms depend on which parts of the brain are involved. Seizures may be short and self-limiting, in which case no pharmacological treatment is needed (only supportive care). They may also occur in clusters of frequent seizures causing more distress or be continuous in nature, known as status epilepticus. Seizures can be generalized (affecting the whole body) or localized to part of the body. They may involve stiffening, jerking, or loss of tone and may, or may, not be associated with loss of consciousness (APPM, 2023b).

Seizures are very distressing for both the child and the family surrounding them. Box 7.10 describes the goal of treatment (Amery, 2016; Hain et al., 2021; New Zealand Child Youth Clinical Networks, 2022e; Paediatric Palliative Care Australia and New Zealand, 2023).

---

**BOX 7.10 SEIZURE STRATEGY**

1. Anticipate, plan and prepare the family for this possibility.
2. Control/reduce the seizures.
3. Reduce family distress.

---

## Assessment

The anticipation of seizures is identified in the "at risk" diagnoses of brain tumours, raised intracranial pressure, intracranial haemorrhage, infection, fever, underlying diagnoses with seizure profiles, neurodegenerative disease, or perinatal hypoxic injury (Hain et al., 2021; New Zealand Child Youth Clinical Networks, 2022e; APPM, 2023b; Paediatric Palliative Care Australia and New Zealand, 2023).

## Management

Preparation of families should include a discussion about the possibility of seizures, what these might look like, first aid (e.g. rolling to recovery position), and pharmaceutical management. Families and other care providers will need training and a visual handout in how to administer first-line medication. A clearly documented Seizure Management Plan may be helpful for families and the varied environments where children are cared for. If seizures occur early in the palliative care journey, consultation with a paediatric neurologist is recommended.

At the end-of-life stage, seizures may be difficult to control and ensuring a low stimulus environment can be an important factor in prevention. Children can develop tolerance to benzodiazepines and rotation management (such as the concept of opioid rotation) may be required. The increased requirement for sedation, including a continuous infusion, for terminal seizures may require clear and compassionate discussion with a family about the goals of care and the ethical doctrine of double effect.

First-line management of seizures in end-of-life care are a palliative emergency (New Zealand Child Youth Clinical Networks, 2022d). Administration of buccal or intranasal benzodiazepines such as Midazolam are recommended (New Zealand Child Youth Clinical Networks, 2022e; APPM, 2023a). There are some children for whom this therapy has little or no effect or who have a paradoxical agitation response. In this case, another medication such as clonazepam or phenobarbitone may be recommended (New Zealand Child Youth Clinical Networks, 2022e; APPM, 2023b; Paediatric Palliative Care Australia and New Zealand, 2023; APPM, 2024).

## PAIN

There is a huge reliance on the expert to know and understand the pain experience of each child receiving palliative care in relation to the unique and specific requirements that children will need to manage their experience of pain. A holistic care approach focusing on collaboration and engagement is paramount due to the unique and specific needs that a family will have. Without early intervention, the trajectory and intensity of a child's pain will activate previously silent pathways, therefore making management and control more challenging. Without effective management and intervention, including management plans, there is potential for higher escalation of analgesic intervention and it may take longer to achieve effective analgesic relief for the patient. An holistic approach focusing on collaboration and engagement is paramount due to the unique and specific needs that a family will have. Long-term consequences may include anticipatory anxiety, a lowering of the pain threshold and sensitisation to future pain, reduced effectiveness of analgesics and increased analgesic requirements subsequently (Wong et al., 2012).

Both a pharmacological and a non-pharmacological and medical approach form the narrative of understanding, intervention and control of distressing symptoms such as pain, due to emotional, psychological, social and spiritual distress, fatigue and fear (Sepúlveda et al., 2002; WHO, 2018b). Access to all available care options is a basic human right, including palliative care and commitment to the relief of pain, more importantly, must be the focus of care (Gwyther et al., 2009). Particular attention must be paid to cultural and spiritual wishes so that care is not solely based on the clinical picture. This creates a holistic care approach, encompassing all "total pain" and allowing a significant focus on non-pharmacological management (Box 7.11).

---

**BOX 7.11 THE ROLE OF THE NURSE**

The role of the nurse is pivotal in advocating, negotiating, and co-ordinating the care of the child, young person and family, managing expectations, and ensuring robust assessment, care planning and management.

---

In this section we will (1) define pain; (2) explore types of pain; (3) describe pain assessment; (4) present pain assessment tools; (5) give guidance on pain management; (6) discuss prescribing; and (7) suggest non-pharmacological interventions.

## 1. Defining pain

Pain is a multidimensional phenomenon in children's palliative care (Figure 7.1).

The WHO (2014) guidelines on the pharmacological treatment of persisting pain in children with medical illnesses refer to "total pain", which therefore needs to be addressed and all elements identified in order to achieve bespoke, competent and confident management. Key issues discussed include the definition, assessment, pharmacological and integrative management of pain, availability of medications,

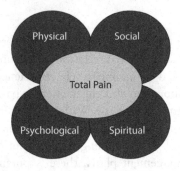

**FIGURE 7.1** Total pain

education, and research (WHO, 2018b). The International Association for the Study of Pain defines pain as "an unpleasant sensory and emotional experience associated with actual or potential tissue damage" (Raja et al., 2020). According to the complete detailed definition, pain is much broader than just physical damage to tissues (Friedrichsdorf, 2010).

## 2. Types of pain

Children requiring palliative care may have mixed somatic pain. This can be acute and visceral, neuropathic, chronic (pain which extends beyond expected time of healing) and psychosocial spiritual pain (total pain). Pain is therefore both physical and psychological, or a combination of both. This must be factored into the nursing assessment. Psychological pain may be emotional or spiritual. Sometimes, psychological pain increases physical pain, and this is referred to as "total pain". It is important to consider the underlying pathology of pain (Box 7.12).

---

**BOX 7.12 THE UNDERLYING PATHOLOGY OF PAIN**

- Musculoskeletal pain: caused by bone, joint and muscle issues (e.g. contractures) and weakness.
- Skin and organ pain: sometimes present in metabolic disease and metastatic cancer. Could also be related to procedures.
- Visceral pain: Most predominantly gastro-intestinal pain. This is even more present in feeding via non-oral routes or issues with constipation (Friedrichsdorf and Bruera, 2018).
- Neuropathic pain: Neuropathic or inflammatory pain.
- Central pain: Often presents in children with central nervous system conditions. Also referred to as neuro-irritability and is not inflammatory in nature. This type of pain can be challenging to manage.
- Dystonia pain: Often seen in children with severe neurological impairment alongside intermittent nausea and vomiting, abdominal distension, feed intolerance and contractures.

---

## 3. Pain assessment

While advances have been made, including publication of the guidelines by WHO (2014; 2020), significant gaps exist in terms of the evidence base, education, and access to essential medications, and both interdisciplinary and international collaboration are required to remove these gaps. There is a global willingness to embrace all aspects of the biopsychosocial model of pain, with active and advancing research in this area. There is collaboration of clinical and scientific research including the exploration of social determinants of pain, which has led to a shift of focus from the biomedical approach to total pain approach. This includes consideration of the thoughts, feelings and social lives of infants and children, their non-verbal pain expression, and the multidimensional features of the total pain experience (Craig, 2020). Paediatric pain management in palliative care must encompass the holistic review and assessment of the child and include sensory, physiological, cognitive, affective, behavioural and spiritual components. All of these are subjective experiences of children and young people, but also are seen and reported by the family around them who watch, experience, feel, see and sense the pain their child is experiencing. This can be, and frequently is, as acute and perhaps sometimes more acute than in the child. We must remember that parents have shared the journey, including the diagnosis, complex and challenging management, and the interactions with many different healthcare professionals. The family experiences the trajectory of the illness, whether this be with or without the consideration of a palliative diagnosis. It is essential to consider this as part of the assessment as this will add an additional layer of fear and anxiety to the circumstances.

This will have a colossal impact on how we, as nurses, manage care and its redirection with a mindful balance and cognisance of the universal needs and resources available to professionals and what we may have as independent nurse practitioners and non-medical prescribers in our pain assessment toolboxes. This is where we can, without clinical variances, international diversities and health inequalities, do away with sophisticated privileges, and use global skills and knowledge which are all within our gift. Such tools include the pain assessment toolbox (Box 7.13).

---

**BOX 7.13 THE PAIN ASSESSMENT TOOLBOX**

- Listening.
- Hearing.
- Seeing.
- Understanding the child's and family's verbal cues and words to describe pain or discomfort.
- Being calm and present.
- Radiating control and support.
- Holding the space, literally or virtually.
- Working through each unique problem.
- Being reassuring and offering reassurance.

- Using the skills of translation.
- Being in the moment without an agenda or time constraints.
- Enabling and empowering the child and the family.
- Understanding strategies implemented by family.
- Understanding the pain, the duration, the onset, the descriptions, the effectiveness of current symptom and pain management.

Consider your approach: if pain is escalating and the child is in acute pain, manage this efficiently using your knowledge and skills to make a rapid assessment and decision without delay. This will reassure and give time to make a more thorough management plan moving forwards. For example, for rapid onset of pain and escalating symptoms, administering a breakthrough or an immediate buccal, sublingual, subcutaneous or intravenous dose while continuing to assess, evaluate and plan the next steps of pain management. When pain is resolving and settling or settled, collaboration with family/carers will be more effective.

Children and young people experience a wider range of life-limiting conditions in comparison to adults. Assessing pain in infants, children and young people living with palliative care needs remains a challenge due to diverse patient conditions, types of pain and often a reduced ability or inability of patients to communicate verbally. Pain assessment considerations must therefore include the child's cognition, dependence and verbal and non-verbal communication, as all will influence their experience and interpretation of pain. The ultimate outcome of total pain management is to minimise pain and painful symptoms, including distressing and anticipatory symptoms while aiming to maximise a quality of life which gives relief, reassurance and confidence to the individual and the family. This will require a trusting and honest approach with a shared understanding that management and control will be a partnership with the healthcare professionals. This will involve regular and honest reviews and communication between the treating teams and the family, as well as a degree of tolerance in finding the most acceptable management for the individual experiencing the pain and the family around them.

The foundation of holistic care is a comprehensive committed collaboration, enabling ongoing assessment and review, open and honest communication, understanding barriers and fears, exposing inappropriate use or non-compliance around ineffective management of analgesics and providing symptom management plans. It is important to continually recognise that holistic care will be governed by the understanding that pain is multi-dimensional. Therefore, successful management of pain requires all dimensions of pain to be understood and addressed (Galloway and Yaster, 2000).

Anticipating symptoms and discussing future management are essential in empowering the child, young person, and the family in maintaining continued trust and understanding of the commitment to maximise quality of life and minimise side effects and unexpected pain and symptoms. Pain is one of the most distressing and prevalent end-of-life symptoms experienced by patients, therefore proactive care planning is paramount (Liben, 1996). As professionals and advocates, we must also consider that pain assessment is a critical first step for adequate pain management across treatment settings (Howard and Liossi, 2014). This is advocated by national and international guidelines. The key in enabling the above is maintaining good communication, while supporting, reviewing, and assessing the longer disease trajectories and extended requirements for children's palliative care.

Assessing and documenting a child's pain are essential for successful pain management. The preferred method for assessment is by self-report as pain is subjective. However, self-reporting may not be appropriate for all children and young people, especially those who are non-verbal or very young. This is when other methods must be implemented, for example, behaviour-based assessment (American Academy of Pediatrics Committee on Psychosocial Aspects of Child and Family Health, 2001). Conversations and review with the family are essential in understanding and reviewing physiologic parameters and support a more informed pain assessment and review. Many methods of pain assessment exist, as mentioned in the pain assessment section above, and ideally should combine patient and family history with assessments by the bedside nurse/community nurse to determine the most appropriate management plan. Assessment of the child in a different care setting, home, hospice, respite and community care, will be an essential component in the review and management pathway and plan. A complex interplay of intrinsic and extrinsic factors will enable management of the total pain, understanding which extrinsic factors affect their total pain outside of the clinical environment. Therefore, core key communication skills are vital and might cue you to think; "what might I see?" (Table 7.3).

**TABLE 7.3** Assessment: what I might see?

| Which physiological signs are evident? | <ul><li>Raised pulse</li><li>Sweating, clammy, shallow breathing</li><li>Positioning and posture</li><li>Sleep disturbance</li><li>Furrowed brow</li><li>Crying and irritability</li><li>Agitated/combative</li><li>Increased sleep</li><li>Reduced mobility</li><li>Reduced appetite/refusal to feed (baby/toddler)</li><li>Nausea +/- vomiting</li><li>Pallor</li><li>Dull eyes</li><li>Flushed skin</li><li>Itching</li><li>Guarding</li></ul> |
|---|---|

*(Continued)*

**TABLE 7.3** Assessment: what I might see? *(Continued)*

| | |
|---|---|
| Which emotional/social changes are evident? | • Low mood<br>• Disengagement (too calm and too compliant, a shift-change from usual behaviour)<br>• Refusal to get up and take part in family life/unwillingness to attend school<br>• Avoidance in key family activities such as mealtimes<br>• Irritability and short-tempered behaviour<br>• Intolerance of siblings<br>• Noise and light intolerance/agitation<br>• Pain assessment<br>  Who is "family" and how is family?: what capacity and support do they have to manage?<br>• Does the family require additional support, an intervention and are other professional bodies/facilities/organisations available to support the family? |
| What is known about the pain? | • Background pain<br>• Breakthrough pain<br>• Incident pain<br>  Allodynia: non-painful stimulus causing pain<br>• Dysesthesia: abnormal sensation (spontaneous or abnormal sensation) (spontaneous or evoked) burning, shooting, tingling, numbness |
| Considerations in pain management<br>• Alternative routes such as buccal, sublingual, intranasal, subcutaneous, intravenous<br>• Opioid switching/rotation<br>• Option of conversion between routes<br>• Indications for use, for example, opioids for dyspnoea, anti-psychotics for symptoms of nausea and vomiting | • Different populations<br>• Sicker/increasing fragility<br>• Polypharmacy<br>• Non typical body weight<br>• Care setting and availability of equipment/disposables/management and governance<br>• Multiple co-morbidities<br>• Infants and children<br>• Availability of nursing support and 24/7 access to "on call"' care |

Effective assessment of pain includes both the measurement of pain severity, with a developmentally appropriate, validated tool, as well as a thorough pain history (exploring the pain quality, characteristics, location, onset, duration, aggravating and alleviating factors, and impact on function) (Gai et al., 2020). What is valuable in managing any level of pain and discomfort is to have clear and defined goal-setting with the carer, family and the patient themselves. It is of paramount importance to be truthful in your approach and clear and transparent in acknowledging that unless you are administering a bolus dose of drug that there will be some delay, up to half an hour in gaining some level of control and pain relief. It is within this time, and beyond, that communication and reassurance are key to maintain trust and understanding and developing a rapport which will be essential in effective management and future confidence-building.

## 4. Pain assessment tools

There are a range of pain assessment tools that measure pain intensity. These incorporate self-assessment (Birnie et al., 2019) and observational approaches (Andersen et al., 2017) considering the wide age range of children and young people and those unable to self-report their pain. Self-assessment tools such as the recommended Faces Pain Scale-Revised can be used with younger children aged from 4 years (Hicks et al., 2001). Children are asked to point to one of six faces that reflects their level of pain. Each face has a corresponding score ranging from 0 which equates to "no pain" to 10 representing "very much pain". The tool is available for download at: https://www.iasp-pain.org/resources/faces-pain-scale-revised/. A visual analogue 0–10 scale without facial images can be used with older children and young people.

Observational tools are useful for young children/infants or non-verbal children. Examples include the recommended FLACC (Faces, Legs, Activity, Cry and Consolability) scales and revised FLACC (Malviya et al., 2006). The revised FLACC tool, for use with children with cognitive impairment, incorporates additional behavioural descriptors such as breath holding and marked increase in spasticity. The Paediatric Pain Profile (Hunt et al., 2004) was developed for children with severe physical and learning impairments. This is a behaviour assessment scale that identifies behavioural cues to when the child is in pain. The Paediatric Pain Profile is available for download at: https://ppprofile.org.uk/. As with all observational tools, robustness of the observations and accuracy of documentation are imperative.

Where formal assessment tools are not available, a simple outline of a person can be drawn and the child or young person being asked to mark where, for example, they are experiencing pain. This can be helpful in minimising the risk of misinterpretation of a child's description or response to pain. Through the additional use of colour, the severity of the pain can also be gauged. For example, the child or young person can be invited to choose a coloured pencil to shade the area on the outline where they feel pain. Their choice of colour and relevance to pain intensity could then be explored.

## 5. Pain management

When palliating children and young people, it is essential that patience, meticulousness, and perseverance are applied to each individual case. This is especially true of those who are very young or non-verbal (Siden et al., 2013). There are several causes of pain that can be reversed to provide more comfort to the child. These include positioning, constipation and poor oral hygiene (Siden, 2018). Managing pain and painful symptoms is the responsibility of the multi-professional team and often requires the input of many disciplines to appropriately and thoroughly manage "pain-like" behaviours. A stepwise (Gai et al., 2020), multi-professional trial and error approach using available assessment tools is needed, along with close communication between clinicians and patients/family members (Table 7.4).

While collaborative decision-making with members of the healthcare team may not always be possible, it is essential to involve the child and family in the decision-making process. Factors for consideration in prescribing which are essential for safe prescribing and working within the parameters of the nursing professional code of conduct and non-medical prescribing must include thoughtful consideration of a thorough history and nursing assessment. Collaboration with the parents and family is essential as well as a visual assessment using non-verbal cues and observation, excellent communication including curious questions and inclusion of the multi-professional approach and management and parallel planning and consideration of the non-pharmacological management. Critical and clinical observations and considerations are dilemmas that must be respectful of the role of a parent in protecting and advocating for their child. A parent will become expert in leading and navigating their child's care, learning how to navigate the systems, processes and possibly multi-professional teams and indeed organisations, if care is shared locally and possibly regionally and indeed nationally. Advocating and protecting on behalf of their child may include treatment options and choices and making decisions regarding weighing the risks and burden of treatment versus the quality of life and impact on the child and family. This will be constant, continued and will reflect the family's cultural choices and religious beliefs and the impact of the illness which will change over time. Each disease has its own biosocial impact and context on the individual

**TABLE 7.4** Pain management (adapted from Anekar et al., 2023; Gai et al., 2020)

| Escalating pain | Uncontrolled pain | Consider: invasive and minimally invasive treatments |
|---|---|---|
| | Level of pain: moderate– severe | Analgesia to consider: opioid +/– non-opioid analgesia +/– adjuvant |
| | Level of pain: mild–moderate | Analgesia to consider: opioid +/– non-opioid analgesia +/– adjuvant |
| | Level of pain: mild | Analgesia to consider: non opioid analgesia +/– adjuvant |

child and family and the disease events and trajectory will influence the decision-making process and highlight the need for engagement and collaboration and a co-production between the child, family and multi-professional individuals and teams in planning safe, effective, and consistent care.

Communication and trust are key as the relationship will be complex and need skill to manage a divergence of assessment when disease progression is evident. There will be a need for the family to normalise this and a need for the professional to manage this effectively and compassionately but address competently the next steps of care and management plans, so that continued engagement is achieved and supported by the family. Synergy and integration of all care providers, inclusion of all care settings and multi-professional teams and a comprehensive care approach will maintain functionality of the symptom management plan. Most importantly, the ultimate goal through engagement and confidence from the family will result in the best outcome and best quality care for the child and young person. Equally, the clinician's decision-making and multi-professional approach will marry with a similar rigorous questioning and reflective theme, acknowledging their professional code of conduct, society's perception of their clinical decision-making, the moral and ethical considerations of treatment versus impact and effect on the child and family and legal and moral beliefs and obligations. Finally, their clinical expertise and experience will influence care and decision-making and wanting to make the right and best choices for the child predominantly with due care and consideration of the family (Bluebond-Langner et al., 2017). Due diligence and consideration of the underlying principles of palliative medicine are required to balance burden and benefit and to have a rational approach with a multi-professional decision-making concept and process, a holistic approach. Beauchamp and Childress (2019) describe four principles which include an obligation to do good, non-maleficence (avoiding harm), respecting autonomy (and valuing the patient and individual and justice as fairness) and giving equal value to patients. These principles underpin the professional obligation to work as a multi-professional team around the child and family, ensuring that care planning is guided by these values and the nurse within their professional capacity is a reflective practitioner with a moral compass and professional commitment to advocate for the child and family and work within the professional scope and code of practice.

## 6. Prescribing: factors affecting prescribing and considerations for practice

Key considerations for practice include pharmacodynamics, the biochemical and physiological effect on drugs on the body and pharmacokinetics, how the body interacts with a substance (Table 7.5).

Opioids must only be used for appropriate indications and prescribed in accordance with prescribing practice and professional bodies, with careful assessments of the benefits and risks (Box 7.14).

**TABLE 7.5** The principles of pharmacokinetics include absorption, distribution, metabolism and elimination (adapted from Grogan and Preuss, 2023)

| | |
|---|---|
| Absorption | *Affecting factors*<br>• The extent to which a drug is absorbed<br>• The maturation of the gastrointestinal tract<br>• Digestion<br>• Absorption |
| Distribution | The route within the bloodstream: fat-soluble or water-soluble<br>Water-soluble: distributes mainly into the bloodstream and aqueous environments<br>Fat-soluble: distributes in fatty tissue/cells with fatty sheaths<br>Fat-soluble drug calculations are made on body weight, the child's weight in relation to age needs to be reviewed. Consider the child's age, weight, fragility and instability<br>Blood-brain barrier: substances in solution and fat-soluble compounds can pass through the barrier but larger molecules are excluded |
| Metabolism | Drug is broken down into active substances<br>Age: newborns and infants have immature liver function so have a higher risk of adverse reaction to drugs with a long half-life. The half-life of a drug is the time it takes for its effectiveness to be reduced by half. When changing opioids, for example, the half-life and time the drug takes to have an effect (time to onset of action) need to be considered, to ensure the child is not over- or under-dosed during the conversion period (Joint Formulary Committee, 2024). |
| Elimination | Metabolism and excretion of the drug through the kidneys and, to a smaller degree, into the bile, saliva, tears, sweat and breast milk<br>Any renal dysfunction, including Immature kidneys of young children, may result in delayed elimination of the drug molecules and drug toxicity concentrations<br>Drug clearance is the volume of blood (or plasma) from which a drug is removed per unit of time |

---

**BOX 7.14 UNDESIRABLE SIDE EFFECTS OF OPIOIDS**

- Drowsiness
- Confusion
- Nausea and vomiting
- Gastrointestinal tract – reduced motility
- Dry mouth
- Pruritus
- Sweating/change in core body temperature
- Respiratory depression
- Reduced oxygen saturation
- Reduced blood pressure

Continuous monitoring, evaluation and assessment must be maintained and communicated within the multi-professional team and organisations participating in active management of the child's care (Box 7.15). Active communication with the family, monitoring the impact on pain and any adverse effects and complying with safe prescribing practice and legislation is essential. A clear plan for the continuation and any adjustments or discontinuation of drugs according to the child's condition must be recorded and shared with the multi-professional team with due diligence in sharing information and guidance with the child and family regarding safe storage and disposal. Barriers to managing effective pain control should be considered by the nurse making the assessment.

---

**BOX 7.15 CONSIDERATIONS**

Has there been any of the following?:

- Denial or lack of acknowledgement of pain.
- A multi-disciplinary team discussion and a decision reached.
- A lack of acknowledgement of psychological, social and cultural aspects of pain.
- Anxiety over side effects or fear of harm.
- Nurse or family misunderstanding or lack of knowledge.
- Lack of acceptance by the family that escalation of analgesia is required.
- Issues surrounding abuse or addiction or fear of this.
- Exclusion of non-pharmacological measures.
- Parental denial, including identifying pain as deterioration.
- Denial by parents, causally linking pain as a sign of deterioration.

Source: adapted from Grégoire and Frager (2006).

---

Holistic assessment of the patient must include observing their physical, emotional, and behavioural changes from the onset of the pain management plan commencing. This must be frequently monitored with clinical observation including face-to-face clinical review and telephone/virtual review, if available. Clinical signs of deterioration will include their emotional, physical, spiritual, religious, cultural and psychological well-being in addition to consideration of the physiological assessment in Box 7.16.

---

**BOX 7.16 ASSESSMENT OF EFFECTIVENESS OF INTERVENTION**

- Age
- Weight
- Oral absorption, capacity and effect, including nausea and vomiting
- Allergies

- Availability of drugs and administration routes
- Concomitant drugs
- Variable gastric and intestinal transit time
- Increased gastric pH (consideration that gastric acid output does not reach adult values until the second year of life)
- Gastrointestinal contents including oral feeds and posturing
- Disease state/progression/organ failure/gut failure, therapeutic interventions (consideration of drug therapy which may affect the absorption process)
- Total body weight (consideration of total body water and extracellular fluid volume, dosing in obesity, permanent/partial immobility and/or non-weight-bearing. Patients requiring children's palliative care may have atypical weight in relation to age and weight or body composition. This means that ideal body weight or adjusted body weight should be used to calculate the doses of certain drugs (APPM, 2024).
- Is the child experiencing end-of-life symptoms?
- Decreased plasma protein may alter binding capacity.
- High circulating bilirubin levels may displace drugs from albumin.
- Metabolic rate in children will be greater than in adults and mature at different times and may be absent at birth. Children may therefore require more frequent dosing or higher doses on an mg/kg basis.
- Renal function and excretion.
- Route of administration and drug regimes.
- Compliance, influenced by the formulation, taste, appearance, and ease of administration.
- Prescribed regimens should be tailored to the child's daily routine (Paediatric Formulary Committee, 2020; APPM, 2024) ensuring that there is adequate information to support the quality, efficacy, safety and intended use of a drug before prescribing it.
- Paediatric doses should be obtained from a paediatric dosage reference text and not extrapolated from the adult dose.
- Adverse drug reaction profiles in children may differ from those seen in adults. The action of the drug and its pharmacokinetics in children, especially in the very young, may be different from that in adults. Drugs are not extensively tested in children.
- Drug safety in the home (Paediatric Formulary Committee, 2020).

Paediatric prescribing progress has been made which is encouraging and has led to better pain and overall symptom management, reducing the burden of poor and inadequate under-prescribing and under-dosing.

## 7. Non-pharmacological interventions

In addition to treatment directed at identified causes of pain, optimal pain management requires a comprehensive approach, combining opioid, adjuvant, and non-pharmacological strategies (Grégoire and Frager, 2006). It is also a major adjuvant therapy in managing the holistic needs of the patients and supporting the family.

Non-pharmacological interventions can be defined as "complementary interventions within the nursing scope of practice". Non-pharmacological interventions can be adapted according to palliative patients' needs and give an element of control and active participation and management of their care planning (van Veen et al., 2024). Complementary therapies allow the parent or carer to proactively participate in the pain management plan, which in turn soothes and comforts both the child and the carer themselves. Examples of these therapies include touch and massage, swaddling, audio therapy and storytelling. The latter two are particularly useful when being touched is too painful or uncomfortable (Cancer Research UK, 2022).

Non-pharmacological interventions can be divided into three categories: physical comforts, distraction, and cognitive behavioural methods (Scrace, 2003). Similarly to pain measurement tools, non-pharmacological interventions need to be adapted to the child's development, capacity, ability, and mobility. Integration and consideration of both are essential in effective and holistic care planning and management. Integrative methods of pain management encompass methods that integrate physical and psychological approaches and include, for example, swaddling, rocking, repositioning hypnosis, relaxation, music therapy and audio therapy.

When caring for patients with pain, it is also important to consider psychosocial factors that will impact how a patient experiences pain. It has been established that anxiety, catastrophising and depression can affect how a patient experiences pain and can aggravate or prolong acute pain (Martin et al., 2007). Such factors as anxiety and mood should be observed, screened, and recorded, either by simple observation of the patient and their interactions, or from direct questions if there is suspicion of severe anxiety or depression. Subsequent strategies must be tailored to each individual patient and severity of symptoms (Martin et al., 2007). Management may include giving the patient a chance to voice their concerns, validate their fears, by reassuring them by reviewing their pain plan. For severe anxiety or depression, a psychiatrist may be consulted for pharmacologic or non-pharmacologic strategies.

There are two ways to classify non-pharmacological interventions: therapeutic input or working mechanisms (Box 7.17) (van Veen et al., 2024).

---

**BOX 7.17 NON-PHARMACOLOGICAL INTERVENTIONS CLASSIFIED BY WORKING MECHANISMS**

1. Mind–body interventions such as meditation, are based on the human mind and affect the human body and physical health.
2. Biologically based treatments involve natural substances, such as herbs or essential oils.
3. Manipulative and body-based practices, such as massage therapy, consist of therapies involving movement or manipulation of one or more parts of the patient's body.
4. Energy therapies, such as Reiki or therapeutic touch, are defined as influencing and applying energy fields to the body.

If appropriate, timely and considered alternatives should be part of the nursing assessment and inclusion of the holistic needs of the child and family, addressing the values, wishes, and needs of patients and their carers. Patients could learn to apply some of the interventions themselves or have them performed by their informal caregiver without the interference of a nurse. The overall benefits empower the child and family to have an immediate influence on the pain which is supportive of their autonomy and overall well-being. These are all crucial factors in addressing pain and symptom management and enabling a proactive and unified approach and therefore giving ownership, control, and choices back to the patient and their family. It can add value to a pain management plan by providing extra relief measures as well as reducing the doses of medication and potential side effect burden. The negative impacts of chronic pain also extend to family members who report a higher burden of care and a detrimental effect on family function (Box 7.18 and Box 7.19).

---

**BOX 7.18 POPPY'S STORY**

At 4 years of age, Poppy has metastatic refractory neuroblastoma. She has had multi-modal treatment including chemotherapy, surgery, radiotherapy, and stem cell transplant. Her disease is progressing, and oral palliative chemotherapy is no longer effective. Her pain is escalating and uncontrolled, she is inconsolable and anxious, and family distress is heightened. In considering the WHO analgesic ladder, consider the classifications of pain and management choices with specific focus on acute, chronic, and chronic primary pain. Chronic primary pain is multifactorial: biological, psychological, and social factors contribute to the pain syndrome.

Care and management must be culturally competent, appropriate, and tailored to the family's values, preferences, and resources. Care expectations must be addressed with honesty and shared decision-making. They must also be adaptive to promote engagement and support Poppy and her family to play an active role in care through informed and shared decision-making. Full assessment of her sleep pattern and physical ability will need addressing as typically children with moderate and severe pain experience physical immobility and disability, heightened emotional distress and anxiety where depression may also be experienced. Assessment is therefore holistic in its approach and focused on the biopsychosocial model of pain which supports the use of multiple modalities to address the management of chronic and complex pain. Adjuvants such as diazepam and or midazolam could also be considered.

First-line agents include gabapentinoids and tricyclic antidepressants (TCAs), with clonidine, methadone, ketamine and cannabinoids could be considered using the guidance of the WHO analgesic ladder if initial therapy fails (see Gai et al., 2020).

---

**BOX 7.19 ABDUL'S STORY**

Abdul is a 14-year-old young man with metastatic Ewings sarcoma of his femur. He has been managing full-time education until recently when his third relapse resulted in increased pain, reduced mobility and psychological distress and anxiety. He is aware that he is not getting better and that his prognosis is poor. Both Abdul and his family are aware that he is palliative. Both parents are engaging in open dialogue with the healthcare professionals and his two younger brothers are also aware that Abdul is getting increasingly worse.

He has been admitted to the teenage and young adults' oncology unit for symptom control and reassessment and is keen to be discharged home as soon as a management plan is established.

The use of gabapentinoids and local topical analgesic patches are supporting the symptom care plan as he is reluctant to take breakthrough opioids as this affects his studies which he is keen to continue. This management plan also supports his quality of life and social and psychological well-being. He is less mobile, and constipation is a symptom he has experienced and is anxious to avoid. He has requested to manage his medication plan, with support and supervision from his parents and has stated that he does not want a burdensome medication regime.

He has shared that he has heightened anxiety at bedtime and is experiencing sleep disturbance, feeling breathless periodically during the day.

To accomplish total pain management, a multimodal approach should be considered which may consist of an opioid, with adjuvant drugs, like anticonvulsants, antidepressants and NSAIDS. Due to its proven analgesic effect in several types of neuropathic pain, its good tolerability, and a rarity of drug-drug interactions, the addition of adjuvants such as ketamine and lidocaine are considerations as the third-line therapy by the WHO pain ladder modified for Acute Pain Management. Adjuncts include non-opioid analgesics such as ketamine, lidocaine, and gabapentinoids (Gai et al., 2020).

There is good evidence that the addition of a benzodiazepine can be effective in managing episodic stressors and insomnia. Benzodiazepines do not relieve breathlessness, but anxiolytics do have a role when anxiety exacerbates breathlessness.

At the end-of-life stage, considerations in the above examples will require compassionate conversations with the family to re-orientate the goal of care planning to achieve maximum quality and minimum distress. This may also reduce the burden of medications and medication regimes to prioritise comfort and reduce anxiety, distress, breathlessness, agitation and pain. Opioid switching should be considered if pain management is no longer effective. There may be a requirement for anxiolytics and/or sedation if seizure activity due to metastatic disease in the brain is evident. This may include continuous infusions with a combination of analgesics, anxiolytics and anti-seizure medication. Parallel holistic care planning must also remain inclusive of comfort care, spiritual care and non-pharmacological interventions and therapies, empowering the family to be pivotal and integral in the child's end-of-life care planning.

## END-OF-LIFE CARE

By "end-of-life care", we are referring to the last hours to days of life. For some children there may not be many changes or signs which herald this but there are some poignant signals which need extra attention, as well as accelerations in support and management. Good practice and planning here say that, by the time this phase occurs, there have already been discussions about place of care, goals of care, use of therapies and the importance of rituals and customs for each family (Hain et al., 2021).

As death draws near, breathing may become noticeably different such as "Cheyne-Stokes" breathing where rapid breaths are followed by apnoea – this can be for a matter of minutes but can also extend for days. The child may have increasingly laboured or shallow breathing with an accompanying dry mouth and lips and additional noises in breathing. It's best to try and avoid the term "death rattle" but for some families they will know this term. While the child is generally unconscious, it is an awful symptom to observe and should be managed promptly. Clarity with the family about these symptoms and what they represent is important preparation and provides opportunity for expression of feelings and our ability to respond and support. They need reassurance that many of these symptoms are not distressing for the child and are an expected part of the dying process.

It is expected that in the last hours to days there will be circulatory changes where the heart rate is slow and irregular and results in the appearance of a cool, pale, cyanotic and sometime sweaty child. Their pupils may become dilated and fixed, with eyes that appear sunken or, in some tumours, bulging. Incontinence may occur as the body functions change and consciousness drops, and this should be planned for with simple attention to linen, disposable draw sheets and continence pads/nappies. These changes require a calm, attentive response and explanation of their end-of-life connections.

Most children will become sleepier or are unconscious at this time, but others may remain alert and responsive. Some can become agitated for a variety of reasons related to unrelieved symptoms, medication side effects, disease progressions and psychological/spiritual distress. Attention to meticulous symptom management and a reassuring environment is paramount, but even so additional sedation for this time may be needed.

## Nursing assessment

A nursing assessment of a child's symptoms at the end-of-life stage is multi-faceted and includes baseline observations, clarification of normal behaviours and responses to pain and a symptom history. The assessment begins on the approach to meeting the child and family, observing, for example, how the child has positioned themselves, their facial expressions and family member interactions. It is important to consider what language might be appropriate for an individual child, which might be informed by their prior experience of pain or the type of words they have previously used to describe their pain. Curious questioning alongside active listening can help elicit a picture of the child's experience of the symptom and aid clarification of the onset, duration, fluctuations and aggravating and alleviating factors. During the assessment itself, a child might not report or may minimise severity of symptoms for a range of reasons, such as fear that this will lead to cessation of treatment or of upsetting a family member. This highlights the need for careful assessment of the wider dimensions such as the severity, frequency, trajectory and impact of a symptom. It is recognised that self-reporting may not always be feasible in children's palliative care, for example, communication can be impacted by the age or health. However, there is evidence to support that both child and proxy, for example, family, reports are valid (Theunissen et al., 1998). While a well-executed assessment will inform clinical decision-making, a nurse's intuition may also play a role. Intuition, a feeling or knowing, draws on knowledge and experience and, when combined with evidence-based practice, can aid assessment and decision-making processes (Melin-Johansson et al., 2017).

## Management

- Engage with calmness, honesty, and reassurance.
- Ensure that families are prepared ahead of time for these symptoms, including with a care pack and a written plan to manage them, and how to call for help.
- Be ready for potential requirement to transition to another care setting per family wishes, coping or clinical burden.
- Ensure that pain and fear/distress are well managed, including the suffering of the family.
- Ensure good regular gentle eye and mouth care.
- Address cyanosis with honesty and reassurance that this is not experienced by the child; but meet the family's need by covering the child with blankets, use warm, blush-coloured pillowcases and gentle washes.
- Position child so that they are lying on their side, with head tilted down if this is comfortable; this may reduce the noise of secretions.
- Reduce artificial hydration to minimise secretions and/or use anti-cholinergic medication to dry residual troublesome secretions up and minimise use of suction.
- Discuss cessation of artificial nutrition sensitively with links to absorption burden, (potential) discomfort and lack of hunger at this time.
- If ventilation devices are in use, careful exploration of what it means to redirect care with additional opioids/sedation may be required.
- Redirection of attention and the soothing role of the calming environment are often important; think about what the child and family can *see, hear, smell, feel* and what adds comfort to that. It may be that there is some favourite music to play, some reassuring prayer as appropriate, reading a much-loved story, making sure that there is a fresh breeze or a warm cuddle rug for the parents, talking to the child about a favourite memory, ensuring that at all times everyone is positioned as comfortably and close as they'd like to be.
- Use of sedation may need to be considered and, at this time, it may be best administered via buccal, intranasal, or parenteral route as the gastro-intestinal system shuts down.
- Provide frequent assessment and intensify support; if at home consider availability of extra nursing respite.
- Prepare for after-death management, ensure that you understand regulations, expectations and customs/rituals, ensure that care team and family are appropriately aware of choices and practicalities.

## SUMMARY

The nurse has a multi-dimensional role which is unique and requires skills which are qualitative and become inherent through learning, reflection and a sound knowledge and research base. Expertise does not always lie within the capabilities and accountabilities of prescribing practice or theorist knowledge but in the fundamental exploratory bedside ability to engage with and support the parent/s or carers to work in collaboration with each other in making the total and holistic assessment. Nurses should draw on their confidence and courage to be alongside the child and family in the quiet moments. This will use core skills and knowledge with experiential reference to learning and acquired knowledge where a trusting, open, honest and professional relationship will be key in managing the palliative care needs of the child and family. Communication is key within the nurse's expertise and management to have the ability to negotiate and navigate both the patient's and the parents; perspective to have a perception and understanding of the family's narrative and need. With professional advocacy, competence and confidence, the nurse will analyse and synthesise these unique and holistic care needs to the multi-professional team, demonstrating and coordinating the specific narrative of their palliative care needs enabling a collaborative multi-professional pathway of care to be delivered, empowering the patient and healthcare professionals. This unique, individualised and intimate knowledge of the child and family will underpin the foundation and continuity of care.

Thorough exploration and inclusion of the parent in the assessment, planning of care and transition enables a sense of hope and further supports the notion and belief of the concept of total pain, revealing that physical, spiritual, emotional, and psychosocial care play a vital role in care planning and evaluating palliative care.

## KEY POINTS

- Clear compassionate communication about goals of care.
- Meticulous assessment.
- Holistic multifaceted management across teams and disciplines.
- Ongoing re-assessment.
- Anticipation and preparation.

## SUGGESTED READING

Amery, J. (2016). *A practical handbook of children's palliative care for doctors and nurses anywhere in the world*. Lulu Publishing Services.

APPM Master Formulary. (2024). 6th edn. Available at: https://www.appm.org.uk/_webedit/uploaded-files/All%20Files/Formulary/Formulary%202024/APPM%20formulary%206th%20edition%202024%20Final%202023-10-26.pdf

Hain, R., Goldman, A., Rapoport, A., Meiring, M. (eds) (2021). *Oxford textbook of palliative care for children*. Oxford University Press.

# REFERENCES

Ahmedzai, S. H., Boland, J. (2010). Constipation in people prescribed opioids. *Clinical Evidence*, 04, 2407.

Akyempon, A. N., Aladangady, N. (2021). Neonatal and perinatal palliative care pathway: A tertiary neonatal unit approach. *BMJ Paediatrics Open*, 5: e000820. https://doi.org/10.1136/bmjpo-2020-000820

American Academy of Pediatrics Committee on Psychosocial Aspects of Child and Family Health. (2001). The new morbidity revisited: A renewed commitment to the psychosocial aspects of pediatric care. *Pediatrics*, 108(5), 1227–1230. https://doi.org/10.1542/peds.108.5.1227

Amery, J. (2016). *A practical handbook of children's palliative care for doctors and nurses anywhere in the world.* Lulu Publishing Services. Available at: https://icpcn.org/wp-content/uploads/2023/01/A-REALLY-PRACTICAL-Handbook-of-CPC.pdf (accessed 6 June 2024).

Andersen, R. D., Langius-Eklöf, A., Nakstad, B., Bernklev, T., Jylli, L. (2017). The measurement properties of pediatric observational pain scales: A systematic review of reviews. *International Journal of Nursing Studies*, 73, 93–101. https://doi.org/10.1016/j.ijnurstu.2017.05.010

Anderson, A. K., Burke, K., Bendle, L., Koh, M., McCulloch, R., Breen, M. (2021). Artificial nutrition and hydration for children and young people towards end-of-life: Consensus guidelines across four specialist paediatric palliative care centres. *BMJ Supportive & Palliative Care*, 11(1), 92–100. https://doi.org/10.1136/bmjspcare-2019-001909

Anekar, A. A., Hendrix, J. M., Cascella, M. (2023). WHO Analgesic Ladder. StatPearls Publishing. Available at: https://www.ncbi.nlm.nih.gov/books/NBK554435/ (accessed 6 June 2024).

APPM (Association for Paediatric Palliative Medicine). (2023a). Clinical guidelines: Agitation. Available at: https://www.appm.org.uk/_webedit/uploaded-files/All%20Files/Clinical%20guidelines/Agitation%20Clinical%20guidelines%20APPM.pdf (accessed 6 June 2024).

APPM (Association for Paediatric Palliative Medicine). (2023b). Clinical guidelines: Seizure. Available at: https://www.appm.org.uk/_webedit/uploaded-files/All%20Files/Clinical%20guidelines/Seizures_Clinical%20guidelines%20APPM.pdf (accessed 6 June 2024).

APPM (Association for Paediatric Palliative Medicine). (2024). APPM Master Formulary (6th edn). Available at:. https://www.appm.org.uk/_webedit/uploaded-files/All%20Files/Formulary/Formulary%202024/APPM%20formulary%206th%20edition%202024%20Final%202023-10-26.pdf (accessed 6 June 2024).

Beauchamp, T., Childress, J. (2019). Principles of biomedical ethics: Marking Its Fortieth Anniversary. *The American Journal of Bioethics*, 19(11), 9–12. https://doi.org/10.1080/15265161.2019.1665402

Benini, F., Orzalesi, M., de Santi, A., Congedi, S., Lazzarin, P., Pellegatta, F., DeZen, L., Spizzichino, M., Alleva, E. (2016). Barriers to the development of pediatric palliative care in Italy. *Annali dell'Istituto superiore di sanita*, 52(4), 558–564. https://doi.org/10.4415/ann_16_04_16

Bergstraesser, E., Hain, R. D., Pereira, J. L. (2013). The development of an instrument that can identify children with palliative care needs: The Paediatric Palliative Screening Scale (PaPaS Scale): A qualitative study approach. *BMC Palliative Care*, 12, 1–14. https://doi.org/10.1186/1472-684X-12-20

Bergstraesser, E., Paul, M., Rufibach, K., Hain, R. D., Held, L. (2014). The Paediatric Palliative Screening Scale: Further validity testing. *Palliative Medicine*, 28(6), 530–533. https://doi.org/10.1177/0269216313512886

Birnie, K. A., Hundert, A. S., Lalloo, C., Nguyen, C., Stinson, J. N. (2019). Recommendations for selection of self-report pain intensity measures in children and adolescents: A systematic review and quality assessment of measurement properties. *Pain, 160*(1), 5–18. https://doi.org/10.1097/j.pain.0000000000001377

Bluebond-Langner M., Hargrave, D., Henderson, E.M., Langner, R. (2017). 'I have to live with the decisions I make': Laying a foundation for decision making for children with life-limiting conditions and life-threatening illnesses. *Archives in Disease in Childhood, 10*(2), 468–471. https://doi.org/10.1136/archdischild-2015-310345

Bowden, V. R., Greenberg, C. S. (2014). *Children and their families: The continuum of nursing care* (3rd edn). Lippincott Williams & Wilkins.

Cancer Research UK. (2022). Using complementary therapies when you are dying. Available at: https://www.cancerresearchuk.org/about-cancer/coping/dying-with-cancer/last-few-weeks-and-days/complementary-therapies (accessed 6 June 2024).

Craig, K. D. (2020). A child in pain: A psychologist's perspective on changing priorities in scientific understanding and clinical care. *Paediatric and Neonatal Pain, 2*, 40–49. https://doi.org/10.1002/pne2.12034

Duc, J. K., Herbert, A. R., Heussler, H. S. (2017). Paediatric palliative care and intellectual disability: A unique context. *Journal of Applied Research in Intellectual Disabilities, 30*(6), 1111–1124. https://doi.org/10.1111/jar.12389

Eilers, J., Berger, A. M., Petersen, M. C. (1988). Development, testing, and application of the oral assessment guide. *Oncology Nursing Forum, 15*(3), 325–330. Oncology Nursing Society.

Eilers, J., Harris, D., Henry, K., Johnson, L. (2014). Evidence-based interventions for cancer treatment-related mucositis: Putting evidence into practice. *Clinical Journal of Oncology Nursing, 18*(6), 80–96. https://doi.org/10.1188/14.CJON.S3.80-96

Feudtner, C., Nye, R., Hill, D. L., Hall, M., Hinds, P., Johnston, E. E., Friebert, S., Hays, R., Kang, T. I., Wolfe, J., Crew, K. (2021). Polysymptomatology in pediatric patients receiving palliative care based on parent-reported data. *JAMA Network Open, 4*(8), e2119730. https://doi.org/10.1001/jamanetworkopen.2021.19730

Friedrichsdorf, S. J. (2010). Pain management in children with advanced cancer and during end-of-life care. *Pediatric Hematology and Oncology, 27*(4), 257–261. https://doi.org/10.3109/08880011003663416

Friedrichsdorf, S. J., Bruera, E. (2018). Delivering pediatric palliative care: From denial, palliphobia, pallilalia to palliative. *Children, 5*(9), 120. https://doi.org/10.3390/children5090120

Gai, N., Naser, B., Hanley, J., Peliowski, A., Hayes, J., Aoyama, K. (2020). A practical guide to acute pain management in children. *Journal of Anesthesia, 34*, 421–433. https://doi.org/10.1007/s00540-020-02767-x

Galloway, K. S., Yaster, M. (2000). Pain and symptom control in terminally ill children. *Pediatric Clinics of North America, 47*(3), 711–746. https://doi.org/10.1016/S0031-3955(05)70234-0

Greenfield, K., Holley, S., Schoth, D. E., Harrop, E., Howard, R. F., Bayliss, J., Brook, L., Jassal, S. S., Johnson, M., Wong, I., Liossi, C. (2020). A mixed-methods systematic review and meta-analysis of barriers and facilitators to paediatric symptom management at end-of-life. *Palliative Medicine, 34*(6), 689–707. https://doi.org/10.1177/0269216320907065

Grégoire, M. C., Frager, G. (2006). Ensuring pain relief for children at the end-of-life. *Pain Research and Management, 11*, 163–171. https://doi.org/10.1155%2F2006%2F608536

Grogan, S., Preuss, C. V. (2023). Pharmacokinetics. StatPearls Publishing. Available at: http://www.ncbi.nlm.nih.gov/books/nbk557744/

Gwyther, L., Brennan, F., Harding, R. (2009). Advancing palliative care as a human right. *Journal of Pain and Symptom Management, 38*(5), 767–774. https://doi.org/10.1016/j.jpainsymman.2009.03.003

Hallyburton, A. (2022). Diagnostic overshadowing: An evolutionary concept analysis on the misattribution of physical symptoms to pre-existing psychological illnesses. *International Journal of Mental Health Nursing, 31*, 1360–1372. https://doi.org/10.1111/inm.13034

Hain, R., Goldman, A., Rapoport, A., Meiring, M. (eds) (2021). *Oxford textbook of palliative care for children.* Oxford University Press.

Hicks, C. L., von Baeyer, C. L., Spafford, P. A., van Korlaar, I., Goodenough, B. (2001). The Faces Pain Scale–Revised: Toward a common metric in pediatric pain measurement. *Pain, 93*(2), 173–183. https://doi.org/10.1016/S0304-3959(01)00314-1

Hockenberry-Eaton, M., Hinds, P., Howard, V., Gattuso, J., O'Neill, J. B., Alcoser, P., Euell, K. (1999). Developing a conceptual model for fatigue in children. *European Journal of Oncology Nursing, 3*(1), 5–11. https://doi.org/10.1016/1462-3889(91)80005-7

Howard, R. F., Liossi, C. (2014). Pain assessment in children. *Archives of Disease in Childhood, 99*(12), 1123–1124. https://doi.org/10.1136/archdischild-2014-306432

Hunt, A., Goldman, A., Seers, K., Crichton, N., Mastroyannopoulou, K., Moffat, V., ... Brady, M. (2004). Clinical validation of the paediatric pain profile. *Developmental Medicine and Child Neurology, 46*(1), 9–18. https://doi.org/10.1111/j.1469-8749.2004.tb00428.x

International Children's Palliative Care Network. (2022). Global levels of service provision. Available at: https://icpcn.org/map-of-services/ (accessed 5 June 2024).

Jassal, S. (2022). Basic symptom control in paediatric palliative care (10th edn). Available at: https://www.togetherforshortlives.org.uk/app/uploads/2022/05/Basic-Symptom-Control-in-Paediatric-Palliaitive-Care-2022.pdf (accessed 6 June 2024).

Joint Formulary Committee. (2024). British National Formulary (online). BMJ and Pharmaceutical Press. Available at: https://bnf.nice.org.uk/

Krasaelap, A. (2023). Understanding pediatric dysphagia: A multi-disciplinary approach. *Current Pediatrics Reports, 11*(4), 1–8. https://doi.org/10.1007/s40124-023-00311-5

Lazzarin, P., Giacomelli, L., Terrenato, I., Benini, F., ACCAPED Study Group. (2021). A tool for the evaluation of clinical needs and eligibility to pediatric palliative care: The validation of the ACCAPED scale. *Journal of Palliative Medicine, 24*(2), 205–210. https://doi.org/10.1089/jpm.2020.0148

Lewis, S. J., Heaton, K. W. (1997). Stool form scale as a useful guide to intestinal transit time. *Scandinavian Journal of Gastroenterology, 32*(9), 920–924.

Liben, S. (1996). Pediatric palliative medicine: Obstacles to overcome. *Journal of Palliative Care, 12*(3), 24–28. https://doi.org/10.1177/082585979601200306

Mahant, S., Cohen, E., Nelson, K. E., Rosenbaum, P. (2018). Decision-making around gastrostomy tube feeding in children with neurologic impairment: Engaging effectively with families. *Paediatrics & Child Health, 23*(3), 209–213. https://doi.org/10.1093/pch/pxx193

Mahant, S., Meiring, M., Rapoport, A. (2021). Feeding, cachexia, and malnutrition in children's palliative care. In R. Hain, A. Rapoport, M. Meiring, A. Goldman (eds), *Oxford textbook of palliative care for children* (pp. 231–243). Oxford University Press.

Malviya, S., Vopel-Lewis, T. E. R. R. I., Burke, C., Merkel, S., Tait, A. R. (2006). The revised FLACC observational pain tool: Improved reliability and validity for pain assessment in children with cognitive impairment. *Pediatric Anesthesia, 16*(3), 258–265. https://doi.org/10.1111/j.1460-9592.2005.01773.x

Marston, J., Boucher, S., Downing, J., Nkosi, B., Steel, B. (2013). International children's palliative care network: Working together to stop children's suffering. *European Journal of Palliative Care, 20*(6), 308–310. https://doi.org/10.1016/j.jpainsymman.2017.03.024

Martin, A. L., McGrath, P. A., Brown, S. C., Katz, J. (2007). Anxiety sensitivity, fear of pain and pain-related disability in children and adolescents with chronic pain. *Pain Research and Management, 12*, 267–272. https://doi.org/10.1155/2007/897395

Melin-Johansson, C., Palmqvist, R., Rönnberg, L. (2017). Clinical intuition in the nursing process and decision-making: A mixed-studies review. *Journal of Clinical Nursing, 26*(23–24), 3936–3949. https://doi.org/10.1111/jocn.13814

Mink, J. W., Zinner, S. H. (2010). Movement disorders II: Chorea, dystonia, myoclonus, and tremor. *Pediatrics in Review, 31*(7), 287–295. https://doi.org/10.1542/pir.31-7-287

Namisango, E., Bristowe, K., Allsop, M.J., Murtagh, F. E. M., Abas, M., Higginson, I. J., Downing, J., Harding, R. (2019). Symptoms and concerns among children and young people with life-limiting and life-threatening conditions: A systematic review highlighting meaningful health outcomes. *The Patient: Patient-Centered Outcomes Research*, 12(1): 15–55. https://doi.org/10.1007/s40271-018-0333-5

Nap-van der Vlist, M. M., Dalmeijer, G. W., Grootenhuis, M. A., van der Ent, K., Van den Heuvel-Eibrink, M. M., Swart, J. F., Nijhof, S. L. (2021). Fatigue among children with a chronic disease: A cross-sectional study. *BMJ Paediatrics Open*, 5(1). https://doi.org/10.1 136%2Fbmjpo-2020-000958

New Zealand Child Youth Clinical Networks. (2022a). Approach to palliative care emergencies. Available at: https://starship.org.nz/guidelines/palliative-care-emergencies-approach-to/ (accessed 6 June 2024).

New Zealand Child Youth Clinical Networks. (2022b). Massive bleeding at the end-of-life. Available at: https://starship.org.nz/guidelines/massive-bleeding-management-of-the-palliative-patient/ (accessed 6 June 2024).

New Zealand Child Youth Clinical Networks. (2022c). Bowel obstruction management in the palliative patient. Available at: https://starship.org.nz/guidelines/bowel-obstruction-management-in-the-palliative-patient/ (accessed 6 June 2024).

New Zealand Child Youth Clinical Networks. (2022d). Breathlessness management in the palliative patient. Available at: https://starship.org.nz/guidelines/breathlessness-management-in-the-palliative-patient/ (accessed 6 June 2024).

New Zealand Child Youth Clinical Networks. (2022e). Seizure management at the end-of-life. Available at: https://starship.org.nz/guidelines/seizure-management-in-the-palliative-patient (accessed 6 June 2024).

Paediatric Formulary Committee. (2020). *BNF for children* (online). BMJ, Pharmaceutical Press and RCPCH Publications. https://bnfc.nice.org.uk/

Paediatric Palliative Care Australia and New Zealand. (2023). *A practical guide to palliative care in paediatrics* (4th edn). Palliative Care Australia. Available at: https://paediatricpalliativecare.org.au/download/5736/ (accessed 6 June 2024).

Papa, S., Mercante, A., Giacomelli, L., Benini, F. (2023). Pediatric palliative care: Insights into assessment tools and review instruments. *Children*, 10(8), 1406. https://doi.org/10.3390/children10081406

Pieper, L., Zernikow, B., Drake, R., Frosch, M., Printz, M., Wager, J. (2018). Dyspnea in children with life-threatening and life-limiting complex chronic conditions. *Journal of Palliative Medicine*, 21(4), 552–564. https://doi.org/10.1089/jpm.2017.0240

Preece, J. (2002). Introducing abdominal massage in palliative care for the relief of constipation. *Complementary Therapies in Nursing and Midwifery*, 8(2), 101–105. https://doi.org/10.1054/ctnm.2002.0610

Raja, S. N., Carr, D. B., Cohen, M., Finnerup, N. B., Flor, H., Gibson, S., Keefe, F. J., Mogil, J. S., Ringkamp, M., Sluka, K. A., Song, X. J., Stevens, B., Sullivan, M. D., Tutelman, P. R., Ushida, T., Vader, K. (2020). The revised International Association for the Study of Pain definition of pain: Concepts, challenges, and compromises. *Pain*, 161(9), 1976–1982. https://doi.org/10.1097/j.pain.0000000000001939

Sanger, T. D., Mauricio, R. D., Gaebler-Spira, D., Hallett, M., Mink, J. W., Task Force on Childhood Motor Disorders. (2003). Classification and definition of disorders causing hypertonia in childhood. *Pediatrics*, 111(1). https://doi.org/10.1542/peds.111.1.e89

Scrace, J. (2003). Complementary therapies in palliative care of children with cancer: A literature review. *Paediatric Nursing*, 15(3), 36. https://doi.org/10.7748/paed2003.04.15.3.36.c846

Sepúlveda, C., Marlin, A., Yoshida, T., Ullrich, A. (2002). Palliative care: The World Health Organization's global perspective. *Journal of Pain and Symptom Management*, 24(2), 91–96. https://doi.org/10.1016/S0885-3924(02)00440-2

Shaw, K. L., Brook, L., Mpundu-Kaambwa, C., Harris, N., Lapwood, S., Randall, D. (2015). The spectrum of children's palliative care needs: A classification framework for children with life-limiting or life-threatening conditions. *BMJ Supportive & Palliative Care, 5*(3), 249–258. https://doi.org/10.1136/bmjspcare-2012-000407

Siden, H. B. (2018). Pediatric palliative care for children with progressive non-malignant diseases. *Children, 5*(2). https://doi.org/10.3390/children5020028

Siden, H. B., Carleton, B. C., Oberlander, T. F. (2013). Physician variability in treating pain and irritability of unknown origin in children with severe neurological impairment. *Pain Research and Management, 18*(5), 243–248. https://doi.org/10.1155/2013/193937

Sisk, B. A., Feudtner, C., Bluebond-Langner, M., Sourkes, B., Hinds, P. S., Wolfe, J. (2020). Response to suffering of the seriously ill child: A history of palliative care for children. *Pediatrics, 145*(1). https://doi.org/10.1542/peds.2019-1741

Sourkes, B. M. (2018). Children's experience of symptoms: Narratives through words and images. *Children, 5*(4), 53. https://doi.org/10.3390/children5040053

Spathis, A., Booth, S., Moffat, C., Hurst, R., Ryan, R., Chin, C., Burkin, J. (2017). The Breathing, Thinking, Functioning clinical model: A proposal to facilitate evidence-based breathlessness management in chronic respiratory disease. *NPJ Primary Care Respiratory Medicine, 27*(1), 27. https://doi.org/10.1038/s41533-017-0024-z

Theunissen, N. C., Vogels, T. G., Koopman, H. M., Verrips, G. H., Zwinderman, K. A., Verloove-Vanhorick, S. P., Wit, J. M. (1998). The proxy problem: Child report versus parent report in health-related quality of life research. *Quality of Life Research, 7,* 387–397. https://doi.org/10.1023/A:1008801802877

Twamley, K., Craig, F., Kelly, P., Hollowell, D. R., Mendoza, P., Bluebond-Langner, M. (2014). Underlying barriers to referral to paediatric palliative care services: knowledge and attitudes of health care professionals in a paediatric tertiary care centre in the United Kingdom. *Journal of Child Health Care, 18*(1), 19–30. https://doi.org/10.1177/1367493512468363

Ullrich, C. K., Mayer, O. H. (2007). Assessment and management of fatigue and dyspnea in pediatric palliative care. *Pediatric Clinics of North America, 54*(5), 735–756. https://doi.org/10.1016/j.pcl.2007.07.006

van Veen, S., Drenth, H., Hobbelen, H., Finnema, E., Teunissen, S., de Graaf, E. (2024). Non-pharmacological interventions feasible in the nursing scope of practice for pain relief in palliative care patients: A systematic review. *Palliative Care and Social Practice, 18.* https://doi.org/10.1177/26323524231222496

WHO (World Health Organization). (2014). *WHO Guidelines on the pharmacological treatment of persisting pain in children with medical illnesses.* WHO.

WHO (World Health Organization). (2018a) Integrating palliative care and symptom relief into paediatrics. A WHO guide for health care planners, implementers and managers. Available at: https://iris.who.int/bitstream/handle/10665/274561/9789241514453-eng.pdf?sequence=1 (accessed 5 June 2024).

WHO (World Health Organization). (2018b). *WHO guidelines for the pharmacological and radiotherapeutic management of cancer pain in adults and adolescents.* WHO.

WHO (World Health Organization). (2020). *Guidelines on the management of chronic pain in children.* WHO.

WHO (World Health Organization). (2023) The WHO definition of paediatric palliative care. Available at: https://www.who.int/europe/news-room/fact-sheets/item/palliative-care (accessed 5 June 2024).

Wolfe, J., Grier, H. E., Klar, N., Levin, S. B., Ellenbogen, J. M., Salem-Schatz, S., ... Weeks, J. C. (2000). Symptoms and suffering at the end-of-life in children with cancer. *New England Journal of Medicine, 342*(5), 326–333. https://doi.org/10.1056/NEJM200002033420506

Wolfe, J., Sourkes, B. M. (2022). *Interdisciplinary pediatric palliative care* (2nd edn). Oxford University Press.

Wong, C., Lau, E., Palozzi, L., Campbell, F. (2012). Pain management in children: Part 1—Pain assessment tools and a brief review of nonpharmacological and pharmacological treatment options. *Canadian Pharmacists Journal/Revue des Pharmaciens du Canada, 145*(5), 222–225. https://doi.org/10.3821/145.5.cpj222

Zinner, S. H., Mink, J. W. (2010). Movement disorders I: Tics and stereotypies. *Pediatrics in Review, 31*(6), 223–233. https://doi.org/10.1542/pir.31-6-223

# CHAPTER 8

# End-of-life care and bereavement

............................................

*Tara Kerr-Elliott, Florence Nalutaaya and Stacey Power Walsh*

## INTRODUCTION

While children's palliative care encourages a broad view on supporting families through their child's diagnosis and living as well as possible for as long as possible, it also incorporates the care of children when they die and supporting their families after the death has occurred. Another essential aspect of children's palliative care is bereavement care, as parents of children with a life-limiting condition grieve throughout their child's life. Feelings of grief and loss often begin for families when their child is diagnosed with a life-limiting condition or becomes unwell (as discussed in Chapter 4). These feelings of grief are likely to be intensified and can be overwhelming, even when the death is anticipated (Together for Short Lives, 2019). Bereavement support encompasses a family's entire experience of their child's death, from anticipating the death, the death itself, and following the death (Department of Health and Children, 2010).

In this chapter we focus on end-of-life care, the care of the body and grief and bereavement, with reference to cultural and spiritual differences and preferences. A case study identifying African cultural and spiritual beliefs will also be presented (see Box 8.2).

---

**LEARNING OBJECTIVES**

The reader will be able to do the following:

1.  Describe the physiological signs commonly seen in expected deaths and changes that occur after death.
2.  Explain the difference between cardiorespiratory and brain death, and describe some of the challenges associated with these.

---

DOI: 10.4324/9781003384861-11

3.  Demonstrate an understanding of the importance of including spiritual and cultural care when a child has died.
4.  Demonstrate a basic understanding of grief and the key principles of bereavement care and memory-/legacy-making.
5.  Illustrate the vast role of the nurse in caring for the child and their family, during the dying and following the death of the child and beyond.

## DEFINITIONS OF DEATH

Until the 1960s, death was diagnosed by confirming that a patient's heart and breathing had ceased, with no heart sounds and with fixed pupils (circulatory death). This remains the most common way of verifying a death, as most deaths occur through the cessation of cardiorespiratory function. However, in 1968, a second definition of death was agreed in response to advances in high-technology care, meaning that patients with brain damage so profound that they will never regain consciousness or survive without life support, could have their hearts and lungs sustained for long periods of time (Wilkinson et al., 2019). Brain death and cardiorespiratory death are considered equivalent on the basis that the brain is required to maintain functioning of a patient as a whole (Truog, 2020). However, while brain death was also considered to be a precursor to rapid and certain cardiorespiratory death, there are increasing numbers of patients, particularly in North America, who continued to survive on life-sustaining treatment for many years after being declared brain dead (Truog, 2020). This is of increasing relevance to children's palliative care, given the increasing numbers of children with life-limiting conditions receiving treatment in paediatric intensive care units (PICUs). Between 2004 and 2015, 57.6% of PICU admissions and 72.9% of deaths in UK PICUs were children with life-limiting conditions (Fraser and Parslow, 2018). However, in some countries, this trend is reversed. In Korea, for example, a small study demonstrated a significant decrease from 72% to less than 30% in the number of children with life-limiting conditions dying in PICU following involvement from a palliative care team (Kwon and Kim, 2023).

While exact definitions may differ slightly around the world, as a concept, brain death is generally accepted in healthcare settings, major medical groups and governments worldwide, using similar clinical testing (Sung, 2023). However, it raises particular challenges for some people, including those with strong religious or cultural views (Ray, 2014). Some families may disagree with the diagnosis of brain stem death such as in the highly publicised case of Jahi McMath (Box 8.1).

---

**BOX 8.1 CASE STUDY 1**

Jahi McMath was a 13-year old girl from California, USA, who suffered serious complications after a tonsillectomy in 2013, resulting in her being diagnosed as brain dead. Her family disputed this on the basis that as Christians, they believed her soul inhabited her body for as long as she had a heartbeat, and that by withdrawing ventilation, the hospital was infringing on the family's right to express their religion. After a lengthy legal battle, her family won the right to transfer her care to New Jersey, a state that allows patients and families to opt out of determination by brain death (Olick et al., 2009). Jahi survived almost five years, mainly cared for at home. She was dependent on a ventilator and enteral feeds. She was given hormones and began menstruating. In 2018, she developed liver failure. Her family declined further interventions and she died from a cardiac arrest. The family have two legal death certificates; one from 2013 in California, and one from New Jersey stating her death occurred in 2018.

Source: Aviv (2018); Truog (2020).

## RECOGNISING DEATH

The majority of children receiving palliative care will ultimately die from cardiorespiratory failure, rather than brain death, regardless of their primary diagnosis. Providing high-quality and timely end-of-life care is dependent upon the ability of clinicians to first recognise death as a potential outcome and then to acknowledge and communicate clearly when death is approaching. This is not always as straightforward as it may sound. Navigating the uncertainty that is increasingly a part of children's palliative care requires significant knowledge, skill, humility and patience. Children with the same diagnosis may have very different clinical outcomes and as medicine continues to advance rapidly, treatments and disease trajectories are increasingly unpredictable.

In Africa, palliative care has been established for over 20 years, but its concept has still not reached all healthcare service providers. Many providers fail to predict the end of life due to a lack of children's palliative care services or integrated models in their hospitals. In Uganda, for example, there is an integrated model of care developing in hospitals but there is still a lack of specialists and only one of very few hospices in the country offers an in-patient service. Primary care teams will often treat children with various aggressive interventions such as resuscitation, chemotherapy, radiotherapy, surgery, intravenous infusions (nutrition drips, albumin, fluids), aiming to prolong life. These interventions can traumatise the child and cause the family to disbelieve the prognosis, increasing the risk of complicated grief. The end of life is also often preceded by desperate attempts to find a cure, *trying* alternative approaches such as traditional medicines or witchcraft and focusing more on cultural rituals than modern medicine. This can result in late reporting to hospitals and fewer treatment options being available due to the more advanced stage of the child's disease.

In practice, and in the literature, the term "actively dying" is commonplace. A universally accepted definition of this term is lacking, but generally seems to refer to the last few days of life (Hui and Mori, 2021). It is important for nurses to understand this process as it has been one of the roles performed by a nurse to be present at the time a patient dies (Montgomery et al., 2017). When the patient is a child, the nurse's role extends to caring for the family as well as the child. Many families find reassurance from a careful and sensitive explanation of the dying process, but this can only happen if nurses understand it themselves and feel confident to communicate this.

## SIGNS OF DYING

It is important to note the difference between "expected" and "unexpected" deaths as not all deaths occur after a period of deterioration with some degree of predictability about the impending phase of death. Depending on their underlying diagnosis, some children may die more suddenly as a result of a catastrophic event such as a cardiac event or haemorrhage. Nurses should be aware of specific procedures that should be followed in the event of sudden, unexpected deaths, especially those relating to children with life-limiting conditions in the location in which they work.

While there are common symptoms of imminent death, not every child will experience each one, and the same symptom may be experienced differently. The five most prevalent symptoms experienced by children in a children's hospital in Australia during their last week of life were lack of energy, feeling drowsy, skin changes, feeling irritable and pain (Drake et al., 2003). The following discussion focuses on the physiological changes more commonly associated with deaths that are anticipated.

## INDICATORS AND SYMPTOMS OF IMMINENT DEATH

### Physical

Change in breathing pattern, skin colour, and reduced appetite, pain, fatigue, sleep disturbances, restlessness, and confusion.

- *Changes in breathing*: the child's respiratory rate may increase or become very slow and may fluctuate between the two. Apnoea is common and may be prolonged. Sighing or moaning, particularly on expiration may occur but does not normally indicate pain or distress unless associated with other signs. Breathing may also be noisy. If the child is deeply asleep, unconscious, or very weak, they may be unable to clear secretions from their airway, leading to gurgling sounds on inspiration and/or expiration (the death rattle).
- *Pain*: pain is a common and very distressing symptom experienced by children with cancer (Agarwal et al., 2022) as discussed in more depth in Chapter 7 on symptom management.
- *Changes in skin colour*: as circulation slows, skin can look pale, cyanosed or speckled.
- *Loss of appetite, fatigue and excessive sleep*: as the disease advances, systems also slow down. The child can become more fatigued, staying in bed.
- *Elimination*: a reduced urine/stool output. See Chapter 7.

### Behavioural

- Increased sleepiness or reduced consciousness.
- Loss of interest in their surroundings can affect their psychosocial well-being.
- Feelings of worthlessness, guilt or self-reproach (Mehler-Wex and Kölch, 2008).

## Psychosocial

- Withdrawal
- Low mood
- Loss of interest
- Joylessness
- Limited activity
- Lack of self-drive
- Easily fatigued
- Reduced self-esteem
- Low self-confidence

(Mehler-Wex and Kolch, 2008).

## CULTURAL PRACTICES AROUND DEATH

Cultural issues refer to the values, norms, habits, beliefs and instructions that flow from a specific worldview and through which patterns of meaning are created. Individual as well as communal approaches to suffering and death are derived from culturally specific community systems and rituals (Stjernsward, 2004; Chaturvedi et al., 2014). Western cultures use coping strategies that are different from those of non-western culture (Barg and Gullate, 2001). In the African context, families present with different cultural norms, for example, some believe in supernatural powers or demigods (Box 8.2). Misconceptions such as relating terminal illnesses to rituals are still evident. See Chapter 2.

---

**BOX 8.2 CASE STUDY 2**

A 9-year-old girl was admitted to a Specialised National Referral Hospital in Uganda with a histological diagnosis of advanced osteogenic sarcoma and lung metastases. A history of being unwell for one and a half years was given, during which time traditional healers were visited and their interventions on the patient's affected limb had resulted in sepsis. The patient presented with a fungating left limb and was in a lot of pain. This had a huge impact on her as she became isolated from local households. Her preference was amputation, but palliative surgery for cosmetic purposes together with pain management were also an offered option.

The delay in seeking medical intervention was attributed to the child's school reporting that, "5 children had been lost to demon attacks". Therefore, traditional medicine was sought at these times. The child attended a boarding school. She reported her sickness started after she had a dream and recounted:

I met a Muslim woman dressed in a black hijab [Muslim attire]. She entered my body I was so frightened, I shouted, and hit a metallic suitcase that hurt my right knee. Since then my leg has never improved.

---

Her mother said, "A lot of money has been used, visiting witcheries and traditional healers to get rid of the demons. Her father has not reported back since last month. He was so depressed when the doctor revealed to us that it was cancer and too advanced to respond to treatment."

### Interventions

The palliative care team was consulted to manage the complex pain and dyspnoea which did not respond to low doses of morphine. The dose was titrated and given alongside antibiotics and oxygen.

Talking therapies were undertaken, with ongoing counselling and information-giving with the mother about the disease and its prognosis. Communication by phone with the patient's father was introduced as their home was upcountry.

The patient requested to be discharged so that she could meet her siblings, but due to a low blood oxygen level, she was not allowed to go home. She wanted to buy them gifts in appreciation of their high achievements at school that term and had kept money from family members and friends who were visiting her in hospital. She asked the Muslim Sheik who also visited her to pray for her.

Her father was spoken to and visited with the siblings. The patient was very happy that day, her siblings appreciated being informed. They asked Allah to make her better.

Spiritual leaders were invited again to a meeting with the family. Myths related to cultural rituals were discussed and addressed.

### Lessons learnt

- End-of-life care can improve a patient's quality of life in the remaining time they have and allow them to die with dignity.
- Children are usually able to express their concerns and these need to be respected.
- Siblings need to be informed and involved in the care; this will help them go through grief (pre-bereavement phase).
- Involving religious leaders creates hope in the patient and reduces suffering.
- Disclosure to the family helps them to plan for all eventualities.
- Involving the family in decision-making improves quality of life.

Culturally specific considerations surrounding death may include:

- Perception and interpretations of symptoms, treatment, pain and suffering.
- Patient's willingness to know the diagnosis and prognosis.
- Doctor's willingness to discuss the disease and progress.
- Decision-making roles between healthcare providers.
- Spiritual and religious rituals and patient's family traditions during palliative and bereavement care.

## SPIRITUAL CONSIDERATIONS

Taking a detailed spiritual history is important as received information can be used to inform care of the child and family. Fisher's model of spiritual health and life orientation has been developed as an assessment tool to aid insight into a child's spiritual well-being (Fisher, 2004). The "Feeling Good, Living Life" tool focuses on the child's relationship with themselves, other people, their environment and God (Fisher, 2004). Children usually search for meaning and purpose as well as connectedness to their life. Health workers should consider the child's spiritual development when assessing their spiritual beliefs; the importance of spirituality in their life, whether they belong to a spiritual community and their perceptions on why their illness has happened to them. Suggested developmental characteristics proposed by Himelstein et al. (2004) are useful when considering a child's spiritual development.

A child may experience stages of grief; feelings of anger towards God or of abandonment by God, hopelessness and spiritual suffering. A referral to, or connection with, the patient's religious/spiritual leaders should be offered. The child's spiritual concerns should be explored in a supportive and respective manner with the aim of finding out what gives hope, peace of mind, meaning and fulfils their spiritual needs (Amery et al., 2009; Halpern, 2014).

Healthcare providers can offer great comfort to children through a compassionate presence, reflective listening, offering empathetic responses, enquiring about spiritual values and beliefs and making referrals to spiritual leaders (Halpern, 2014).

## COMMUNICATION AT END OF LIFE

The best way to manage end-of-life symptoms is to anticipate and prepare both the family and the patient (Amery et al., 2009), although the involvement of children and young people in decision-making as death approaches differs across cultures. Discussions will include about the place of death, in hospital or home. In the African context, if a child is in hospital, they will be kept in a cubicle for patients in critical care, where frequent reviews are done, ongoing counselling is offered as well as support provided to the family at intervals. If death is to happen at home, family meetings are held before the child is discharged from hospital. Family members are taught basic nursing care and how to manage any devices such as a nasogastric tube, and what to expect from the anticipated plan. The child's condition is monitored through telephone contact.

In the African setting the majority of families are unable to afford medical costs, for example, when a bone marrow transplant might be required to treat myeloid leukaemia or Sickle Cell Disease. Decision-making for a child or young person under the age of 18 years is by a proximal decision-maker, who must be a family member, such as a parent, older sibling, relative or guardian. Plans are usually made without the involvement of the child (see Chapters 4 and 9).

Effective communication is central to all healthcare. Issues relating to communication have formed the majority of complaints to the UK National Health Service over recent years (Parish, 2023). Sensitive, compassionate and timely communication is arguably the most important aspect of the nurse's role and of particular importance when a child is dying (see Chapter 4). Families may differ in how much information they wish to receive and discuss in advance, requiring nurses to be attentive, responsive and adaptable. Good communication leads to families feeling empowered by having the knowledge to make informed decisions about care (Tsey et al., 2009).

Nurses also need to be able to communicate with the sick child and their siblings and peers. Talking with children in this context can be complex. Nurses need to assess the child's personal and unique preferences, giving consideration to the child's developmental understanding, confidentiality and the culture of the family unit of which they are part (see Chapter 4).

Communication is linked to culture and language and there will be nuances to what may be considered best practice around the world. However, general principles of timing, sensitivity and compassion are likely to be important everywhere. The terminology used when discussing dying and death should also be considered. In some cultures, particularly in western countries, death has become a taboo subject and consequently, as we have become less familiar with it, we have lost the vocabulary that describes it (Koksvik, 2020). As referenced in Chapter 4, euphemisms such as "passed", "lost", "poor outcome" may be used with kind intention and clear understanding on the part of the person using them, but can lead to confusion and missed opportunities for families to make timely important decisions and plans. British palliative care doctor, author and speaker, Dr Kathryn Mannix, encourages us to use the "D-words" with dignity; naming dying and death, hence facilitating open and honest discussion, reducing misunderstanding and subsequently reducing fear (Adams et al., 2017).

## Barriers to effective communication

Barriers to effective communication between the child and the health service care provider have been identified (Zurca et al., 2017). These include the health service provider not having time or being worried about taking up a child's or family's time; concern around upsetting the child and not knowing how to respond to their emotional reactions. Fear of being asked questions that are difficult or unanswerable, or saying the wrong thing, can also be a barrier to effective communication (see Chapter 9).

---

**LEARNING ACTIVITY**

- Reflect and spend a few minutes considering what has informed your attitudes and beliefs towards death. You do not need to share this with anyone else unless you wish to.
- Think about your own personal and professional experiences, the way death was or wasn't talked about and any religious views you might have.
- Reflect on why this is important, for example, how might an increase in self-awareness impact our practice as nurses supporting families when a child is dying?
- How well is spiritual care incorporated into clinical care where you work? Do you know where to go to find more resources and support?

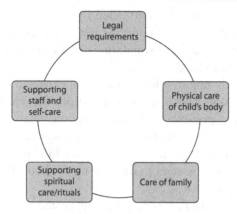

**FIGURE 8.1** The nurse's role in care after death

Source: adapted from Black et al. (2020).

## CARE AFTER DEATH

The role of the nurse in providing care after death can encompass several different tasks, as illustrated in Figure 8.1.

## Legal requirements

Legal requirements following the death of a child will be country-specific. In this chapter, practices in England are described, where every death (for babies over the age of 24 weeks) must be verified (confirmed), certified and registered.

In England, verification has traditionally been the role of a medical doctor, but it is increasingly being undertaken by experienced nurses who have completed further training. Verification of death is the procedure of determining whether a patient has died and involves performing physiological assessments to confirm this. Certification of death describes the process of completing the Medical Certificate of Cause of Death (MCCD) and can only be done by a Medical Practitioner who attended the child before their death (Stationery Office, 1953). All MCCDs are discussed with a Medical Examiner. Medical Examiners are senior medical doctors whose role includes agreeing the cause of death proposed by the doctor completing the MCCD and discussing the cause of death with the bereaved family. Once the MCCD has been completed, the death needs to be registered at a register office. This needs to take place within five working days of the death and must be done before a funeral can take place.

In Ireland, a registration of death is encouraged within three months, however, a period of 12 months is allocated for a family to register a death (Citizens Information, 2023). Registering a death outside of this time frame requires the family to contact the General Register Office (Citizens Information, 2023). Registering a stillbirth is optional in Ireland. It is important to know that each country has their own definition of what constitutes a stillborn, depending on the baby's weight and/or gestation. If a stillborn baby in Ireland has not been registered within 12 months, the hospital, midwife or medical practitioner who attended the birth may be asked to register it (Citizens Information, 2021). It is important healthcare professionals are aware of national guidelines relating to time stipulations when registering a death to ensure families are accurately informed.

Post-mortems are only required for a sudden, unexpected death where the cause is not clear. Countries will have different stipulations for when a coroner, an independent public official responsible for investigating unexplained deaths, will request a post-mortem. For example, a post-mortem might be required if a person has not been seen within a month of their death (Citizens Information, 2023). However, families may request a post-mortem to find out more about the child's illness, cause of death or for research purposes.

The death of every child in England, whether expected or unexpected, is reviewed by a Child Death Overview Panel as part of the Child Death Review Process. The overall purpose of this is to understand why children die, ensure any learning takes place and potentially identify ways to prevent future deaths (HM Government, 2018).

## Supporting the family

Talking with the family about who they would like to be present at the time of death can be useful, for example, siblings may wish to be present. The death of a child is likely to be a time of many intense emotions for families. Nurses should provide skilled, sensitive and timely communication and information, incorporating cultural and spiritual dimensions of care (Together for Short Lives, 2019). It is important to verbalise when the child dies so the family are aware and also to inform the wider team who have been involved in the child and family's care. If the death is expected, there is no rush to *do* anything. In fact, it is often helpful for nurses to encourage families just to *be with* their child at this time. Again, families will make different choices about what they want to do at this time, but many will not have thought about this in advance. Nurses should not be afraid to ask the family what they would like to do, and if it seems appropriate, gently make suggestions such as lying in the bed with the child, or holding their hand. Some families may want to sleep before doing anything. We do know from the limited literature that exists that many parents reflect positively on having time to be with their child after death (Barrett et al., 2022).

## Care of the child after death

It is important that the family are given time with their child following their death. When the family is ready, they may wish to help wash and dress their child. Nurses are required to be aware of policies and guidelines specific to their own area of work in terms of removal of lines and medical equipment and, how, when and to where, the child is transferred.

Nurses should also have a basic understanding of the physical changes that occur after death (Box 8.3), to support and reassure families. For some families, adherence to religious or cultural practices will be important.

**BOX 8.3 DETERIORATION OF THE BODY: WHAT NURSES NEED TO KNOW AND WHY**

- *Algor mortis* refers to the cooling of the body that begins once the heart stops beating. Without intervention the body will cool slowly over a few hours. This is affected by factors such as the environmental temperature and clothing. Nurses may need to sensitively suggest to families that they remove layers of clothing or blankets from the child. The more of the body surface that is exposed, the quicker the child's body will cool.

- *Eyes* that are open at the time of death can be closed by gently pressing down on the eyelids. Over time the eyes may appear sunken, and families may benefit from reassurance that this is normal.

- The child's *skin* will become pale and potentially also dry. Parents may apply moisturiser to the skin and balm to the child's lips if they would like to, but as the skin is likely to become more fragile after death, it should be explained that this needs to be done gently and carefully.

- *Lividity* refers to discoloration of the skin that occurs after death. As blood is no longer circulating around the body, gravity causes it to pool in the lowest parts of the body. For example, if the child is lying on their back, this is where lividity will be seen. It appears as dull red patches and as the rest of the skin is paler, it can be very noticeable, but it does vary. The family might need reassurance that these patches are not bruising. Nurses should consider this when positioning the child after death. For example, placing the child's head in the midline will prevent discoloration of the child's cheeks that may occur if their head is turned to one side.

- *Rigor mortis* is the term used to describe the stiffening of muscles that occurs within a few hours of death. It fades around two days after death. This knowledge may be helpful for nurses if parents request that their child's clothing is changed or if they are considering memory-making activities such as taking handprints or casts.

- *Bodily fluids* may leak from orifices any time after death, but this is more likely during moving and handling. Urinary and faecal leakage is common, as are secretions from the nose or mouth. Nurses may want to ensure a supply of incontinence pads, wipes and clean linen is available, and should be ready to gently prepare families, particularly if they plan to move or hold their child.

- *Bleeding* does not occur commonly but is a potential occurrence, particularly if the child had a bleeding disorder or had been taking anticoagulants. Nurses might consider the use of dark linen if bleeding is likely and be ready to intervene using suction or padding the orifice from which the bleeding occurs.

Source: Adapted from Together for Short Lives (2019).

There is huge variation across countries and religions in terms of how quickly funerals take place, and choices between burial, whether below or above ground, or cremation. In the UK, it is not uncommon for non-Muslim funerals to take up to three weeks to arrange. During this time the child's body may be cared for in a mortuary, either in a hospital or community funeral directors, or in a bereavement suite within a children's hospice or hospital. Many areas also offer the use of portable cooling technologies to enable the child to be cared for at home after death although currently there is variation in practices across the country. Most commonly, cooling mattresses are placed underneath the child or cold cots are provided for babies, which use electricity to circulate cooling fluid to regulate the child or baby's temperature. Bereavement suites and cooling mattresses offer families the chance to spend more time with their child after death.

---

**LEARNING ACTIVITY**

- Do you know what your local policy says about care of a child after death? If not, do you know who to talk to or how you can find out?
- Do you know where and how children are normally cared for in the area you work?
- What do you think about when you think of a mortuary? How does that make you feel?
- Have you ever visited a mortuary? If not, consider arranging to visit your local one, to meet the staff and find out what is possible for families.

---

## Staff support

The emotional impact of working in palliative care is well documented (Together for Short Lives, 2019). While it is important that managers and leaders provide opportunities for reflection, education and supervision, it is equally important that individual nurses take responsibility for accessing what is offered to them. Nurses should contribute towards the development of a working culture in which staff are encouraged to acknowledge when they might be struggling to cope with the emotional demands of their work. Nurses should also look out for signs of stress among their colleagues, particularly those who are less experienced.

The use of debriefs and pre-briefs (reflective discussions after and before a child dies) can be helpful and may be held within one team or across teams and different agencies (Neilson et al., 2011). These aim to provide a time of reflection, and an opportunity to provide and receive emotional support and to learn from each experience (Together for Short Lives, 2019).

## BEREAVEMENT AND GRIEF

Bereavement and grief are terms used inconsistently and interchangeably in the literature. Bereavement has been described as the loss of someone significant through death and the emotional experience created by this bereavement is referred to as grief (Granek, 2010; Chang et al., 2012; Shear and Skritskaya, 2012). Another definition is that bereavement is the term that describes the loss and grief in response to death, describing the emotional, psychological, physical, behavioural and functional reactions (McGuinness, 2009; Zisook and Shear, 2009). The latter allows for a broader use of the terms to represent everyday losses people experience, be it, for example, a loss of opportunities or functional abilities (Zisook and Shear, 2009). While bereavement is a natural human experience and one that many individuals can relate to, it can be hugely debilitating, causing a considerable amount of emotional pain (Schut and Stroebe, 2005; Department of Health and Children, 2010). There is an individuality of grief influenced by personal and cultural differences, backgrounds, and orientations (Moon Fai and Gordon Arthur, 2009).

## Grief

Grief theories date back as early as the sixteenth century. Burton ([1651] 1938) refers to grief as transitory melancholy and context-specific, at the time of a bereavement, and also transitory, arising upon occasions of sadness, sorrow or fear. Rush did not identify grief as an illness, however, he suggested that those bereaved can experience a physical illness and/or memory loss and recommended treatment of opium use, bloodletting and purging to assist in their recovery (Rush, 1947). During this era it was believed that bereavement could cause mental illness and even premature death (Granek, 2010). Shand (1914) made further progress on this and argued for the existence of four stages of grief reactions. These included active aggression towards the outside world, depression and lacking energy, suppression through self-control and frenzied and frantic activity. Shand acknowledged the need for social support and spoke about the need for a continued relationship with the deceased and trauma associated with sudden death (Shand, 1914). In contrast, Freud ([1917] 1963) during this time made known his belief that those bereaved needed to detach their emotional energy from the deceased and direct this energy into more acceptable areas of their lives. The need to sever the relational bond to the deceased became a Freudian notion called "grief work" (Moon, 2016). Although Freud noted that he never intended to pathologise grief or refer to medical treatment, much of his work has been interpreted as this, believing that those who did not do their "grief work" could develop a psychiatric illness (Freud et al., 1957; Freud, [1917] 1963). He addressed this misinterpretation, stating that the grief felt after a loss of a loved one was natural, time-consuming and a process that is never truly resolved and which had potential to lead to a psychiatric illness (Freud, [1917] 1963). Lindemann (1944) used empirical studies of bereaved parents to explore the physical and psychological symptoms evident after grief and developed a list of normal and abnormal grief symptoms with reference to grief as a medical illness. He suggested that grief symptoms presented in a systematic way. This led to the belief that grief could be predicted and therefore managed and treated by psychiatrists. He also advocated for the automatic involvement of a psychiatrist as intervention will be required to ensure the bereaved stay on course with their grief work and to monitor if they are overly or insufficiently grief-stricken (Lindemann, 1944). He further claims comfort measures provided by a religious order, social workers or family members are not adequate and their involvement should only extend to recommending a psychiatrist. Like some of his American counterparts, Parkes in the UK provided a rationale for the pathologisation of grief and the involvement of psychiatrists for its treatment (Parkes, 1964a; 1964b; 1965; 1971). Parkes, under the supervision of John Bowlby (1907–1990) (founder of the Attachment Theory) began the notion that those bereaved had higher mortality rates and physical symptoms requiring medical attention. Parkes provided "sound empirical methods" on which future studies were based to study this phenomenon, which further supported his view that grief was a complex process requiring medical support (Parkes, 1964a; 1964b; 1965; 1971). This created an opportunity for subsequent studies to concentrate on the symptoms and provided researchers with the ability to measure grief. Other well-known names in the world of grief studies are Stroebe et al. (1988), who focused on the symptoms of grief and implemented quantitative approaches to measure, diagnose and manage them.

During the nineteenth century, one of the most influential "gurus" in dying and death and grief, was Elisabeth Kübler-Ross (1926–2004), who created five stages of grief. These five stages were a pattern of adjustment created for the person facing their death, adopted and applied to those experiencing the death of a loved one (Kübler-Ross et al., 1982). Her work has received much criticism over the years relating to ethical issues and the rigor of her work (Parkes, 2013). Furthermore, her failure to recognise the involvement of John Bowlby in discovering these "stages of grief" previously caused questions to be asked of her work (Parkes, 2013). However, she remains the most-quoted author in addressing the bereavement process, with her work contributing to a clearer understanding of bereavement and grief for health professionals, families and all who handle and/or experience mourning (Parkes, 2013). A major contribution was her ability to make a fearful topic like death into an ordinary topic which could be discussed without fear. Kübler-Ross (2005) in her book, *On Grief and Grieving*, addressed the controversy over her five stages. She highlighted that they were never intended to be linear or solely represent what those bereaved experienced, instead they were to reflect a framework that facilitates learning in how to live without the one we lost. In her own words, "They are responses to loss that many people have, but there is not a typical response to loss, as there is no typical loss. Our grief is as individual as our lives" (Kübler-Ross, 2005, p. 7).

The five stages of grief include denial, anger, bargaining, depression, and acceptance, and it was hoped that with these stages would come knowledge to equip those bereaved to cope with life and loss (Kübler-Ross, 2005).

Although these theories offer a particular perspective on how parental bereavement is examined, they remain limited in their ability to encompass the range of affected areas in a bereaved parent's life and in their potential for individual approaches aligned to where the parents are on their post-bereavement trajectory (Barrera et al., 2009).

## Anticipatory grief

As previously discussed in Chapter 4, parents experience grief commencing at the initial diagnosis and at every subsequent deterioration. This type of grief is referred to as anticipatory grief. Anticipatory grief was first recognised by Lindemann (1944) and he hypothesised that pre-death grieving would facilitate coping and reduce grieving following the death of the loved one (Lindemann, 1944; Nielsen et al., 2016). Anticipatory grief arose from the Freudian notion of "grief work" and it was felt that the fear of losing the loved one led to the person detaching the bonds to prepare for this loss (Nielsen et al., 2016). This concept has significantly evolved, however, and more recent studies suggest that care-givers are witness to the patient's losses to a terminal illness, such as loss of future plans, uncertainties and deterioration (Nielsen et al., 2016). These can place the carer in a vulnerable position, experiencing grief and psychological stress leading up to and following the death (Nielsen et al., 2016). It is widely accepted that grief during care-giving contributes to a complex process, one where there is a reaction to multiple losses rather than a lone response to the loss created by the actual death (Evans, 1994). In demonstrating the individuality of how grief is experienced and its incomparable nature, to the contrary of Lindemann's (1944) original hypotheses, it is identified that there is no positive effect of grief before death on the bereaved.

## Continuing bonds

The concept of continuing bonds is a psychological perspective that challenges traditional notions of grief and bereavement. Developed by clinical psychologists Dennis Klass, Phyllis Silverman and Steven Nickman, continuing bonds theory suggests that the relationship with a deceased loved one can persist and evolve after death, rather than being severed (Klass et al., 1996). Contrary to earlier views and Freud's notion of "grief work" and "letting go", a bereaved parent's ability to reconstruct their relationship with their deceased child and integrate this memory into their inner and social worlds in a way that is meaningful to them, is now considered central to parental bereavement and adjustment (Klass and Walter, 2001; Davies, 2004). The continuing bonds theory acknowledges that maintaining a connection with the deceased can be a healthy and adaptive way for individuals to cope with their loss. Key principles of the continuing bonds concept include an ongoing relationship between those bereaved and their loved one who has died, memories and rituals, internal representations, narrative reconstruction, and spiritual and symbolic connections.

Parents are encouraged to keep possessions and physical objects that link them to and evoke memories of their deceased child, so they keep a sense of their child intact and contribute to the sense of an enduring connection (Davies, 2004). These memories support families to recount their feelings, thoughts and events following a bereavement, assisting them to make changes and adjust while giving meaning to their loss and maintain an ongoing connection to their loved one (Davies, 2004). This ability to derive meaning from the death of their loved one is characterised by a renewed sense that life is worthwhile and purposeful and has been related to the achievement of post-bereaved growth (Calhoun and Tedeschi, 2004). It is recommended that families talk to their dead child, talk about the deceased child to others in their social world and take meaning from how their child continues to be part of their ongoing life, contributing to a sense of continuity rather than finality (Davies, 2004). This continuing bond brings solace and consolation to the bereaved person.

In essence, the continuing bonds concept emphasises that grief is a dynamic and ongoing process that doesn't necessarily require severing the emotional ties with the deceased. Instead, individuals can find ways to integrate the loss into their lives while maintaining a sense of connection and meaning. This perspective allows for a more personalised and flexible approach to coping with grief.

Legacy-making, defined as memory-making, actions or behaviours aimed at remembrance (Foster et al., 2009), has been shown to enhance coping and improve grief outcomes for bereaved parents and siblings (Akard et al., 2018; Schaefer et al., 2020), enabling a continued bond with the deceased. Clarke and Connolly (2022) reported the overwhelmingly positive impact parents experienced from memory-making. It offered them tangible and precious mementos that were created by them and their deceased child. The process of memory-making itself provides families with precious quality time together (Tan et al., 2012; Clarke and Connolly, 2022).

## Parental grief

Losing a child is a tragedy and evokes a significant emotional response (Hughes and Goodall, 2013). Assisting families through bereavement is an essential part of comprehensive end-of-life care (O'Shea and Bennett Kanarek, 2013). Parents express their grief not only at losing a child but also as the loss of a part of themselves that was invested in future aspirations (Butler et al., 2015). Parental grief is a more intense and overwhelming type of grief (Davies, 2004) and bereaved parents are consequently at higher risk of long-term psychosocial morbidities (Rando, 1983) and depressive symptoms and episodes (American Psychiatric Association, 2000; Goodenough et al., 2004; Li et al., 2005; Rogers et al., 2008; Rosenberg et al., 2012). Short-term grief reactions such as disruptions in occupational, social, and family roles are generally associated following a child bereavement (Stebbins et al., 2007; Rogers et al., 2008; Barrera et al., 2009). However, in a study conducted by Rogers et al. (2008), disruptions in parents' normative functioning were unfounded, and it was suggested that this was reflective of recovery that enabled parents to return to roles and activities. However, in this study, these parents continued to report negative emotions, suggestive of the fact that parents' grief reactions may not be evident as they return to normative functioning in social roles and that therefore they may not be recognised by others (Rogers et al., 2008). Social support is of utmost importance in aiding parental coping and providing parents with practical and emotional sustenance to "keep going" through uncertainty and distress (Price et al., 2011). There is conflicting research with regards to the impact of a child bereavement on relationships. Some studies suggest bereaved parents are more at risk of marital problems than those without a child bereavement (Bohannon, 1991; Goodenough et al., 2004; Rogers et al., 2008). However, many of these studies don't take into consideration the high divorce rates in the region in which the study is undertaken, or methodological limitations such as a lack of a control group and potential selection bias.

Parents can experience a similar range of emotions following the death of their child as those described in Chapter 4 when they receive the diagnosis and begin grieving at the loss of their healthy child. These can vary from anger, numbness, shock, constant pain, sadness, loneliness, and guilt (The Irish Hospice Foundation, 2020a). These emotions can present physically in the parent. Parents have reported an overwhelming feeling of exhaustion, lower concentration and attention levels exacerbated from the inability to sleep or eat (The Irish Hospice Foundation, 2020a). It is important to note, bereaved parents rarely experience and express grief in the same manner (Rando, 1991; Pohlkamp et al., 2019), and this, alongside the lack of strength and ability to provide support to each other, can create challenges with comforting one another (Rando, 1991). There is evidence, however, that identifies resilience in couples, where parents describe a stronger and closer relationship, resulting from the loss of their child (Barrera et al., 2009; Bergstraesser et al., 2014).

## Sibling grief

The impact a child death has on the siblings is a complex one influenced by the child's age, developmental age, understanding about death, position in the family and family dynamics. Bereaved siblings have been referred to as the "forgotten mourners" and are often overlooked as the focus remains on the unwell child and the parents (Buckle and Fleming, 2011; Rajendran et al., 2024). Siblings are expected to adjust to the loss of the sibling relationship and the subsequent changes in parenting and family dynamics because of the loss (Buckle and Fleming, 2011; Rajendran et al., 2024). Changes in parenting can result in a loss of emotional support or lack of parental figure and can impact on the sibling's daily lives (Fullerton et al., 2017; Chin et al., 2018; Rajendran et al., 2024). Children can experience emotion and behavioural difficulties as they face challenges in expressing their needs; feeling left out or angry at the child who died (The Irish Hospice Foundation, 2020b). They are heavily influenced by those around them, learning through observation how to grieve and act (Fullerton et al., 2017; Chin et al., 2018; Rajendran et al., 2024). Children can have strong emotions, then appear to return to normality and routine quickly, but frequently return to the strong emotions (The Irish Childhood Bereavement Network, 2018). As a result, child bereavement can negatively impact their relationships with their parents, within their family and their friends (Fullerton et al., 2017; Chin et al., 2018; Rajendran et al., 2024).

Parents may find it difficult to understand others' individual ways of grieving (i.e. their child's and/or their partner's), however, when differences between the expression of grief within the family are embraced and accepted, it has been noted that families have an improved way of coping with the loss together (The Irish Hospice Foundation, 2020a). Additionally, it is noteworthy to address and acknowledge bereaved grandparents as they experience the pain of not only the loss of a grandchild but the pain of their own child's bereavement (Nehari et al., 2007).

Grief, distress and persistent sadness are normal responses to the death of a loved one, but these usually diminish over time as the loss is integrated into the bereaved person's life (Arizmendi and O'Connor, 2015). When there are problems with the adaptation process, where grief symptoms are persistent and prolonged, resulting in chronic debilitation interfering with daily functioning, it becomes of concern and is classified as complicated grief (Shear et al., 2013; Shear, 2015; Zisook and Reynolds, 2017). This disorder is diagnosed through assessing the symptoms, the effect of these on the body and the length of time following the actual death of their loved one (Shear et al., 2011). It is suggested that grief itself is not the single cause of complicated grief, but the impact of predisposing factors such as previous loss, avoidant coping style, and underlying psychiatric disorders (Moon, 2016).

The bereaved are at higher risk of ill health when unable to cope with their grief and loss (Tatsuno et al., 2012; Keegan, 2013; Johnson, 2015). The experience of a child bereavement can present as emotional distress, reduced quality of life and anxiety (Eilertsen et al., 2013) but can also allow post-traumatic growth for families through creating an opportunity for them to find meaning after the loss (Barrera et al., 2009). In addressing both of these potential outcomes, it is recommended that support services are available to families as required (Department of Health and Children, 2010). This support includes formal and informal approaches ranging from a caring listener to more specialist and professional care, while honouring the need to respect and support the family's natural coping (Department of Health and Children, 2010).

## BEREAVEMENT CARE AND SUPPORT

Bereavement care encompasses compassionate and sensitive communication, information sharing, and opportunities created for families to talk (Health Service Executive, 2022). When delivered effectively, bereavement care is delivered in accordance with spiritual, cultural and social values addressing varying levels of need (Ryan et al., 2014). It helps to regain emotional stability (Tatsuno et al., 2012) and so the quality of bereavement support has a major impact on the parents' grieving process (Widger et al., 2009). Parents and families can require a range of immediate and longer-term support to help them with their bereavement (O'Connell et al., 2016; Cullen et al., 2018; Nuzum et al., 2018) with their needs ascending from basic to more complex needs (Health Service Executive, 2022). All those bereaved will have a need for compassion and acknowledgement of the death. Some individuals may require additional support outside their natural network of family, peers, and community, such as counselling or a more specialist therapeutic service (The Irish Hospice Foundation, 2020c). The provision of support can therefore be delivered by various sources including family, friends, and their community, to more formal support services provided by healthcare professionals (Koopmans et al., 2013), depending on the individual's need.

The Irish Hospice Foundation developed the National Collaborative project, a framework for adult bereavement care in Ireland. The framework outlines the support and services required to effectively meet the varied levels of needs experienced by those who are bereaved, and the knowledge and skills required by those providing the support (The Irish Hospice Foundation, 2020c).

Healthcare providers can have a major influence on the experiences of families during the life and during and after the death of the child (Butler et al., 2015). Helping families develop continuing bonds often requires professional support when parents have trouble in talking about their deceased child to family members and the wider social world, which can result in loneliness and isolation (Davies, 2004; Clarke and Connolly, 2022). In response to this, healthcare professionals can support parents and families through therapeutic interventions such as listening and conversational remembering and referring families to support groups made up of those who have suffered the same loss (Davies, 2004). Furthermore, healthcare professionals can introduce the idea of memory-making and legacy intervention to contribute to a sense of continued bonds (Akard et al., 2018; Clarke and Connolly, 2022; Schaefer et al., 2020).

## THE NURSE'S ROLE IN BEREAVEMENT SUPPORT

Health professionals have a critical role in supporting bereaved parents (Davies, 2004). Follow-up care is necessary to identify and support parents and families through the grief reactions, such as anxiety, depression, and to improve their psychological well-being (Royal College of Obstetricians and Gynaecologists, 2010; O'Connell et al., 2016; Meaney et al., 2017; Nuzum et al., 2018). Due to the nature of bereavement care, a bereavement follow-up is best provided by a healthcare professional who had a pre-existing relationship with the family and their child prior to the child's death (Darbyshire et al., 2013). Parents report that expressing emotions and memories was easier knowing the healthcare professional had been on their journey with them and led them to feeling more understood (Darbyshire et al., 2013). It is suggested that nurses are best placed to provide bereavement support as they frequently care directly for the child and family and are present from active treatments aimed at cure, right through to palliative and end-of-life care (Pearson, 2010; Aschenbrenner et al., 2012; Chan et al., 2013). Nurses are in a position to spend extended periods with the patient and their families, providing an opportunity to influence the care experience (Aschenbrenner et al., 2012) and build a therapeutic relationship (Chang et al., 2012). This therapeutic relationship has been identified as the most important aspect within the role of bereavement care (Chang et al., 2012). In the absence of bereavement follow-up care by healthcare professionals with whom families had a close relationship, the family's grief and loss expanded to not only that of the child, but the loss of the relationships with the healthcare professionals who had supported them (Widger et al., 2009; Laws, 2011). Similarly, Jackson et al. (2023) reported that in the absence of efficient communication, support and continuity of care, parents' stress was exacerbated, resulting in parental isolation.

## ROLE OF VOLUNTARY SUPPORT GROUPS
## IN BEREAVEMENT SUPPORT

It is important to note that bereaved parents and families often require ongoing support that surpasses that of the hospital admission, with parents developing high levels of distress in the absence of formal follow-up care and supports (Boyle et al., 2015; Health Service Executive, 2020). The negative emotions and amplified grief associated with the lack of appropriate follow-up care or social acknowledgement are well documented in the international literature (Cacciatore, 2010; Royal College of Obstetrics and Gynaecology, 2010; Koopmans et al., 2013; Boyle et al., 2015; Burden et al., 2016; Meaney et al., 2017). This inadequacy of care has resulted in an over-reliance on voluntary support groups to respond to the unmet holistic needs of bereaved parents (Boyle et al., 2015; Health Service Executive, 2022).

Voluntary support groups have long played an important role in healthcare in responding to the unmet needs of individuals and policy worldwide (Clarke and Quin, 2007; Enjolras et al., 2018; Day et al., 2019; Power et al., 2021). Voluntary peer-support bereavement organisations have been acknowledged for their invaluable role (Health Service Executive, 2022) with parents reporting positive outcomes from sharing their experience with those with similar experiences and circumstances (Department of Health and Children, 2010; Aho et al., 2012; Cacciatore et al., 2018). However, while voluntary support groups play a vital role in filling gaps in healthcare provision and are motivated to respond to bereaved parents' holistic needs, they potentially lack the knowledge and skills necessary to meet these needs (Department of Health and Children, 2010; Power et al., 2020; Power et al., 2021).

In Ireland, the National Standards for Bereavement Care Following Pregnancy Loss and Perinatal Death, developed in 2016 and implemented over a two-year programme, were designed to enhance bereavement care services for parents who experience a pregnancy loss or perinatal death (Health Service Executive, 2022). These guidelines acknowledge the important role that both healthcare professionals and voluntary organisations play in supporting those bereaved. A two-way sharing of information and a collaborative approach are ideal to facilitate a holistic approach to supporting those bereaved to meet their individual needs (Power et al., 2021).

## SUMMARY

The need for nurses to be knowledgeable and skilled in identifying dying and death and to care for the child and their family at end of life and beyond is essential within children's palliative care. Communication that clearly informs children and families about the impending death is necessary to prepare families for what potentially lies ahead and to assess and develop a plan of care to respond to the needs and choices of the family. Nursing care is required to reflect and respect the diverse and multicultural needs of patients and their families. Therefore, the care at end of life and subsequent bereavement care must be holistic, individual, and delivered in accordance with spiritual, cultural and social values. Furthermore, this care must reflect local and national guidelines and policy, ensuring legal requirements are met when caring for a dead body. While grief is a natural human experience, parental grief is unique and results in intense reactions and overwhelming sadness. Siblings' grief is more complex as it is heavily influenced by the child's age and development. Nursing care that encourages legacy-/memory-making can assist parents and siblings in their grief, encouraging them to talk about their deceased child, facilitating their continuing bonds. A collaborative and multi-disciplinary team approach is most beneficial to ensure ongoing care of the child and family during and following the death of the child.

## KEY POINTS

- Nurses at the bedside of the dying child are required to be skilful, knowledgeable and up-to-date with local and national guidelines/requirements when caring for the child and family during and after the death.
- The holistic child- and family-centred care delivered during the dying and death of the child needs to reflect that of the child and family's cultural, spiritual and religious preferences to ensure their individual needs are met.
- Clear communication is of utmost importance ensuring:
  - families understand when death is imminent and are made aware of when the death occurs
  - healthcare professionals are aware of the child's/parents' wishes, preferences and concerns
  - those involved in caring for the child with the life-limiting condition are informed of the child's death and families are provided with bereavement care and support to meet their individual needs.
- Memory-making is a powerful aid in facilitating families to continue a bond with their deceased child/sibling and should be encouraged. The delivery of compassionate and sensitive communication, information sharing, and opportunities created for families to talk, positively impacts on the parents'/family's grieving process and ability to regain emotional stability.

## REFERENCES

Adams, A. M. N., Mannix, T., Harrington, A. (2017). Nurses' communication with families in the intensive care unit: A literature review. *Nursing in Critical Care*, 22(2), 70–80. https://doi.org/10.1111/nicc.12141

Agarwal, S., Singh, V. P., Sangwan, A., Mishra, S. (2022). Refractory cancer pain in young child at end-of-life: Can we alleviate the suffering? *Indian Journal of Cancer*, 59(2), 265–268. https://doi.org/10.4103/ijc.IJC_635_20

Aho, A. L., Paavilainen, E. Kaunonen, M. (2012). Mothers' experiences of peer support via an Internet discussion forum after the death of a child. *Scandinavian Journal of Caring Science*, 26, 417–426. https://doi.org/10.1111/j.1471-6712.2011.00929.x

Akard, T. F., Duffy, M., Hord, A., Randall, A., Sanders, A., Adelstein, K., Gilmer, M. J. (2018). Bereaved mothers' and fathers' perceptions of a legacy intervention for parents of infants in the NICU. *Journal of Neonatal-Perinatal Medicine*, 11(1), 21–28. https://doi.org/10.3233/NPM-181732

American Psychiatric Association. (2000). *Diagnostic and statistical manual of mental disorders* (4th edn, text rev.). APA.

Amery, J. M., Rose, C. J., Holmes, J., Nguyen, J., Byarugaba, C. (2009). The beginnings of children's palliative care in Africa: Evaluation of a children's palliative care service in Africa. *Journal of Palliative Medicine*, 12(11), 1015–1021. https://doi.org/10.1089/jpm.2009.0125

Arizmendi, B. J., O'Connor, M. F. (2015). What is "normal" in grief? *Australian Critical Care*, 28(2), 58–62. https://doi.org/10.1016/j.aucc.2015.01.005

Aschenbrenner, A. P., Winters, J. M., Belknap, R. A. (2012). Integrative review: Parent perspectives on care of their child at the end-of-life. *Journal of Pediatric Nursing*, 27(5), 514–522. https://doi.org/10.1016/j.pedn.2011.07.008

Aviv, R. (2018). What does it mean to die? *New Yorker*, 5 February. Available at: https://www.newyorker.com/magazine/2018/02/05/what-does-it-mean-to-die (accessed 4 June 2024).

Barg, F. K., Gullatte, M. M. (2001). Cancer support groups: Meeting the needs of African Americans with cancer. *Seminars in Oncology Nursing*, 17(3), 171–178. https://doi.org/10.1053/sonu.2001.25946

Barrera, M., O'Connor, K., D'Agostino, N. M., Spencer, L., Nicholas, D., Jovcevska, V., Tallet, S., Schneiderman, G. (2009). Early parental adjustment and bereavement after childhood cancer death. *Death Studies*, 33(6), 497–520. https://doi.org/10.1080/07481180902961153

Barrett, L., Fraser, L., Noyes, J., Taylor, J., Hackett, J. (2022). Understanding parent experiences of end-of-life care for children: A systematic review and qualitative evidence synthesis *Palliative Medicine*, 37(2), 178–202.

Bergstraesser, E., Inglin, S., Hornung, R., Landolt, M. A. (2014). Dyadic coping of parents after the death of a child. *Death Studies*. https://doi.org/10.1080/07481187.2014.920434

Black, R., Kerr-Elliott, T., Judge-Kronis, L., Sebire, N. (2020). Care after death: For the baby and their family, including post-mortem examination. In A. Mancini, J. Price, T. Kerr-Elliot (eds), *Neonatal palliative care for nurses* (pp. 229–324). Springer.

Bohannon, J. R. (1991). Grief responses of spouses following the death of a child: A longitudinal study. *Omega: Journal of Death and Dying*, 22(2), 109–121. https://doi.org/10.2190/QCX3-36WQ-KJTQ-3N1V

Boyle, F. M., Mutch, A. J., Barber, E. A., Carroll, C., Dean, J. H. (2015). Supporting parents following pregnancy loss: A cross-sectional study of telephone peer supporters. *BMC Pregnancy and Childbirth*, 15, 1–10. https://doi.org/10.1186/s12884-015-0713-y

Buckle, J. L., Fleming, S. J. (2011) *Parenting after the death of a child: A practitioner's guide*. Routledge.

Burden, C., Bradley, S., Storey, C., Ellis, A., Heazell, A. E., Downe, S., Siassakos, D. (2016). From grief, guilt, pain and stigma to hope and pride: A systematic review and meta-analysis of mixed-method research of the psychosocial impact of stillbirth. *BMC Pregnancy and Childbirth*, 16, 1–12. https://doi.org/10.1186/s12884-016-0800-8

Burton, R. ([1651] 1938). *The anatomy of melancholy* (6th edn). Tudor Publishing Corporation.

Butler, A., Hall, H., Willetts, G., Copnell, B. (2015). Parents' experiences of healthcare provider actions when their child dies: An integrative review of the literature. *Journal for Specialists in Pediatric Nursing*, 20(1), 5–20. https://doi.org/10.1111/jspn.12097

Cacciatore, J. (2010). The unique experiences of women and their families after the death of a baby. *Social Work in Health Care*, 49(2), 134–148. https://doi.org/10.1080/00981380903158078

Cacciatore, J., Blood, C., Kurker, S. (2018). From "silent birth" to voices heard: Volunteering, meaning, and posttraumatic growth after stillbirth. *Illness, Crisis & Loss*, 26(1), 23–39. https://doi.org/10.1177/1054137317740799

Calhoun, L. G., Tedeschi, R. G. (2004). The foundations of posttraumatic growth: New considerations. *Psychological Inquiry*, 15(1), 93–102. https://doi.org/10.1207/s15327965pli1501_03

Chan, H. Y. L., Lee, L. H., Chan, C. W. H. (2013). The perceptions and experiences of nurses and bereaved families towards bereavement care in an oncology unit. *Supportive Care in Cancer*, 21(6), 1551–1556. https://doi.org/10.1007/s00520-012-1692-4

Chang, E., Bidewell, J., Hancock, K., Johnson, A., Easterbrook, S. (2012). Community palliative care nurse experiences and perceptions of follow-up bereavement support visits to carers. *International Journal of Nursing Practice, 18*(4), 332–339. https://doi.org/10.1111/j.1440-172X.2012.02046.x

Chaturvedi, S. K., Strohschein, F. J., Saraf, G., Loiselle, C.G. (2014). Communication in cancer care: Psycho-social, interactional, and cultural issues. A general overview and the example of India. *Frontiers in Psychology, 5*, 107404. https://doi.org/10.3389/fpsyg.2014.01332

Chin, W. L., Jaaniste, T., Trethewie, S. (2018). The role of resilience in the sibling experience of pediatric palliative care: What is the theory and evidence? *Children, 5*(7), 97. https://doi.org/10.3390/children5070097

Citizens Information. (2021). Registering a stillbirth. Available at: https://www.citizensinformation.ie/en/birth-family-relationships/miscarriage-and-stillbirth/registering-stillbirth/

Citizens Information. (2023). Registering a death. Available at: https://www.citizensinformation.ie/en/death/practical-arrangements-after-a-death/registering-a-death/#:~:text=To%20register%20a%20death%2C%20you,it%20to%20the%20registry%20office (accessed 4 June 2024).

Clarke, J., Quin, S. (2007). Professional carers' experiences of providing a pediatric palliative care service in Ireland. *Qualitative Health Research, 17*(9), 1219–1231. https://doi.org/10.1177/1049732307308316

Clarke, T., Connolly, M. (2022). Parents' lived experience of memory making with their child at or near end-of-life. *American Journal of Hospice and Palliative Medicine, 39*(7), 798–805. https://doi.org/10.1177/10499091211047838

Cullen, S., Coughlan, B., McMahon, A., Casey, B., Power, S., Brosnan, M. (2018). Parents' experiences of clinical care during second trimester miscarriage. *British Journal of Midwifery, 26*(5), 309–315. https://doi.org/10.12968/bjom.2018.26.5.309

Darbyshire, P., Cleghorn, A., Downes, M., Elford, J., Gannoni, A., McCullagh, C., Shute, R. (2013). Supporting bereaved parents: A phenomenological study of a telephone intervention programme in a paediatric oncology unit. *Journal of Clinical Nursing, 22*(3–4), 540–549. https://doi.org/10.1111/j.1365-2702.2012.04266.x

Davies, R. (2004). New understandings of parental grief: Literature review. *Journal of Advanced Nursing, 46*(5), 506–513. https://doi.org/10.1111/j.1365-2648.2004.03024.x

Day, C., Grimson, J., Madden, D. (2019). Report of the Independent Review Group established to examine the role of voluntary organisations in publicly funded health and personal social services. Department of Health.

Department of Health and Children (2010). Palliative care for children with life-limiting conditions in Ireland: A national policy. Available at: https://assets.gov.ie/43328/0dbcb20b794c481ea00f9f858b9faa04.pdf (accessed 4 June 2024).

Drake, R., Frost, J., Collins, J. J. (2003). The symptoms of dying children. *Journal of Pain and Symptom Management, 26*(1), 594–603. https://doi.org/10.1016/s0885-3924(03)00202-1

Eilertsen, M. E. B., Eilegård, A., Steineck, G., Nyberg, T., Kreicbergs, U. (2013). Impact of social support on bereaved siblings' anxiety: A nationwide follow-up. *Journal of Pediatric Oncology Nursing, 30*(6), 301–310. https://doi.org/10.1177/1043454213513838

Enjolras, B., Salamon, L. M., Sivesind, K. H., Zimmer, A. (2018). *The third sector as a renewable resource for Europe: Concepts, impacts, challenges and opportunities.* Springer Nature. https://doi.org/10.1007/978-3-319-71473-8

Evans, A. J. (1994). Anticipatory grief: A theoretical challenge. *Palliative Medicine, 8*(2), 159–165. https://doi.org/10.1177/026921639400800211

Fisher, J. (2004). Feeling good, living life: A spiritual health measure for young children. *Journal of Beliefs & Values, 25*(3), 307–315. https://doi.org/10.1080/1361767042000306121

Foster, T. L., Gilmer, M. J., Davies, B., Barrera, M., Fairclough, D., Vannatta, K., Gerhardt, C. A. (2009). Bereaved parents' and siblings' reports of legacies created by children with cancer. *Journal of Pediatric Oncology Nursing*, 26(6), 369–376. https://doi.org/10.1177/1043454209340322

Fraser, L. K., Parslow, R. (2018). Children with life-limiting conditions in paediatric intensive care units: A national cohort, data linkage study. *Archives of Disease in Childhood*, 103(6), 540–547.

Freud, S. ([1917] 1963). Mourning and melancholia. (Johan Riviere, Trans.). In *General Psychology Theory*. Collier.

Freud, S., Strachey J., Freud, A. (1957). *The standard edition of the complete psychological works of Sigmund Freud* (pp. 152–170). Hogarth Press.

Fullerton, J. M., Totsika, V., Hain, R., Hastings, R. P. (2017). Siblings of children with life-limiting conditions: Psychological adjustment and sibling relationships. *Child: Care, Health and Development*, 43(3), 393–400. https://doi.org/10.1111/cch.12421

Goodenough, B., Drew, D., Higgins, S., Trethewie, S. (2004). Bereavement outcomes for parents who lose a child to cancer: Are place of death and sex of parent associated with differences in psychological functioning? *Psycho-Oncology*, 13(11), 779–791. https://doi.org/10.1002/pon.795

Granek, L. (2010). Grief as pathology: The evolution of grief theory in psychology from Freud to the present. *History of Psychology*, 13(1), 46. https://psycnet.apa.org/doi/10.1037/a0016991

Halpern, J. (2014). From idealized clinical empathy to empathic communication in medical care. *Medicine, Health Care and Philosophy*, 17, 301–311. https://doi.org/10.1007/s11019-013-9510-4

Health Service Executive. (2020). Bereavement and grief: Levels of bereavement support. Available at: https://hli.ie/bereavementgrief/levels (accessed 4 June 2024).

Health Service Executive (2022). Bereavement care following pregnancy loss and perinatal death. Ireland. Available at: https://www.hse.ie/eng/services/list/3/maternity/bereavement-care/national-standards-for-bereavement-care-following-pregnancy-loss-and-perinatal-death.pdf (accessed 4 June 2024).

Himelstein, B. P., Hilden, J. M., Boldt, A. M., Weissman, D. (2004). Pediatric palliative care. *New England Journal of Medicine*, 350(17), 1752–1762 https://doi.org/10.1056/nejmra030334

HM Government. (2018). Child Death Review: Statutory and Operational Guidance (England). Available at: https://assets.publishing.service.gov.uk/media/637f759bd3bf7f154876adbd/child-death-review-statutory-and-operational-guidance-england.pdf (accessed 4 June 2024).

Hughes, K. H., Goodall, U. A. (2013). Perinatal bereavement care: Are we meeting families' needs? *British Journal of Midwifery*, 21(4), 248–253. https://doi.org/10.12968/bjom.2013.21.4.248

Hui, D., Mori, M. (2021). Physiology of dying. In N. I. Cherny, M. T. Fallon, S. Kaasa, R. K. Portney, D.C. Currow (eds), *Oxford textbook of palliative medicine* (6th edn). Oxford University. Press. https://doi.org/10.1093/med/9780198821328.003.0103

Jackson, P., Power-Walsh, S., Dennehy, R., O'Donoghue, K. (2023). Fatal fetal anomaly: Experiences of women and their partners. *Prenatal Diagnosis*, 43(4), 553–562. https://doi.org/10.1002/pd.6311

Johnson, A. (2015). Analysing the role played by district and community nurses in bereavement support. *British Journal of Community Nursing*, 20(6), 272–277. https://doi.org/10.12968/bjcn.2015.20.6.272

Keegan, O. (2013). Submission to the Oireachtas Committee on Health and Children: Public Hearing on End-of-Life Care, *Bereavement Care*, Briefing Document: The Irish Hospice Foundation.

Klass, D., Silverman, P., Nickman, S. L. (1996). *Continuing bonds: New understandings of grief.* American Psychological Association Press.

Klass, D., Walter, T. (2001). Processes of grieving: How bonds are continued. In M. S. Stroebe, R. O Hansson, W. Stroebe, H. Schut (eds), *Handbook of bereavement research: Consequences, coping, and care* (pp. 431–448). American Psychological Association. https://doi.org/10.1037/10436-018

Koksvik, G. H. (2020). Neoliberalism, individual responsibilization and the death positivity movement. *International Journal of Cultural Studies, 23*(6), 951–967. https://doi.org/10.1177/1367877920924426

Koopmans, L., Wilson, T., Cacciatore, J., Flenady, V. (2013). Support for mothers, fathers and families after perinatal death. *Cochrane Database of Systematic Reviews, 6.* https://doi.org/10.1002/14651858.CD000452.pub3

Kübler-Ross, E. (2005). *On grief and grieving: Finding the meaning of grief through the five stages of loss.* Simon & Schuster Inc.

Kübler-Ross, E., Furth, G. M., Elliott, M. P. (1982). *Living with death and dying.* Souvenir.

Kwon, J. E., Kim, Y. H. (2023). Changes in the end-of-life process in patients with life-limiting diseases through the intervention of the Pediatric Palliative Care Team. *Journal of Clinical Medicine, 12*(20), 6588. https://doi.org/10.3390/jcm12206588

Laws, T. (2011). Book review. *Contemporary Nurse, 39*(2), 287–288. https://doi.org/10.1080/10376178.2011.11002567

Li, J., Laursen, T. M., Precht, D. H., Olsen, J., Mortensen, P. B. (2005). Hospitalization for mental illness among parents after the death of a child. *New England Journal of Medicine, 352*(12), 1190–1196. https://doi.org/10.1056/NEJMoa033160

Lindemann, E. (1944). Symptomatology and management of acute grief. *American Journal of Psychiatry, 101*(2), 141–148. https://doi.org/10.1176/ajp.101.2.141

McGuinness, B. (2009). Grief in the workplace: Developing a bereavement policy. *Bereavement Care, 28*(1), 2–8. https://doi.org/10.1080/02682620902746037

Meaney, S., Corcoran, P., Spillane, N., O'Donoghue, K. (2017). Experience of miscarriage: An interpretative phenomenological analysis. *BMJ Open, 7*(3), e011382.

Mehler-Wex, C., Kölch, M. (2008). Depression in children and adolescents. *Deutsches Ärzteblatt International, 105*(9), 149. https://doi.org/10.3238%2Farztebl.2008.0149

Montgomery, K. E., Sawin, K. J., Hendricks-Ferguson, V. (2017). Communication during palliative care and end-of-life: Perceptions of experienced pediatric oncology nurses. *Cancer Nursing, 40*(2), E47–E57. https://doi.org/10.1097/NCC.0000000000000363

Moon, P. J. (2016). Anticipatory grief: A mere concept? *American Journal of Hospice and Palliative Medicine, 33*(5), 417–420. https://doi.org/10.1177/1049909115574262

Moon Fai, C., Gordon Arthur, D. (2009). Nurses' attitudes towards perinatal bereavement care. *Journal of Advanced Nursing, 65*(12), 2532–2541. https://doi.org/10.1111/j.1365-2648.2009.05141.x

Nehari, M., Grebler, D., Toren, A. (2007). A voice unheard: Grandparents' grief over children who died of cancer. *Mortality, 12*(1), 66–78. https://doi.org/10.1080/13576270601088475

Neilson, S. J., Kai, J., MacArthur, C., Greenfield, S. M. (2011). Caring for children dying from cancer at home: A qualitative study of the experience of primary care practitioners. *Family Practice, 28*(5), 545–553. https://doi.org/10.1093/fampra/cmr007

Nielsen, M. K., Neergaard, M. A., Jensen, A. B., Bro, F., Guldin, M. B. (2016). Do we need to change our understanding of anticipatory grief in caregivers? A systematic review of caregiver studies during end-of-life caregiving and bereavement. *Clinical Psychology Review, 44*, 75–93. https://doi.org/10.1016/j.cpr.2016.01.002

Nuzum, D., Meaney, S., O'Donoghue, K. (2018). The impact of stillbirth on bereaved parents: A qualitative study. *PLoS One, 13*(1), e0191635. https://doi.org/10.1371/journal.pone.0191635

O'Connell, O., Meaney, S., O'Donoghue, K. (2016). Caring for parents at the time of stillbirth: How can we do better?. *Women and Birth*, 29(4), 345–349. https://doi.org/10.1016/j.wombi.2016.01.003

Olick, R. S., Braun, E. A., Potash, J. (2009). Accommodating religious and moral objections to neurological death. *The Journal of Clinical Ethics*, 20(2), 183–191.

O'Shea, E. R., Bennett Kanarek, R. (2013). Understanding pediatric palliative care: What it is and what it should be. *Journal of Pediatric Oncology Nursing*, 30(1), 34–44. https://doi.org/10.1177/1043454212471725

Parish, R. (2023). *Informed choice or informed voice? A consideration of the impact of proposed NHS service developments on divided communities* (Doctoral dissertation, Cardiff University).

Parkes, C. M. (1964a). Effects of bereavement on physical and mental health: A study of the medical records of widows. *British Medical Journal*, 2(5404), 274. https://doi.org/10.1136%2Fbmj.2.5404.274

Parkes, C. M. (1964b). Recent bereavement as a cause of mental illness. *The British Journal of Psychiatry*, 110(465), 198–204. https://doi.org/10.1192/bjp.110.465.198

Parkes, C. M. (1965). Bereavement and mental illness. 2. A classification of bereavement reactions. *British Journal of Medical Psychology*, 38,13–26. https://doi.org/10.1111/j.2044-8341.1965.tb00957.x

Parkes, C. M. (1971). Determination of outcome of bereavement. *Proceedings of the Royal Society of Medicine*, 64, 279. https://doi.org/10.1177/003591577106400320

Parkes, C. M. (2013). Elisabeth Kübler-Ross, *on death and dying*: A reappraisal. *Mortality*, 18(1), 94–97 https://doi.org/10.1080/13576275.2012.758629

Pearson, H. (2010). Managing the emotional aspects of end-of-life care for children and young people. *Paediatric Nursing*, 22(7), 31–35. https://doi.org/10.7748/paed2010.09.22.7.31.c7951

Pohlkamp, L., Kreicbergs, U., Sveen, J. (2019). Bereaved mothers' and fathers' prolonged grief and psychological health 1 to 5 years after loss: A nationwide study. *Psycho-Oncology*, 28(7), 1530–1536. https://doi.org/10.1002/pon.5112

Power, S., Meaney, S., Cotter, R., O'Donoghue, K. (2020). Education priorities for voluntary organisations supporting parents experiencing perinatal loss: A Delphi survey. *International Journal of Palliative Nursing*, 26(4), 156–166. https://doi.org/10.12968/ijpn.2020.26.4.156

Power, S., O'Donoghue, K., Meaney, S. (2021). Experiences of volunteers supporting parents following a fatal fetal anomaly diagnosis. *Qualitative Health Research*, 31(5), 835–846. https://doi.org/10.1177/1049732320987834

Price, J., Jordan, J., Prior, L., Parkes, J. (2011). Living through the death of a child: A qualitative study of bereaved parents' experiences. *International Journal of Nursing Studies*, 48(11), 1384–1392. https://doi.org/10.1016/j.ijnurstu.2011.05.006

Rajendran, P., Jarasiunaite-Fedosejeva, G., İsbir, G. G., Shorey, S. (2024). Healthy siblings' perspectives about paediatric palliative care: A qualitative systematic review and meta-synthesis. *Palliative Medicine*, 38(1), 25–41. https://doi.org/10.1177/02692163231217597

Rando, T. A. (1983). An investigation of grief and adaptation in parents whose children have died from cancer. *Journal of Pediatric Psychology*, 8(1), 3–20. https://doi.org/10.1093/jpepsy/8.1.3

Rando, T. A. (1991). Parental adjustment to the loss of a child. In D. Papadatou, C. Papadatos (eds), *Children and death* (pp. 233–253). Taylor & Francis. https://doi.org/10.4324/9780203782262

Ray, K. (2014). The case of Jahi McMath: Race, culture, and medical decision-making. *Voices in Bioethics*, 1. https://doi.org/10.7916/vib.v1i.6509

Rogers, C. H., Floyd, F. J., Seltzer, M. M., Greenberg, J., Hong, J. (2008). Long-term effects of the death of a child on parents' adjustment in midlife. *Journal of Family Psychology*, 22(2), 203–211. https://doi.org/10.1037%2F0893-3200.22.2.203

Rosenberg, A. R., Baker, K. S., Syrjala, K., Wolfe, J. (2012). Systematic review of psychosocial morbidities among bereaved parents of children with cancer. *Pediatric Blood & Cancer*, 58(4), 503–512. https://doi.org/10.1002/pbc.23386

Royal College of Obstetricians and Gynaecologists. (2010). Termination of pregnancy for fetal abnormality in England, Scotland and Wales. Available at: https://www.rcog.org.uk/media/21lfvl0e/terminationpregnancyreport18may2010.pdf (accessed 4 June 2024).

Rush, B. (1947). Medical inquiries and observation upon the diseases of the mind. *Occupational Therapy*, 26, 177–180.

Ryan, K., Connolly, M., Charnley, K., Ainscough, A., Crinion, J., Hayden, C., Wynne, M. (2014). *Palliative care competence framework 2014*. Health Service Executive (HSE).

Schaefer, M. R., Wagoner, S. T., Young, M. E., Madan-Swain, A., Barnett, M., Gray, W. N. (2020). Healing the hearts of bereaved parents: Impact of legacy artwork on grief in pediatric oncology. *Journal of Pain and Symptom Management*, 60(4), 790–800. https://doi.org/10.1016/j.jpainsymman.2020.04.018

Schut, H., Stroebe, M.S. (2005). Interventions to enhance adaptation to bereavement. *Journal of Palliative Medicine*, 8(suppl. 1), s-140. https://doi.org/10.1089/jpm.2005.8.s-140

Shand, A. F. (1914). *The foundations of character: Being a study of the tendencies of the emotions and sentiments* (2nd edn). Macmillan.

Shear, M. K. (2015). Complicated grief. *New England Journal of Medicine*, 372(2), 153–160. https://doi.org/10.1056/NEJMcp1315618

Shear, M. K., Ghesquiere, A., Glickman, K. (2013). Bereavement and complicated grief. *Current Psychiatry Reports*, 15(11), 1–7. https://doi.org/10.1007/s11920-013-0406-z

Shear, M. K., Simon, N., Wall, M., Zisook, S., Neimeyer, R., Duan, N., Keshaviah, A. (2011). Complicated grief and related bereavement issues for DSM-5. *Depression and Anxiety*, 28(2), 103–117. https://doi.org/10.1002/da.20780

Shear, M. K., Skritskaya, N. A. (2012). Bereavement and anxiety. *Current Psychiatry Reports*, 14(3), 169–175. https://doi.org/10.1007/s11920-012-0270-2

Stationery Office. (1953). Births and Deaths Registration Act. Available at: https://www.legislation.gov.uk/ukpga/Eliz2/1-2/20 (accessed 4 June 2024).

Stebbins, J. W., Batrouney, T., Victoria, C. F. (2007). *Beyond the death of a child: Social impacts and economic costs of the death of a child*. Compassionate Friends Victoria.

Stjernswärd, J. (2004). Foreword: Instituting palliative care in developing countries—an urgently needed and achievable goal. *Journal of Pain & Palliative Care Pharmacotherapy*, 17(3–4), xxix–xxxvi. https://doi.org/10.1080/J354v17n03_a

Stroebe, M. S., Stroebe, W., Hansson, R. O. (1988). Bereavement research: An historical introduction. *Journal of Social Issues*, 44(3), 1–18. https://doi.org/10.1111/j.1540-4560.1988.tb02073.x

Sung, G.(2023). Brain death/death by neurological criteria: International standardization and the world brain death project. *Critical Care Clinics*, 39(1), 215–219. https://doi.org/10.1016/j.ccc.2022.08.005

Tan, J. S., Docherty, S. L., Barfield, R., Brandon, D. H. (2012). Addressing parental bereavement support needs at the end-of-life for infants with complex chronic conditions. *Journal of Palliative Medicine*, 15(5), 579–584. https://doi.org/10.1089/jpm.2011.0357

Tatsuno, J., Yamase, H., Yamase, Y. (2012). Grief reaction model of families who experienced acute bereavement in Japan. *Nursing & Health Sciences*, 14(2), 257–264. https://doi.org/10.1111/j.1442-2018.2012.00688.x

The Irish Childhood Bereavement Network. (2018). Families. Available at: https://www.childhoodbereavement.ie/families/ (accessed 4 June 2024).

The Irish Hospice Foundation. (2020a). Losing a child. Available at: https://hospicefoundation.ie/i-need-help/i-am-bereaved/losing-a-child/ (accessed 4 June 2024).

The Irish Hospice Foundation. (2020b). Children's grief. Available at: https://hospicefoundation.ie/i-need-help/i-am-bereaved/types-of-grief/childrens-grief/ (accessed 4 June 2024).

The Irish Hospice Foundation. (2020c). Adult Bereavement Care Pyramid. A national framework. Available at: https://hospicefoundation.ie/wp-content/uploads/2021/02/Adult-Bereavement-Care-Framework-Pyramid-Booklet.pdf (accessed 4 June 2024).

Together for Short Lives (2019). Caring for a child at end-of-life: A guide for professionals on the care of children and young people before death, at the time of death and after death. Available at: https://www.togetherforshortlives.org.uk/app/uploads/2019/11/TfSL-Caring-for-a-child-at-end-of-life-Professionals.pdf (accessed 4 June 2024).

Truog, R. D. (2020). Defining death: Lessons from the case of Jahi McMath. *Pediatrics*, *146*(Suppl.1), S75–S80. https://doi.org/10.1542/peds.2020-08180

Tsey, K., Harvey, D., Gibson, T., Pearson, L. (2009). The role of empowerment in setting a foundation for social and emotional wellbeing. *Australian e-journal for the Advancement of Mental Health*, *8*(1), 6–15. https://doi.org/10.5172/jamh.8.1.6

Widger, K., Steele, R., Oberle, K., Davies, B. (2009). Exploring the supportive care model as a framework for pediatric palliative care. *Journal of Hospice & Palliative Nursing*, *11*(4), 209–216. https://doi.org/10.1097/NJH.0b013e3181aada87

Wilkinson, D., Herring, J., Savulescu, J. (2019). *Medical ethics and law: A curriculum for the 21st century*. Elsevier Health Sciences.

Zisook, S., Reynolds C. F. (2017). Complicated grief. *Focus. American Psychiatric Publisher*, *15*(4), 12s–13s. https://doi.org/10.1176/appi.focus.154S14

Zisook, S., Shear, K. (2009). Grief and bereavement: What psychiatrists need to know. *World Psychiatry*, *8*(2), 67–77. https://doi.org/10.1002%2Fj.2051-5545.2009.tb00217.x

Zurca, A. D., Fisher, K. R., Flor, R. J., Gonzalez-Marques, C. D., Wang, J., Cheng, Y. I., October, T. W. (2017). Communication with limited English-proficient families in the PICU. *Hospital Pediatrics*, *7*(1), 9–15. https://doi.org/10.1542/hpeds.2016-0071

# PART III

## Specialist

# CHAPTER 9

# Managing complexity

..............................................

*Karen Carr, Jitka Kosikova, Tara Kerr-Elliott and Bernadette Basemera*

## INTRODUCTION

Children's palliative care is an intricate and multifaceted field that encompasses a myriad of challenging and sensitive aspects, each of which plays a vital role in the holistic care of children with life-limiting conditions.

In order to identify and discuss complexities within children's palliative care, it is first necessary to ensure we are clear on what we mean by the term "complexity". The theory of complexity and the study of complex systems are a huge topic, but for the purposes of this chapter, we will use the complexity definition of health proposed by Rambihar and Rambihar (2009, p. 338): "Health is an ever-changing emergent property of the complex and dynamic interactions in the web of causation and change that lead individuals and communities towards or away from well-being, disease and infirmity." As such, we will consider complexities arising from decision-making, ethics, including differences in law across countries, complexity in managing physical and psychological symptoms and the challenges associated with bringing these together during the process that is Advance Care Planning. The unique dynamics in the relationships of families, children, nurses and other members of the healthcare team will be explored as we consider the complexity of communication and negotiations.

We acknowledge the intricate tapestry of components that influence the care provided to these vulnerable patients and their families. We explore the complexity of communication within different cultures and the role of healthcare professionals in managing this. We address the imperative of supporting others in high-profile, complex, and controversial cases and the ethical considerations that arise on the "edge of life".

DOI: 10.4324/9781003384861-13

---

**LEARNING OBJECTIVES**

Readers will be able to do the following:

1.  Apply basic ethical principles that are relevant when making decisions with and for very sick children.
2.  Analyse cultures and patterns of communication in managing complex issues and in children's palliative and end-of-life care. This will include the importance of early and ongoing discussions regarding Advance Care Planning which are fundamental in enabling children and their families to make informed decisions about their future medical care. We also analyse the intricate dilemmas for healthcare professionals posed by ethical considerations.
3.  Assess, plan for and implement complex symptom management, including the management of different interacting symptoms encountered in children's palliative and end-of-life care.
4.  Analyse and evaluate the nurse's role, both as an individual and a professional, in self-care and in supporting others to manage reactions to complex and/or multiple interacting issues.

---

Throughout this chapter, we will emphasise the critical importance of child- and family-centred, multi-disciplinary and compassionate approaches in children's palliative care, highlighting the interconnectedness of the themes presented. These themes underscore the intricate nature of the field and the multifaceted approach required to provide the best possible care for children with palliative care needs and their families.

## COMPLEXITY OF COMMUNICATION CULTURES

Each healthcare worker is a trained individual with specific knowledge related to their field of expertise. As nurses, our work involves constant communication with others, such as our colleagues, patients and families. That means talking, asking questions, also listening and at the same time evaluating the verbal and non-verbal messages we are receiving, translating and comparing them to our system of personal and work-related values. Each profession has its unique styles of communication and understanding of the world. One of the key points of keeping the atmosphere of mutual understanding is to acknowledge the differences and create, and treasure, the communication culture within nurses, within our teams, within our facilities, or among other healthcare providers (Larson et al., 2014; Yamasaki et al., 2017).

Mayer (2016) looks at different countries and their cultures from the point of nine coping strategies that people in each culture incorporate while growing up. She compares strategies in communication, giving negative feedback, decision-making, building trust, leadership and hierarchy, and perception of time. The culture we grew up in equips us with strategies that guide us when facing varieties of tasks, both personal and work-related.

Complexity of communicating culture is spread through all the above-mentioned aspects. As Mayer emphasises, the important thing is not to stick to culture or country stereotypes, but to acknowledge the differences and be aware of from which side of the line we look at the communication strategy. It brings us to a better understanding of each other and helps us avoid conflicts.

She divided countries according to the way we have tendencies to communicate in each country. In *High context* cultures, people often use stories for explanation and communication and expect others to understand the message. The other side of the imaginary line are countries using *Low context* communication, where people have a tendency to formulate messages in simple sentences, and finish with verbal clarifications, conclusions and recapitulations (Mayer, 2016).

By understanding our strategies in each aspect of the culture map (Mayer, 2016), we learn about ourselves and, funnily enough, we may realise that we do not have to always belong to the nation or country we were raised in. If we replace the countries with different healthcare professions or specialties, we come to understand how easily one message can be misunderstood by our colleagues or among the interdisciplinary team (Box 9.1).

---

**BOX 9.1 THE HEART STORY FROM YEMEN**

On my first mission in Yemen in 2008, I was part of a team assessing the children with heart conditions. Our task was to complete the diagnostic process and prepare them, when it was indicated, for intervention during the next round in four months. Coming from Europe, the culture was quite new for me, and I was expecting that parents would make decisions based on the same values as in my home country, the Czech Republic. I was surprised when parents left their baby, Leyla, in hospital, with the explanation that we would take better care of her. I did not understand why they acted this way and the question in my head was popping out: "How they could do that? Don't they love their child?" Later that day we managed to sit down with my local colleague and Leyla's parents and he asked them what difficulties they were having and what would help them in the next four months. They calmly answered that they loved their little girl so much, and they had already lost one girl. They feared that they didn't have sufficient money and skills to take care of Leyla, and they understood that she would not survive till our next visit in four months.

Only then we realised it was a misunderstanding. What I have learned is: that understanding the reasons will help me to plan the next steps according to family needs and local possibilities. The most important lesson for me was not to forget to ask.

Source: Jitka Kosikova, paediatric nurse, specialist in intensive care, palliative care, humanitarian worker for Doctors Without Borders.

---

The first step to make communication effective is to acknowledge that we speak in different styles: some use more stories, others conclusions and summary points or checklists. Being able to use strategies and a combination of skills will help us to minimise situations of misunderstanding and lower risks of severe conflicts in the complex healthcare system.

It might seem a difficult task to manage the complexity of communication in our workplace, but the tips mentioned in Box 9.2 can guide you through the steps of what to think about to ensure a good communication flow in a complex environment and, moreover, save you time.

---

**BOX 9.2 ENSURING A GOOD FLOW OF COMMUNICATION IN COMPLEX ENVIRONMENTS**

- Make it simple and accessible:

  - Have a system in place, and know where to find the relevant information.
  - Decide who has access to the information about patients and families and think about why he/she needs it.
  - Think about what topics the system needs to cover, e.g. contents of conversation with families, patients, or your colleagues.

- Standardisation:

  - Write a list of frequently used palliative care words we use and their accurate meaning, e.g. palliative. This will ensure clear communication and better understanding, e.g. in many teams there is misunderstanding that palliative care means actively dying.
  - Standard naming of interactions, e.g. family meetings, team meetings.
  - Understanding the meaning of care helps us to work as individuals in predictable ways.
  - Standards are useful for common interactions, e.g. steps and questions we go through at the first meeting with a child and a family.

- Make it organised:

  - Use checklists, they are useful tools that help us not to skip tasks or areas in communications, e.g. conversation with the patient and the family for the first time.
  - Think about the structure of team meetings and the planning of care.
  - Use summaries of communication with interdisciplinary teams, primary health teams, etc.
  - Write down the summaries of understanding from the information or patients' and family stories.

Source: Larson et al. (2014), Amery (2016), Nimmon and Regehr (2018).

---

## ETHICAL PRINCIPLES ARE KEY TO CHILDREN'S PALLIATIVE CARE

Decisions are made on behalf of and in conjunction with children every day, but for those living with palliative care needs, these decisions can often be particularly challenging with no obvious "correct" option. Where a child is unable to be the sole decision-maker, either because of their age or ability to understand, their parents are usually best placed to decide on their behalf. However, this may not always be straightforward in the context of legal, ethical, societal and healthcare-related complexities.

Ethics is a broad term covering the study of both the nature of morals and also specific moral choices (Varkey, 2021). A basic understanding of the four pillars of medical ethics and related principles will help nurses supporting children and their families when making decisions which are not straightforward or associated with an obvious "right or wrong" course of action.

## The four pillars of medical ethics

1. *Beneficence*: Professionals have a responsibility to act in ways that benefit the child, to "do good".
2. *Non-maleficence*: The obligation to "do no harm". In practical terms, this requires professionals to consider the benefits of potential interventions with burdens.
3. *Autonomy*: Every person has an intrinsic and unconditional worth and should therefore have the power to make rational and moral decisions, and should also be allowed to exercise their capacity for self-determination (Guyer, 2003). Applying this to children, if they are capable of understanding their situation, their input should be taken into account and their wishes and preferences considered.
4. *Justice*: The fair and equitable treatment of all people. Distributive justice is most applicable to clinical ethics and refers to the fair, equitable and appropriate distribution of healthcare (Varkey, 2021). This, however, is often complicated by the structure of healthcare systems which vary across the globe.

While there are numerous opportunities for ethical dilemmas in children's palliative care to arise, certain principles occur frequently and are therefore discussed in more detail below.

## Best interests

Relating to the key ethical principle of beneficence, the paramount consideration in any decision regarding a child's end-of-life care has traditionally been the *best interests* of the child. This includes considering the child's well-being, comfort, and minimising suffering. In some cases, what is perceived as best for the child may differ between the parents and the medical professionals.

When determining the best interests for a child, careful consideration must be paid to the following (adapted from Hauer, 2013):

- the chances of survival
- harms versus benefits of potential treatments
- evidence predicting short- and long-term outcomes of treatment
- long-term implications for the child's suffering and ability to derive pleasure and meaning from life.

It is vital that the child is viewed as a whole person and that best interests decisions do not focus only on what is medically right for the child. Families, including the child wherever possible, can be encouraged to consider the values the child may have developed alongside their goals, likes, dislikes, priorities and any religious beliefs.

It is important to add that the use of "best interests" as a standard in decision-making has become controversial and more recently several bioethicists have argued that a criterion of "significant harm" should be employed instead, particularly when there is significant and irresolvable disagreement (McDougall and Notini, 2014). Wilkinson (2019) summarises this debate in simple terms: when there is disagreement between parents and professionals about healthcare treatment for a child, should the parents be overruled based on "an assessment of what would be *best* for the child, or only if what the parents propose would be *harmful* for the child?". Particular criticisms of the best interest standards often focus on the argument that it is often not possible to know what is the *best* option for an individual child (Wilkinson, 2019). When disagreements occur, there are usually compelling different views about what is *best* for the child.

## Autonomy

In the context of children's palliative care, autonomy becomes much more complex. Children may or may not have the mental and emotional ability to make decisions for themselves and the extent to which they can do so will also depend on the law and the culture in which they live.

In England and Wales, the following key points apply with regard to decision-making:

- Who are those with legal "parental responsibility" for the child.
- Young people aged 16 or 17 years old can consent to treatment on their own with no legal requirement to seek separate consent from their parents. The treatment can legally take place even if the parents refuse consent.
- Young people under the age of 16 can consent to treatment *if* they are deemed to have capacity to fully understand the decision.
- Young people aged 16 or 17 years cannot refuse a treatment that is either life-saving or will prevent serious harm. The same applies to children under the age of 16 who are deemed to have capacity.

Relational autonomy encourages us to consider and respect the child as an individual with their own autonomy, while also recognising their dependence on their family and others (Weaver et al., 2022). The interests of the child and of their parents often overlap and are interdependent (Wilkinson, 2019). Serious childhood illness can impact wider family relationships, finances, physical and emotional well-being, and the ability to achieve at work or school (Weaver et al., 2022). However, the sociological perspective of childhood encourages us to see children as agents, creating meaningful lives through interactions with others, not just within their family, but also with peers and within wider society (Mayall, 2002). Importantly, the ability of children to exercise their own agency or autonomy usually changes as the child grows and develops but, clearly, this can be complicated by the impact of living with palliative care needs.

It is often claimed that parents are uniquely positioned to advocate on behalf of their children and should, therefore, be recognised as the "next best" decision-maker when a child is too young, or cognitively incapable to do so themselves (Weaver et al., 2022).

However, the idea that parents have a fundamental ethical right to make medical decisions for their children is challenged by others, such as Archard et al. (2023), who state that "the child is neither an extension of nor the property of the parent" (p. 5). They point out that while "most parents are moved to do what they think is best for their children ... being moved to do what you think is best is not being moved to do what is, in fact, best" (p. 7). Safeguarding children at all times is of paramount importance and nurses must play an important role in this. Sometimes, actual or potential harm can clearly be identified, and in this case, nurses should follow local safeguarding procedures. At other times, as the discussions in this chapter highlight, the threshold for *harm* is more complex and, when this is the case, nurses are often the professionals who spend the longest amount of time caring for children and should ensure they actively participate in discussions and decision-making in the wider multi-disciplinary team.

As another example, in the Czech Republic, while involving parents is also considered to be a foundation for decision-making, the reality is sometimes different. The Ministry of Health has declared that children have the right to be accompanied at all times by a parent, however, in practice, parents are often prohibited from being present on paediatric wards. Reasons given include "lack of space" or concern that "daily ward routines" may be disrupted. In response, the Czech Helsinki Committee has begun a movement to change this, entitled "Being Together is Normal" (Klinika Paliativní mediciny 1 (2024), https://helcom.cz/tiskova-konference-k-projektu-byt-spolu-je-normalni/, cited in Desai et al., 2018).

While the degree to which parents' rights and responsibilities are balanced may be more nuanced across different countries and legal systems, there is consideration for child protection and welfare across the world and as such, the *rights* of parents are limited, albeit to different degrees in different countries. The World Health Organization recognises children under the age of 18 as being vulnerable and in need of welfare and protection measures and, as stated by Wilkinson et al. (2020), "it is unquestionably good for there to be clear processes within society to intervene if parents are making decisions that would be risky or harmful for the child" (p. 171).

## Truth-telling

One of the most problematic dilemmas for healthcare providers caring for children, when death is a potential outcome, occurs when parents request that the child is not told either their diagnosis, prognosis or both (see Chapter 3, page 76, on closed/open awareness and mutual pretence, adapted from Grinyer, 2012). This request normally arises from a well-intentioned desire to protect their child but appears to conflict with some of the key ethical principles already discussed, most specifically respect for the child's autonomy. How can a child be an active participant in making decisions if they are not told the truth? However, professionals also often fear that overriding this request risks damaging trusting relationships between themselves and the family, and also between the child and their parents.

An autonomous patient also has the right to forgo disclosure of diagnosis and problematic information, but again in practice this can be challenging when working with children and young people. It requires experienced clinicians skilled in communicating to navigate these situations.

Again, the concept of truth-telling or full disclosure differs across different countries and cultures which may vary in their approach to this (Varkey, 2021). However, the United Nations' Convention on the Rights of the Child (United Nations, 1989) highlights the importance of truth-telling and open discussion as modes of protecting a child's rights. However, in the context of children's palliative care, when treatment outcomes may be unclear and prognosis uncertain, defining the "truth" can be complex (Coyne et al., 2016). Gillam et al. (2022) consequently suggest that it may be more helpful to consider the idea of speaking "truthfully". This involves aiming to share our understanding of the situation, allowing us to acknowledge uncertainty and to say "I don't know" when this is appropriate.

While general consensus among both clinicians and ethicists continues to maintain that children "have the right" to "honest" information in a way that is developmentally appropriate for them, some have proposed that it is more helpful to address questions of truth-telling in terms of whether a child's interests are likely to be promoted or threatened by being told the truth (Gillam et al., 2022). This would clearly require careful consideration, excellent communication skills and the ability to analyse the needs of each individual within a unique family unit. Box 9.3 presents Hamida's story.

---

**BOX 9.3 HAMIDA'S STORY**

Hamida was a 13-year-old girl whose family had moved to England from Somalia several years previously. She was from a Muslim family and had three siblings, one of whom had died after a Bone Marrow Transplant (BMT) for the same condition.

She had already had one BMT and was now going through her second, experiencing a significant symptom burden and complications, including graft failure.

She became acutely unwell and required admission to the intensive care unit for sepsis. A week later she was transferred back to the BMT ward, but this experience had been traumatic for both Hamida and her parents as this was the same intensive care unit in which her sister had died.

Back on the ward, Hamida began to deteriorate again and her parents were told that, although active treatment could continue, death was the most likely outcome.

Hamida was expressing increasing anxiety, refusing to be left alone and seeking constant reassurance from nurses and other staff. Her parents, however, refused any psychological support for either Hamida or themselves and stated they did not want her to be told that curative treatment was unlikely.

As Hamida became sicker, she displayed fear and distress, asking staff if she was going to die and begging not to go back to intensive care. Her parents maintained their position that they did not want her to be told and also refused to engage in discussions about goals of care and resuscitation. Hamida was readmitted to the intensive care unit despite asking not to and, after suffering a cardiac arrest, died after multiple resuscitation attempts.

After her death, Hamida's parents, while clearly devastated, maintained that they did not regret the decisions they had made, and reflected that she "died a good death" with many people trying to save her, trying to give her every opportunity to live, and that they had not "given up on her". The staff teams, on both intensive care and the BMT ward, expressed high levels of emotional distress and moral injury, illustrating the complexity of decision-making in these circumstances.

## Support for ethical decision-making

Once again, this will vary geographically. Many countries have well-established bioethics services offering support to healthcare professionals and families facing complex decisions, but others do not.

In the UK, the number of Clinical Ethics Committees (CEC) has been increasing steadily in recent years but, during the COVID-19 pandemic, the numbers accelerated further (Slowther et al., 2004; Brierley et al., 2021). These are multi-disciplinary groups which include lay members that aim to provide support for ethical decision-making within a healthcare setting and can be a helpful resource. The UK Clinical Ethics Network was formed in 2001 to provide support for these committees, including offering a wealth of advice and case studies.

The Nuffield Council on Bioethics (2023) has recommended that guidance should be produced on how to ensure that the parents' and the child's views are taken into account and that parents are supported to provide input into CEC meetings. Currently, there is variation in practice in terms of whether parents and children are invited to be present at reviews, and this is likely to be an area of debate, focus and development over the next few years.

## SUPPORTING OTHERS IN HIGH-PROFILE, COMPLEX AND CONTROVERSIAL CASES: EDGE OF LIFE

Making life or death decisions for children can be profoundly distressing for all involved, and ensuring parents are part of this process can be complex, requiring sensitive communication skills, knowledge of ethical and legal frameworks, ensuring medical expertise and consensus and parental rights and responsibilities are carefully balanced.

Given the complexity of care, medical advances, changes in societal expectations and highly emotive and sensitive decisions, it is unsurprising that conflict can arise. In cases where there is a difference of opinion between medical professionals and parents, efforts should be made to facilitate collaborative decision-making. This can involve open and honest discussions, involving a multi-disciplinary team, and seeking mediation if necessary. Consideration should be given to the cultural and religious beliefs of the parents. These beliefs can significantly influence their decisions about end-of-life care, and healthcare professionals should receive training in how to incorporate these into decision-making conversations.

Compassionate and transparent communication between medical professionals and parents is essential. This will often require the clinicians to acknowledge that the potential outcomes for a particular child are uncertain. This can help build trust and facilitate shared decision-making.

In cases of disagreement, parents have the right to seek second opinions from other medical professionals to ensure that they have explored all available options and are making informed decisions.

Irresolvable differences occasionally occur, even when all the parties are well intentioned, communicating openly and making use of additional resources such as second opinions and mediation services. In the UK in particular, complex cases involving conflict between families and healthcare teams are being played out publicly in the media, invariably causing increased distress and enhancing the need for support for all involved. Parents may turn to social media for support and approval, however, this support is often driven by emotion with facts about the medical issues becoming distorted (Xafis and Bromley, 2020).

It is not only the mainstream and social media that can impact these cases. Parents may seek help from or be approached by other third parties. A judge in a recent UK court case in 2023 expressed "profound concern" about the use of "manipulative litigation tactics" after the family involved in the case was supported by a religious group (Halliday, 2023). The Paediatric Critical Care Society in the UK has stated: "While it's crucial to respect the rights of all parties involved and ensure the child's best interests are upheld, it's equally important to consider the potential impacts of prolonged legal disputes on both the families and healthcare staff" (Halliday, 2023).

In December 2022, the UK Government commissioned an independent review looking into disagreements that arise in the care of critically ill children and concluded that, regardless of severity or duration of a disagreement, everyone involved is at risk of profound and enduring adverse impacts (Nuffield Council on Bioethics, 2023).

Support mechanisms for those involved need to take a multi-pronged approach. There will be no "one-size-fits-all" way of providing support and this is an area of current focus, with some options being briefly discussed below.

## Child

When disagreements become high profile, the child can suffer further as their care and treatment are no longer the sole focus as the time, energy and resources are then directed towards resolving conflict. As Xafis and Bromley (2020, p.94) say: "external pressures in relation to a specific patient can cause both parents' and healthcare professionals' focus to shift *from* the patient to issues *about* the patient".

When a child has capacity to understand their situation, their views and hopes should be sought in a developmentally appropriate way. It is also good practice to appoint an independent person who can advocate for the child, promoting their autonomy.

## Parents

The inevitable emotional and psychological harm experienced by parents due to their child's illness and treatment can be exacerbated by disagreements with their team, sometimes resulting in a complete loss of trust in the healthcare team.

Parents should be provided with appropriate advocacy and support throughout the decision-making process, including access to counselling and resources to help them cope with the emotional and practical challenges they face.

## Healthcare professionals

The potential for moral distress among staff involved in these cases is significant. Jameton (2013) describes moral distress as a response one has to an ethical or moral judgement about care that is different from that of the people who are in charge. High-profile cases increase the potential for moral distress as the dilemmas and conflict that professionals are facing are debated at all levels of society globally, while the teams involved are, of course, unable to comment or reply due to professional issues and patient confidentiality. This includes, of course, not commenting on social media posts relating to the case. Nurses must ensure they adhere not only to their employers' policies and procedures but also the applicable nursing codes and legal restrictions, wherever they are located. For nurses in the UK, for example, this would be the Nursing and Midwifery Council's "Code" of professional standards (NMC, 2018).

The experience of witnessing a child's case reported widely in the media can cause anxiety and distress to healthcare professionals who see their work become distorted in the public eye. Obviously, this is greatest for those involved with that child but the potential for distress extends beyond the treating team. The Nuffield Council on Bioethics (2023) recommended that all staff involved in these cases "are made aware of, supported and encouraged to access a variety of sources of emotional and psychological support" (p. 56). This support may include access to psychological support and clinical supervision, as well as improving the access and quality of communication training for professionals, but it is likely that this needs developing, further research and investment.

## Impact at public health level

The impact of media interference in these cases reaches further than those directly involved, and can lead to misconceptions about children's palliative care, creating mistrust in healthcare professionals in society (Xafis and Bromley, 2020). Education is important here. Public conceptions of children's palliative care often focus on themes of unbearable suffering, tragedy, dying, death and conflict (see Chapter 3), all of which contribute to barriers to timely referral of palliative care. Early referral to palliative care services has been clearly identified as one strategy for preventing conflict in these cases escalating in the first place.

Strategies, such as the project by HEARD, funded by the True Colours Trust in the UK, are one way of attempting to "change hearts and minds" in regards to children's palliative care. HEARD is a specialist communications charity which is seeking to shift the narrative about children's palliative care and provide an alternative view to the story presented in the media when clinical cases make the headlines (for more information, see the Suggested Resources at the end of this chapter).

## CHILDREN'S ADVANCE CARE PLANNING CONVERSATIONS

Globally, paediatric advance care planning discussions are becoming ever more necessary as interventions, technology and treatment trials present increasing choices for families (Jacobs et al., 2023). Advance Care Planning (ACP) discussions should be considered a vital component to providing quality palliative care and in ensuring the child's treatment and care decisions align with child and family needs, values and preferences. Here we are using the term "advance care planning" but, in some places, terms such as "future care", "wishes" or "goals of care discussions" might be used to reflect a focus on the child's and family's hopes, desires and wishes for the child requiring palliative care.

Children's advance care planning discussions must take into account general aspects related to childhood, such as developmental stages, ongoing development, levels of understanding; legalities such as legal age of child (parental rights/responsibility), minor's capacity to consent (Gillick competency/Fraser guidance; NSPCC, 2024) and nurses as surrogate decision-makers, tri/multipartite decision-making responsibility and influence of parents. Alongside these there are many specific issues related to the individual child and their diagnosis and prognostic situation. Uncertain prognosis is common and becoming complicated with medical and technological advances and new interventions offering options where in the past no choice existed. Child death in many societies nowadays is uncommon and becoming more difficult to accept (Burton, 2022). With these challenges in mind, it may be helpful to review Chapter 4 in this text on breaking bad news, or another source on how to communicate bad news or unwanted information.

Advance Care Planning (ACP) is NOT a single intense conversation, it is a communication *process* over time which gives families and, where appropriate, the child/

young person the opportunity to consider care, treatment and realistic options. Discussions may, or may not, result in decision-making or in recording of choices or decisions recorded within the child's notes/formal ACP documentation (Burton, 2022). Documentation is beneficial for communication clarity between nurses and the wider team, however, the sole aim to have written reports can be off-putting to families. Some countries have specifically designed documentation such as that from the Child and Young Person's Advance Care Plan Collaborative UK (CYPACP, 2023).

Advance care discussions should consist of distinct aspects: goals during life, emergency planning, decisions regarding life-sustaining treatments, options at end of life and after death. The focus should be on enabling a good quality of life for the child and family (good palliative care).

There is a misunderstanding that ACP discussions are only about end-of-life decisions (Carr et al., 2022). However, ACP discussions should be based on all aspects of the child's life and reflect the child's and family's values and what is important to them. Wishes impacting the child's life quality, such as time with friends, being at home, memory-making, for example, grandparents holding a newborn, family photographs, etc., may be equally important to the child/family rather than making a decision about life-sustaining treatment options, place of care, place of death and care after death. Professionals are responsible for enabling families to become aware of the choices and thereafter supporting families to achieve the agreed "goals of care".

It is advocated that ACP discussions should begin early in the illness trajectory. Parents and health professionals prefer early phased discussions (Carr et al., 2021; 2022), with parents stating that they feel more in control and "listened to" and professionals report more clarity of parent wishes. However, initiation of these discussions is challenging, and evidence suggests these discussions start at crisis points or close to the end of life (Carr et al., 2022). Factors such as unpredictable illness trajectory, perceived parental non-acceptance and worry about parental reactions delay professionals from initiating the discussions. Parents have worries about initiating the discussions and often feel professionals avoid them (Carr et al., 2021). Children's advance care planning is a sensitive and potentially complicated process which needs to be individually context-driven and tailored to the specific parent and child situation. There are specific legal issues addressing competence, age of consent to interventions, acceptance of or refusal of treatment which are impacted by an individual child's circumstances, e.g. experience with treatments to date or the implications of the decision to be made.

It is the responsibility of the nurse to enable opportunities for these discussions to start early in the illness trajectory. A number of resources have been developed to assist nurses and parents/ill children get conversations started and communicate wishes (see Suggested Resources at the end of the chapter). A synopsis of the information from these resources is presented in Table 9.1.

**TABLE 9.1** Who, where and when

| | |
|---|---|
| Who? | • Who starts? Parent, child or professional? Parents are wary of starting these discussions and expect the professional to take the lead. Parents are dependent on nurses being willing, able and brave enough to start discussions and pick up on parental cues. Professionals await parent cues for "permission" to open the conversation and also to have discussions with the child.<br><br>• Who should lead? The professional must be trusted by the parent/child to be focused on the child's best interests. It is important the health professional is self-aware and has good communication skills, and an appropriate level of comfort with extreme emotions. Rapport with parents is important though this does not always require a long-term relationship with the family.<br><br>• Who should be present? Parent(s), or child (where appropriate), trusted competent professional. Thereafter, any professional and family support individuals must be requested and agreed by the family. Caution is required not to overwhelm or outnumber the family. |
| Where? | A private place where parents and family feel safe to ask questions and be emotional without fear of interruption or being overheard. |
| When? | When in the illness trajectory? Preferably the discussions should start early enough in the child's illness trajectory. Timely initiation allows for progressing at the parents'/child's pace and enables a phased approach, where the professional can in due course broach more difficult topics and end-of-life issues at a stage when the family indicate readiness. Initiation early allows the family more time to ask questions and process the situation. Families not willing to make decisions regarding major aspects of advance planning, such as treatment limitation, should be offered the option to participate in discussions at reasonably regular opportunities, and their choice to "not make decisions" recorded and shared as it is the communication around these discussions which is paramount. Early discussions increase the time the family has to think and consider options so that ultimately, where possible, the family and professional are in agreement regarding future plans and decisions, or in the worst scenario, that health professionals are aware early of potential disagreements. Early awareness enables appropriate introduction of mediation.<br><br>When in the day/admission, etc.? Conversations may be proactive or reactive. Proactive allows for planning whereas reactive is "grasping the moment". If the nurse does not have time when a parent indicates readiness, the importance of the topic should be acknowledged and a new time agreed. The nurse must ensure they return as arranged. Parents and nurses should be strong – these conversations require energy.<br><br>How much time? Enough to have an in-depth discussion and for parents to have questions answered. Limited when parents clearly need to stop. Agreed time for further conversations should be arranged. Gauge each case individually, e.g. the situation where a parent has travelled for hours to be available while balancing other home/family/work responsibilities may be different to a couple being available daily on the ward. |

## What should be said in ACP and *how* should it be said?

The following can help in planning an ACP discussion:

- Prepare:
  - Plan ahead and identify any personal gaps in knowledge regarding diagnosis, prognosis, treatment options, communication skills and specifics regarding the child and family.
  - Gather the information required. Be aware of local resources. Understand the process of ACP locally.
  - Professionals must communicate well between each other and agree on roles, responsibilities, and processes for information sharing, as this is vital whether decisions are made or not. Professionals must also be aware of the complexity of communication cultures (see section above).
  - Inform parents about the concept of advance planning discussions.
  - Ask parents who they would prefer to have the discussion with and help them identify a professional they are comfortable talking to.
  - Start early and remember advance care planning is more than one conversation.
  - Involve a trained facilitator (if available).
- Seek permission:
  - Invite the parent/child to share what is important to them.
- Explore:
  - Assess information preferences of the parent/child.
  - Explore parents'/child's understanding of current stage of illness.
- Align parents'/child's and professionals' understanding:
  - Inform parents/child of medical and nursing knowledge of current illness stage and predicted care changes.
  - Listen to parents/child regarding their current lived experience.
- Key discussions:
  - The process of communication and discussing should assist parents/child to be aware of what lies ahead, and the potential decisions they will be supported to make prior to being under pressure in a crisis.
  - Goals, fears, worries, family support, cultural requirements, how they communicate to child, siblings and extended family are all important to discuss.
  - Parallel planning is important where the prognosis is unclear, i.e. planning both for recovery/rehabilitation and for death/bereavement alongside each other.
  - Addressing, in a sympathetic manner, what lies ahead, what is predictable and what is possible.
  - Educating parents of interventions, such as resuscitation, and what this really involves before a deterioration or crisis occurs.
  - Informing parents/child of realistic options, such as the potential for chosen place of death to be home, hospital or a children's hospice.

- Informing parents of support available to them.
- Review:
  - Summarise succinctly.
  - Check parental/child understanding.
  - Inform parents/child of the process.
  - Arrange the next meeting.
- Documentation:
  - Whether advance care discussions result in an advance care preference and/or decisions regarding aspects of care or not, discussions must be logged in medical and nursing notes and, where available, in dedicated documentation.
- Dissemination of information:
  - Be clear on the process for dissemination to ensure other professionals are aware of progress, decisions, changes.
  - Use electronic sharing, when available.
  - Provide parents with original document.
  - Ensure parents are aware of who to contact if changes are to be made.
- General:
  - Keep conversation person-/child-centred and focus on maintaining discussion and decisions in the child's best interest.
  - Maintain an openness to change.
- Vital point:
  - These discussions have an emotional toll on professionals and the family, therefore appropriate support should be available for all involved.

## INCLUDING CHILDREN

Advance care discussions should include the child/young person when they are capable of understanding the options and choices and the benefits and consequences of decisions, i.e. have the capacity to understand their situation. The child's ability, stage of development and experience regarding personal illness and treatments impact the capacity of the individual child in participating in advance care planning. In addition to this, there is variation within and between countries regarding involvement of the child, e.g. in the Czech Republic, it is the law that from 14 years old children must "have a voice" when any treatments have an impact on their physical integrity, basically to all procedures, and nurses have to inform the parents about this law.

Children may benefit from ACP conversations that are sensitive to their age, cognitive development and emotional needs. Engaging in these conversations early can empower children to express their preferences, offer a sense of control, and ensure their values and goals are considered in decision-making processes. However, initiating ACP conversations with children presents several challenges. These include concerns about the child's emotional well-being, the child's comprehension of complex medical scenarios, and the need to involve parents or guardians in the process. Concerns of involving the child are also closely linked to relational autonomy and

**TABLE 9.2** Strategies to involve children in ACP

| Strategy | Implementation |
| --- | --- |
| Tailoring the conversation to the child's developmental stage | Discussions should be age-appropriate, taking into account the child's cognitive abilities and emotional readiness (IMPACT, 2023) |
| Involving the child's support network | Parents, guardians, and other trusted individuals should be engaged to ensure a comprehensive approach to ACP |
| Ongoing education and communication | Consistent communication and periodic re-assessment of the child's wishes are key to maintaining a relevant ACP |
| Providing a safe and supportive environment | A non-threatening, empathetic atmosphere is crucial to help children express their thoughts, fears and preferences |
| Using age-appropriate tools and resources | Visual aids, storybooks and interactive materials can make the process more accessible and engaging for children |
| Tailoring the conversation to the non-verbal child | Consider how a child can be assisted to participate, e.g. augmented and alternative communication strategies and equipment |

truth-telling, as discussed previously in this chapter, and are undoubtedly a reflection of how children are seen or thought of in a community, i.e. we don't think children of X age can make their own decision, despite the abilities of the child and the poor predictive value of age. Healthcare providers, educators and parents must collaborate to address these challenges. Tools to facilitate ACP conversations with adolescents and children exist such as My CHOiCES™ (Zadeh et al., 2015) and IMPACT (IMPACT, 2023). Some strategies can be employed to assist with involving children, see Table 9.2.

## EDUCATION

ACP education and training are variable between and within countries with limited input to undergraduate nursing education. The focus tends to be post-registration multiprofessional education on the implementation of ACP conversation and documentation, such as in the United Kingdom – CYPACP – Child & Young Persons Advance Care Plan Collaborative, in Canada, the Serious Illness Communication Program for Advance Care Planning in Children, Adolescents, and Young Adults with Serious Illness (DeCourcey et al., 2021), and in the Netherlands, Implementing Pediatric Advance Care Planning Toolkit (IMPACT) (Fahner et al., 2021).

The Children's Palliative Care Education Standard Framework and Self-Audit Tool is recommended to standardise professional education in advance care planning for children (Children's Palliative Care Education and Training UK and Ireland Action Group) (CPCET, 2023).

## THE RELATIONSHIPS OF CARERS, CHILDREN AND NURSES (HEALTHCARE STAFF): TRIPARTITE NEGOTIATIONS

For humans, there are two basic needs: safety and control (McLeod, 2007). While we work with children and their parents, the task of keeping the child safe and protecting them is becoming the most important one for their parents. However, there are many aspects and times they cannot control, nor may be controlled. This includes the place of care such as hospital, home, respite, holidays or school. This also influences who will be with them, such as professionals, other parents, other children, and who cannot be with them such as their friends, school mates and other family members. All this creates an environment in which children and parents have limited power and cannot control and create a safe space for their child and themselves. That also means the option of saying "STOP" or "NO", and choosing and expressing who they trust are restricted.

Decisions children and parents make are based on these needs and also on their own values. Getting to know a family's values is one of the communication skills nurses must become adept at. Nurses spend a lot of time with the child and their parents, and this gives them the opportunity to listen to their conversation, their fears and enables opportunities to ask questions and understand about their values, needs and fears. In these conversations, nurses can become translators using paraphrases from parent to child and more often from child to parents (Voss and Raz, 2016) (Box 9.4).

---

**BOX 9.4 CAUGHT IN ROUTINE TO PLEASE PARENTS**

At the hospice, we were taking care of a 9-year-old boy with leukaemia. He went to hospital once every ten days for a transfusion, which was done in an outpatient setting and this meant he and his parents only had to spend up to 4 hours in hospital. To limit the time in hospital, before the visit, we took the blood samples at home, and they went when the transfusion was ready for him. The parents of this child were always there with us during the visits and directed the conversation. One day, it happened that I stayed with the child alone. He used this time to tell me one sentence, "I see lots of suffering each time I go to hospital, and I am better at home." It opened up space for me to ask more and understand what he really meant by saying this. I later communicated to his parents that his wish was to stay at home, where he feels safe. At first, they were surprised that he had never told them that he didn't like hospitals. They felt that they needed to go there, because that would be something helping him to feel better. They always bribed him with some toy to make the visit better and bearable, as they were trying to make it a fun trip.

During my next visit, they told me that they had asked the child about the trips to hospital and gave him the option not to go there, if that was his wish. They had one month together at home with fun times to go to the park, to play with his brother, to watch movies and simply be together. After he passed away, his parents reflected that when they had a conversation about values and wishes, and let their son guide them in what he needed and where he felt safe, it gave them one beautiful month together as a family.

Source: Jitka Kosikova, paediatric nurse, specialist in intensive care, palliative care, humanitarian worker for Doctors Without Borders.

## ASSESSING AND UNDERSTANDING VALUES

Underpinning the communication, and vital to advance care planning (ACP), are some core values (Figure 9.1).

Rosenberg and Chopra (2015) in their book, *Nonviolent Communication*, present four steps of communication techniques that help us to gain further understanding of people's values (Figures 9.2.(a)–9.2(d)).

We all can have difficulty assessing others' values, priorities and wishes. This relates to our own values, priorities and wishes. From time to time, it can cause conflict between us as professionals, and also between parents and their children, as values can vary and are unique to the individual. All healthcare professionals can use meditation techniques not only to facilitate the conversations between parents and children, but also between professional healthcare and social care workers and all the above-mentioned groups. Meditation is often used in planning the future care or when dealing with complaints or conflicts of interest (Moore, 2014). Getting "no" as an answer is the beginning, not the end, often it is a demonstration of feelings rather than the result of considerations of all the pros and cons (Voss and Raz, 2016, p. 34).

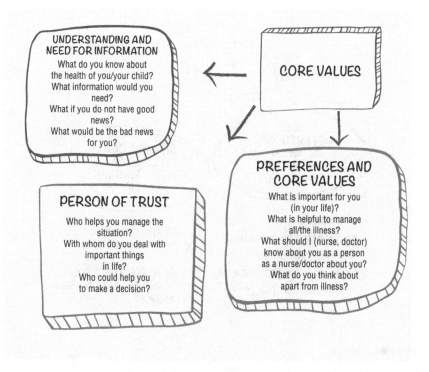

**FIGURE 9.1** Core values and understanding

Source: Klinika paliativni mediciny 1. (2024), cited in Desai et al. (2018).

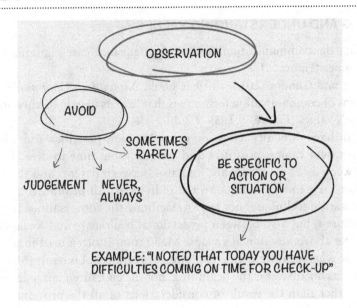

**FIGURE 9.2(A)** Observation

Source: adapted from Rosenberg and Chopra (2015).

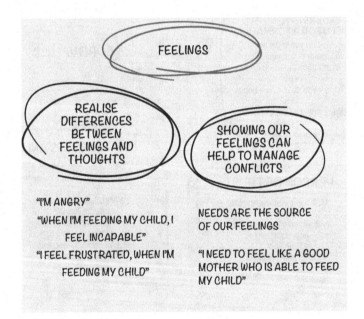

**FIGURE 9.2(B)** Feelings

Source: adapted from Rosenberg and Chopra (2015).

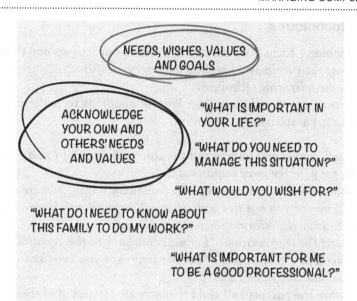

**FIGURE 9.2(C)** Needs, wishes, values and goals

Source: adapted from Rosenberg and Chopra (2015).

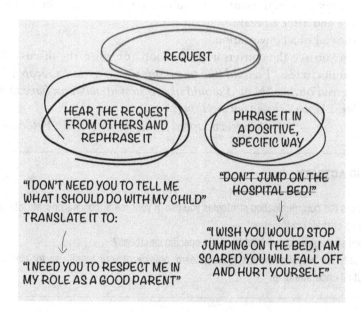

**FIGURE 9.2(D)** Request

Source: adapted from Rosenberg and Chopra (2015).

## Mediation techniques

1. Active listening – focus is on the context, not on our feelings and thoughts:
   - Naming their feelings: *"I see you are angry, confused ..."*
   - Using the mirroring technique.
   - Confirmation of understanding: We use questions to understand the core meaning, paraphrase or conclusion.
2. Paraphrase:
   - To confirm that you understand the core meaning: *"If I understand it correctly, for you, the most important ..."*
   - To soften the negative impact of the communication: *"You are saying that it is difficult for you not to know what will happen with your child, and you need to have the information written down."*
   - To direct the conversation: *"Let me come back to this point/fact ..."*
   - To interrupt a long speech: *"Let me interrupt you here and ensure that I understand everything..."*
   - To assure the parents and child that you are interested in their story/situation and their feelings: *"I see that this information surprised you"*, or *"I see that you worry about your parents."*
3. Conclusion: Summarising helps during difficult and long conversations to anchor each of the parties. We use it:
   - At the beginning, if we are continuing from a previous conversation.
   - Before and after a break.
   - At the end of a conversation.
   - When you see the conversation is chaotic or when the discussion is going round in circles: *"I would like to summarise ..."*, *"Let's recap"*, *"Till now, we agreed on..."*, *"Now, I would like to sum up what we have talked about so far... Have I forgotten anything?"*

                    *Source: adapted from Moore (2014); Patockova (2013).*

---

**LEARNING ACTIVITY**

- Assess the communication strategies you use in your team (conclusions, structures, storytelling or their combination).
- What strategies do you tend to use in specific situations?
- Identify the ways/methods you (your team, outside of your team) use for clarification of mutual understanding.

---

## MANAGING COMPLEX SYMPTOM INTERACTIONS IN CHILDREN'S PALLIATIVE CARE FOR CHILDREN WITH LIFE-LIMITING CONDITIONS

With empathy and affection, nurses provide holistic care to children with palliative care needs and their families. Children's palliative care is more complex because we are working with children rather than young adults. In most instances, having precise knowledge and skills in caring for children with complex issues is significantly beneficial. It requires a lot of patience and courage in dealing with children who have life-threatening and life-limiting conditions especially those with more complex symptoms.

Children's symptom management can be complex and difficult, but when nurses are able to do it correctly, it considerably enhances the quality of life (see Chapter 7). Symptom assessment should begin from the diagnosis of a life-threatening condition and continue throughout the course of the disease. Treatment techniques for each symptom are determined by the symptom's reversibility, disease trajectory, and family care goals. Non-pharmacological as well as pharmacological treatments should be used. The healthcare team and the parents/caregivers should make decisions together. Whenever possible, cultural norms and customs should be respected and followed. However, in certain cultures this may conflict with the nurses' beliefs and research-based palliative care education, such as the Taiwanese may not discuss dying aloud as they believe this will bring bad luck, or Buddhists may refuse their child medications which may "cloud" their mind near death (Givler et al., 2023). Palliative care should be holistic, covering not only the physical but also the spiritual, emotional, and social components of the patient's life.

When working with children living with palliative care needs, it is essential to ensure adequate and continuous assessment of the child's and the family's needs, as well as the quality of care. This assessment, however, can be challenging due to the wide range of patients in terms of age, developmental stage, and medical condition. Physical, psychological, social, and spiritual needs are all included.

Children living with palliative care needs experience a range of physical and psychosocial symptoms which can be challenging to manage. Complex symptom interactions require a holistic approach which addresses the interplay of the various symptoms, treatment effects and side effects, considers the unique needs of each child and acknowledges the impact that child and family psychological harmony or discord has on the physical symptoms.

There are increasing numbers of children with multiple acute and chronic health problems potentially affecting multiple organs (Marcus et al., 2022). The outcome of this is the need for supportive healthcare throughout the child's life from many professionals, with knowledge and skills encompassing many areas such as basic nursing care, medical care, the use of complex medical technology, specialist nursing care, psychological support of the child, siblings and parents. There is a need not only to support parents but also to teach them to care for their child and maintain a functional home in the midst of the practicalities and stresses involved in caring for a child with complex needs.

In Chapter 7, we looked specifically at individual symptoms, and guidelines on symptom management are readily available (Jassal, 2022). However, it is vital to recognise that it is often the combination of many physical and psychological symptoms, alongside the situational impact on the family, available support services and individual levels of resilience, which makes symptom management in children's

**TABLE 9.3** SBAR communication

| | |
|---|---|
| **S** = Situation | • Identify yourself and the address/unit you are calling from |
| | • Identify the patient by name and the reason for your report |
| | • Describe your concern |
| **B** = Background | • Give the reason for the patient's admission |
| | • Explain significant medical history |
| | • Inform of the patient's background, e.g. current medications |
| **A** = Assessment | • Vital signs |
| | • Clinical impressions, concerns |
| **R** = Recommendation | • Explain what you need: be specific about the request and time frame |
| | • Make suggestions |
| | • Clarify expectations |
| Readback | • Making sure you have been understood. It is important that the receiver of the information "reads back" a summary of the information to ensure accuracy and clarity |

Source: NHS Institute for Innovation and Improvement (2010).

palliative care more complex. This complexity renders the child at a high risk of adverse medical and developmental outcomes and the child and family in danger of negative psychosocial impacts. All professionals involved with the child and family have a role in assessing and managing symptoms and their interactions (Sreedhar et al., 2020). However, nurses have a key role in symptom management. With their provision of direct care, alongside parents, nurses are in a prime position to observe and assess the effectiveness of therapies, interventions and medication. The nurse has a responsibility to act on what is happening with the child symptomatically. The nurse must use their knowledge, skills and experience to use prescribed medications and therapies appropriately to alleviate troublesome symptoms. When symptoms are not responding to the interventions recommended, the nurse must know when and how to contact specialist nurses and other appropriate health professionals in a timely manner to ensure the child is appropriately cared for. Use of the SBAR (S = Situation, B = Background, A = Assessment, R = Recommendation), approach is recommended to ensure effective communication which requires a prompt response from the receiver (NHS Institute for Innovation and Improvement, 2010), see Table 9.3.

### Example

**S:** This is Jenna Jones, Community Children's Nurse. I am calling from a patient's home. The patient is Samuel Foster, address 7 Rowan Lane, Bigtown. My contact number is …

Samuel is 7, has a diagnosis of medulloblastoma and is receiving palliative care at home. Overall deterioration over the past 10 days in keeping with his diagnosis. I believe he is in pain.

**B:** He has been on a syringe driver containing Diamorphine and Midazolam for the past 5 days. In the past 12 hours, he has required three doses of break-through medication. Syringe driver not due to be changed for another 8 hours.

**A:** Currently he is very restless and crying out. Pulse 125, Temp 36.8. Last bowel motion 36 hours ago. Intake minimal. His parents are very anxious. Site and driver checked, and medication being delivered as prescribed. Pain assessment has gone from 4/10 two hours ago to 9/10.

**R:** I need a home visit by a doctor or specialist nurse with prescribing authority to assess Samuel and update prescription administration chart and start the new prescription in syringe driver as soon as possible.

Readback expected:

**S:** Samuel Foster, address 7 Rowan Lane, Bigtown. You are Nurse Jenna Jones and your contact number is …

Samuel is 7, has medulloblastoma and is receiving palliative care. He is in pain.

**B:** He has a syringe driver with Diamorphine and Midazolam. In the past 12 hours he has required three doses of breakthrough medication. Syringe driver not due to be changed for another 8 hours.

**A:** He appears in severe pain.

**R:** You need a doctor or specialist nurse with prescribing authority as soon as possible to assess Samuel and write up a new prescription, and to get increased analgesia commenced in syringe driver quickly.

The nurse must be alert to changes in the child physically, psychologically and behaviourally which may indicate the need to change management. The nurse must know what symptoms to expect with the child's prognosis/condition, and also the effects and side effects prevalent with the treatments being used. Nurses must also know about normal childhood development so they can recognise and deal appropriately with each stage when combined with a life-limiting condition Complexities increase further in the pre-verbal and non-verbal child. It becomes the nurse's responsibility to ensure that assessment of symptoms is carried out effectively and that there is a consistency between assessments.

Open communication with parents or adult carers who know the child well, a clearly discussed and well-written history of the child's "normal" behaviour and their specific communication idiosyncrasies, e.g. common signs of discomfort, pain, hunger, boredom, anger, etc, are vital. In all cases, but particularly complex cases, the need to discuss actual and potential symptoms with specialist palliative care nurses and medical professionals and share this with parents is crucial. This enables the nurses and families to understand what is expected. In-depth open-minded assessment and thereafter a diagnostic process tailored to the individual child are important. A thorough, efficient approach is essential, contemplating aspects such as, "Is this expected with the prognosis? Is this a side effect of current/new medication? Is this a new symptom or worsening of an existing one? Could this be a symptom any child at this developmental stage may experience, e.g. gum ache when a new tooth is erupting? Maybe a common childhood ailment, e.g. chicken pox?"

The complexity of not only making the diagnosis but then finding the cause is common in children with medical complexity, e.g. constipation may be caused by a lack of movement in an immobile child, poor fluid intake, dietary content, medication side effects, hence the history is vital – "Is this a new or existing symptom? When did it start? Were there other changes in care associated with the new/aggravated symptom?" Often finding the source of the problem is elusive and a trial of treatment, e.g. regular analgesia, could be commenced to identify if irritability is caused by pain.

## KEY STRATEGIES FOR MANAGING COMPLEX SYMPTOM INTERACTIONS IN CHILDREN'S PALLIATIVE CARE

- *Comprehensive assessment*: Alongside the holistic assessment described above, conduct a thorough assessment of the child's symptoms. This assessment should include physical symptoms (such as pain, nausea and shortness of breath), psychological symptoms (anxiety, depression), and other concerns (spiritual, social, and cultural). Include the family/carers in the child assessment. Adequate and continuous assessment of the child's and the family's needs is essential. Assessment, however, can be challenging due to the wide range of patients in terms of age, developmental stage and medical condition. There is a considerable need in current clinical practice to identify and deploy validated tools with a wide range of goals, such as referring patients to the most appropriate children's palliative care service, assessing the severity of the child's and the family's needs, and monitoring the quality of care provided.
- *Family assessment*: Multi-disciplinary collaboration. Involve and work closely with the available multi-disciplinary team, including doctors, nurses, social workers, psychologists and other specialists. Collaborative efforts help to ensure a comprehensive approach to managing multiple symptoms. Work as a team and use all available technologies to communicate clearly, regularly and effectively.
- *Prioritise symptom management*: Children living with palliative care needs often experience complex symptoms that require specialised care. Therefore, expertise in managing pain and symptoms is crucial in ensuring the child's comfort and quality of life. Identify and address the underlying causes of symptoms whenever possible. Address the symptom expected with the condition or expected with the current medication. Treatment techniques for each symptom are determined by the symptom's reversibility, disease trajectory and family care goals. Anticipate and, where possible, avoid symptoms due to side effects, e.g. constipation related

to morphine (see Chapter 4 and Chapter 7). Prioritise symptoms based on their severity and impact on the child's quality of life. This helps in focusing on the most critical symptoms, while also considering the child's preferences.

- *Medication management*: Use evidence-based guidelines for medication management. Ensure that medications are administered in a way that optimises symptom relief, while simultaneously minimising potential side effects and drug interactions.

- *Proactive monitoring*: Continuously monitor and reassess symptoms, as their severity and nature may change over time. Regular assessments help detect new symptom interactions and evolving needs. Educate parents/carers on what to observe and monitor.

- *Non-pharmacological interventions*: Work with parent/carers/child to explore non-pharmacological interventions, such as physical therapy, occupational therapy, relaxation techniques, or complementary therapies like massage, play, pet or music therapy, to complement pharmacological treatments.

- *Psychological support*: Address the psychosocial aspects of symptom interactions by providing emotional support, counselling and coping strategies to both the child and the family. Anxiety, depression and distress can significantly exacerbate physical symptoms. Support the child and family and ensure they are referred to appropriate additional services and encourage them to develop their own healthy coping strategies (Verberne et al., 2019).

- *Family involvement*: Involve the child's family in symptom management discussions and decision-making. Their insights and observations are invaluable in understanding the child's experience and tailoring care plans.

- *Clear communication*: Maintain open and honest communication with the child and the family. Discuss expected and potential symptoms and management options throughout the course of the illness. Ensure the child and the family are aware of potential outcomes to ensure informed decision-making (Fraser et al., 2020).

- *Ethical considerations*: Be prepared to navigate complex ethical dilemmas that may arise when managing symptom interactions, especially in cases where aggressive treatment options may have limited benefit. Trials of new treatments are experiments, they may not save this child, may even hasten or change the death, but they may eventually improve outcomes for others. Parents must be made aware of this.

- *Self-care*: While supporting families, nurses should not neglect themselves. McCloskey and Taggart (2010) pinpointed several work-related stressors of particular relevance to children's palliative care which included the ethical conflicts that exemplify the role, and the specific emotional demands of this type of nursing.

In children's palliative care, managing complex symptom interactions is an ongoing process that demands a child-centred, family-supportive, multi-disciplinary and empathetic approach. By addressing physical, psychological, and social aspects of care, healthcare providers can improve the overall quality of life for children with palliative care needs and their families.

## SUMMARY

As a children's palliative care nurse, the role involves managing the multifaceted and often emotionally charged complexities of caring for children living with palliative care needs. Expertise, compassion, and the ability to collaborate with healthcare teams and families are essential in delivering holistic, child-centred care.

In the past decade, the ethical disputes have undoubtedly become more complex and public. Support should be strategic and multifaceted with the onus not just on the caregiver but the institutions and governing bodies (Grauerholz et al., 2020).

## KEY POINTS

- Assessing the culture of others helps us to understand each other and be able to work and care for a variety of patients from different cultures.
- Be brave: do not be afraid to address difficult topics.
- When individual cases involve conflict or become high profile, it is vital to consider the impact on all involved and continue to develop support mechanisms that are varied and flexible.
- A basic understanding of key ethical issues can help nurses when supporting families making complex decisions.
- Advance care planning is a communication process over time and must be started early to avoid complex decision-making in times of crisis.
- Nurses are often translators from child to the parents and vice versa. Therefore, it is important for every nurse to incorporate good communication and facilitation skills to help them to identify the values, wishes and fears.
- Prioritise symptoms based on their severity and impact on the child's quality of life.

## SUGGESTED RESOURCES

- Australia
  - Royal Children's Hospital, Melbourne. Comprehensive information for professionals on advance care planning within the palliative care section (RCH Melbourne, 2023). Available at: https://www.rch.org.au/rch_palliative/for_health_professionals/Advance_Care_Planning/
- The UK
  - CYPACP (Child & Young Persons Advance Care Plan and Child and Young Person's Advance Care Plan Collaborative). Resources and documents to assist with advance care planning discussions between professionals, patients and their families such as *Collaborative planning for end-of-life decisions-Best practice guidance to enhance the process of advance care planning for a child or young person* (CYPACP, 2023). Available at: http://cypacp.uk

- Royal College of Paediatrics and Child Health. "Making decisions to limit treatment in life-limiting and life-threatening conditions in children: a framework for practice" (Larcher et al., 2015).
- Heard toolkit for communicating about children's palliative care. Available at: https://heard.org.uk/articles/childrens-palliative-care-project-page
- Canada
  - Serious illness conversation guide for use in paediatrics (van Breemen, 2018).
- The Netherlands
  - IMPACT – Kenniscentrum kinderpalliatieve zorg – Resources to support children, parents and health professionals. Available atL https://kinderpalliatief.nl/impact/en/uk-en-us (IMPACT, 2023).

## REFERENCES

Amery, J. (2016). *A really practical handbook of children's palliative care for doctors and nurses anywhere in the world.* Lulu Publishing Services. Available at: https://icpcn.org/wp-content/uploads/2023/01/A-REALLY-PRACTICAL-Handbook-of-CPC.pdf (accessed 23 May 2024).

Archard, D., Cave, E., Brierley, J. (2023). How should we decide how to treat the child?: Harm versus best interests in cases of disagreement. *Medical Law Review*, 32(2), 158–177. https://doi.org/10.1093/medlaw/fwad040

Brierley, J., Archard, D., Cave, E. (2021). Clinical ethics support: Addressing legal uncertainties. *Journal of Medical Ethics* (online blog). Available at: https://blogs.bmj.com/medical-ethics/2021/02/04/clinical-ethics-support-addressing-legal-uncertainties/

Burton, L. (ed.). (2022). *Care of the child facing death* (9th edn). Routledge.

Carr, K., Hasson, F., McIlfatrick, S., Downing, J. (2021). Parents' experiences of initiation of paediatric advance care planning discussions: A qualitative study. *European Journal of Pediatrics*, 181, 1185–1196. https://doi.org/10.1007/s00431-021-04314-6

Carr, K., Hasson, F., McIlfatrick, S., Downing, J. (2022). Initiation of paediatric advance care planning: Cross-sectional survey of health professionals reported behaviour. *Child: Care, Health and Development*, 48(3), 423–434. https://doi.org/10.1111/cch.12943

Coyne, I., Amory, A., Gibson, F., Kiernan, G. (2016). Information-sharing between healthcare professional, parents and children with cancer: More than a matter of information exchange. *European Journal of Cancer Care*, 25(1), 141–156. https://doi.org/10.1111/ecc.12411

CPCET (Children's Palliative Care Education and Training UK and Ireland Action Group) and Child and Young Person's Advance Care Plan Collaborative, (2023), ICPCN. Available at: https://icpcn.org/wp-content/uploads/2023/09/CPCET-Standard-Framework-for-Advance-Care-Planning-for-Children.pdf (accessed 14 May 2024).

CYPACP (Child and Young Person's Advance Care Plan Collaborative), (2023). Collaborative planning for end-of-life decisions: Best practice guidance to enhance the process of advance care planning for a child or young person. Available at: https://cypacp.uk/wp-content/uploads/2023/11/CYPACP-Guidance-Nov-2023.pdf (accessed 23 May 2024).

DeCourcey, D. D., Partin, L., Revette, A., Bernacki, R., Wolfe, J. (2021). Development of a stakeholder driven serious illness communication program for advance care planning in children, adolescents, and young adults with serious illness. *The Journal of Pediatrics*, 229, 247–258. e8. https://doi.org/10.1016/j.jpeds.2020.09.030

Desai, A. V., Klimek, V. M., Chow K., Epstein, A. S., Bernal, C., Anderson, K., Okpako, M., Rawlins-Duell, R., Kramer, D., Romano, D., Goldberg J. I., Nelson, J. E. (2018). 1-2-3

Project: A quality improvement initiative to normalize and systematize palliative care for all patients with cancer in the outpatient clinic setting. *Journal of Oncology Practice*, 14(12), e775–e785, https://doi.org/10.1200/JOP.18.00346

Fahner, J., Rietjens, J., van der Heide, A., Milota, M., van Delden, J., Kars, M. (2021). Evaluation showed that stakeholders valued the support provided by the Implementing Pediatric Advance Care Planning Toolkit. *Acta Paediatrica*, 110(1), 237–246. https://doi.org/10.1111/apa.15370

Fraser, L. K., Bluebond-Langner, M., Ling, J. (2020). Advances and challenges in European paediatric palliative care. *Medical Sciences*, 8(2), 20. https://doi.org/10.3390/medsci8020020

Gillam, L., Spriggs, M., McCarthy, M., Delany, C. (2022). Telling the truth to seriously ill children: Considering children's interests when parents veto telling the truth *Bioethics*, 36, 765–773. https://doi.org/10.1111/bioe.13048

Givler, A., Bhatt, H., Maani-Fogelman, P. A. (2023). The importance of cultural competence in pain and palliative care. StatPearls Publishing. Available at: https://www.ncbi.nlm.nih.gov/books/NBK493154/ (accessed 23 May 2024).

Grauerholz, K. R., Fredenburg, M., Jones, P. T., Jenkins, K. N. (2020). Fostering vicarious resilience for perinatal palliative care professionals. *Frontiers in Pediatrics*, 8, 572933. https://doi.org/10.3389/fped.2020.572933

Grinyer, A. (2012). *Palliative and end-of-life care for children and young people: Home, hospice and hospital*. Wiley-Blackwell.

Guyer, P. (2003). Kant on the theory and practice of autonomy. *Social Philosophy and Policy*, 20(2), 70–98. https://doi.org/10.1017/s026505250320203x

Halliday, J. (2023). Medics quitting jobs over "distress caused by right-wing Christian group". *Guardian*. Available at: https://protect-eu.mimecast.com/s/6Sq0C5LJZspoV21Fz3DD-?domain=theguardian.com (accessed 23 May 2024).

Hauer, J. M. (2013). *Caring for children who have severe neurological impairment*. Johns Hopkins University Press.

IMPACT. (2023). Implementing Pediatric Advance Care Planning Toolkit. Kenniscentrum Kinderpalliatieve zorg. Available at: https://kinderpalliatief.nl/impact/en/children (accessed 23 May 2024).

Jacobs, S., Davies, N., Butterick, K. L., Oswell, J. L., Siapka, K., Smith, C. H. (2023). Shared decision-making for children with medical complexity in community health services: A scoping review. *BMJ Paediatrics Open*, 7(1). https://doi.org/10.1136/bmjpo-2023-001866

Jameton, A. (2013). A reflection on moral distress in nursing together with a current application of the concept. *Bioethical Inquiry*, 10(3), 297–308. https://doi.org/10.1007/s11673-013-9466-3

Jassal, S. S. (ed.) (2022). *Basic symptom control in paediatric palliative care: Together For Short Lives* (10th edn). Available at: https://www.togetherforshortlives.org.uk/app/uploads/2022/05/Basic-Symptom-Control-in-Paediatric-Palliative-Care-2022.pdf (accessed 23 May 2024).

Klinika Paliativní medicíny 1. (2024). LF.UK a VFN, Zaklady komunikace a paliativni mediciny pro 3. Rocnik [Basics of communication and palliative medicine for 3rd year]. Být spolu je normální. Available at: https://helcom.cz/tiskova-konference-k-projektu-byt-spolu-je-normalni/. https://www.wikiskripta.eu/sites/www.wikiskripta.eu/images/a/a4/Hodnotova_anamneza.png (accessed 27 June 2024).

Larcher, V., Craig, F., Bhogal, K., Wilkinson, D., Brierley, J. (2015). Making decisions to limit treatment in life-limiting and life-threatening conditions in children: A framework for practice. *Archives of Disease in Childhood*, 100(Suppl.), s1–s6. https://doi.org/10.1136/archdischild-2014-306666

Larson, D. B., Froehle, C. M., Johnson, N. D., Towbin, A. J. (2014). Communication in diagnostic radiology: Meeting the challenges of complexity, *American Journal of Roentgenology*, 203(5). https://doi.org/10.2214/AJR.14.12949

Marcus, K. L., Kao, P. C., Ma, C., Wolfe, J., DeCourcey, D. D. (2022). Symptoms and suffering at end-of-life for children with complex chronic conditions. *Journal of Pain and Symptom Management*, 63(1), 88–97. https://doi.org/10.1016/j.jpainsymman.2021.07.010

Mayall, B. (2002). *Towards a sociology of childhood: Thinking from children's lives.* Open University Press.

Mayer, E. (2016). *The culture map: Decoding how people think, lead, and get things done across cultures.* Perseus Books.

McCloskey, S., Taggart, L. (2010). How much compassion have I left? An exploration of occupational stress among children's palliative care nurses. *International Journal of Palliative Nursing*, 16(5), 233–240. https://doi.org/10.12968/ijpn.2010.16.5.48144

McDougall, R. J., Notini, L. (2014). Overriding parents' medical decisions for their children: A systematic review of normative literature. *Journal of Medical Ethics*, 40, 448. https://doi.org/10.1136/medethics-2013-101446

McLeod, S. (2007). Maslow's hierarchy of needs. *Simply Psychology*, 1,1–18. https://www.simplypsychology.org/maslow.html

Moore, C. W. (2014). *Mediation process: Practical strategies for resolving conflict* (4th edn). John Wiley & Sons Inc.

NHS Institute for Innovation and Improvement. (2010). Safer care: SBAR: situation background assessment recommendation implementation and training guide. Available at: https://www.england.nhs.uk/improvement-hub/wp-content/uploads/sites/44/2017/11/SBAR-Implementation-and-Training-Guide.pdf (accessed 23 May 2024).

Nimmon, L., Regehr, G. (2018). The complexity of patients' health communication social networks: A broadening of physician communication. *Teaching and Learning in Medicine*, 30(4), 352–366. https://doi.org/10.1080/10401334.2017.1407656

NMC (Nursing and Midwifery Council). (2018). *The Code: Professional standards of practice and behaviour for nurses, midwives and nursing associates.* Available at: https://www.nmc.org.uk/standards/code/ (accessed 30 May 2024).

NSPCC (National Society for the Prevention of Cruelty to Children). (2024). Gillick competency and Fraser guidelines. Available at: https://learning.nspcc.org.uk/child-protection-system/gillick-competence-fraser-guidelines (accessed 19 September 2024).

Nuffield Council on Bioethics. (2023). Disagreements in the care of critically ill children. Report presented to Parliament pursuant to Section 177(2) of the Health & Care Act 2023. Available at: fromhttps://www.nuffieldbioethics.org/publications/disagreements-in-the-care-of-critically-ill-children-2 (accessed 23 May 2024).

Patockova, D. (2013). *Nejlepsi je domluvit se aneb pruvodce mediacnim procesem,* (1st edn). ALFOM.

Rambihar, V. S., Rambihar, V. (2009). Complexity science may help in defining health. *BMJ*, 338. https://doi.org/10.1136/bmj.b32

RCH Melbourne. (2023). Advance care planning. Available at: https://www.rch.org.au/rch_palliative/for_health_professionals/Advance_Care_Planning/ (accessed 12 December 2023).

Rosenberg, M. B., Chopra, D. (2015). *Nonviolent communication: A language of life.* Puddle Dancer Press.

Slowther, A., Johnston, C., Goodall, J., Hope, T. (2004). Development of clinical ethics committees. *British Medical Journal*, 328, 950. https://doi.org/10.1136%2Fbmj.328.7445.950

Sreedhar, S. S., Kraft, C., Friebert, S. (2020). Primary palliative care: Skills for all clinicians. *Current Problems in Pediatric and Adolescent Health Care*, 50(6), 100814. https://doi.org/10.1016/j.cppeds.2020.100814

United Nations. (1989). Convention on the rights of the child. Available at: https://www.unicef.org.uk/what-we-do/un-convention-child-rights/ (accessed 24 May 2024).

van Breemen, C. (2018). Adapting the serious illness conversation guide for use in pediatrics. *Journal of Palliative Medicine*, 21(12), 1683. https://doi.org/10.1089/jpm.2018.0515

Varkey, B. (2021). Principles of clinical ethics and their application to practice. *Medical Principles and Practice*, 30, 17–28. https://doi.org/10.1159%2F000509119

Verberne, L. M., Kars, M. C., Schouten-van Meeteren, A. Y. N., van den Bergh, E. M. M., Bosman, D. K., Colenbrander, D. A., Grootenhuis, M. A., van Delden, J.J.M. (2019). Parental experiences and coping strategies when caring for a child receiving paediatric palliative care: A qualitative study. *European Journal of Pediatrics*, 178, 1075–1085. https://doi.org/10.1007/s00431-019-03393-w

Voss, C., Raz, T. (2016). *Never split the difference: Negotiating as if your life depended in it.* HarperCollins USA.

Weaver, M. S., Boss, R. D., Christopher, M. J., Gray, T. F., Harman, S., Madrigal, V. N., Michelson, K. N., Paquette, E. T., Pentz, R. D., Scarlet, S., Ulrich, C. M., Walter, J. K. (2022). Top ten tips palliative care physicians should know about their work's intersection with clinical ethics. *Journal of Palliative Medicine*, 25(4), 656–661. https://doi.org/10.1089/jpm.2021.0521

Wilkinson, D. (2019). In defence of a conditional harm threshold test for paediatric decision-making. In I. Goold, J. Herring, C. Auckland (eds), *Parental rights, best interests and significant harms: Medical decision-making on behalf of children post Great Ormond St vs Yates.* Hart Publishing.

Wilkinson, D., Herring, J., Savulsecu, J. (2020). *Medical ethics and law* (3rd edn). Elsevier.

Xafis, V., Bromley, K. (2020). Ethical concepts in neonatal palliative care. In A. Mancini, J. Price, T. Kerr-Elliott (eds), *Neonatal palliative care for nurses.* Springer.

Yamasaki, J., Geist-Martin, P., Sharf, B. F. (2017). *Storied health and illness: Communicating personal, cultural, and political complexities.* Waveland Press.

Zadeh, S., Pao, M., Wiener, L. (2015). Opening end-of-life discussions: How to introduce Voicing My CHOiCES™, an advance care planning guide for adolescents and young adults. *Palliative Support Care*, 13(3), 591–599. https://doi.org/10.1017/s1478951514000054

# CHAPTER 10

# Learning to design, deliver and evaluate children's palliative care education

..........................................

*Susan Neilson and Alexandra Daniels*

## INTRODUCTION

Across regulated professions, nursing is the largest professional group involved in palliative care in most developing countries (Martins Pereira et al., 2021). However, to provide exemplary care to children receiving palliative care and their families, education and training of those involved at all levels are essential. Inclusion of children's palliative care in undergraduate and postgraduate nursing, although recommended, is not always mandatory in curricula (Benini et al., 2022; Martins Pereira et al., 2021).

Children's palliative nursing care education and training should encompass the whole age range of childhoods; from neonatal (including pre-birth), child, young people and transition to adult care services. As well as generic palliative care education and training, there is a need for targeted specialities education and training, for example, in neonatal palliative care (Mancini et al., 2013; Twamley et al., 2013; Murakami et al., 2015). The recommended three levels of training range from the palliative care approach (aimed at both students and professionals), general children's palliative care (aimed at those involved in palliative and end-of-life care but not as their main role) to specialist (those for whom palliative and end-of-life care is their main role) (Downing et al., 2013). Recognition of the role of community health workers and volunteers in palliative care provision (Arias-Casais et al., 2019; WHO, 2020a) highlights the need for education and training at the public health level. There is also the recognised need to train carers of children with palliative and end-of-life care needs (Downing and Ling, 2012). The required knowledge, skills, competencies and moral beliefs, and palliative care attitudes for those working in children's palliative care are well recognised (Liben et al., 2008; Braun et al., 2010; Hain et al., 2012).

DOI: 10.4324/9781003384861-14

Core competencies are measurable knowledge, skills and competencies that inform the work being undertaken; they can be enhanced through training (Parry, 1996). The European Association of Palliative Care (EAPC) identifies core competencies within the three-tiered approach to education: (1) the palliative care approach; (2) general palliative care; and (3) specialist palliative care (Gamondi et al., 2013, Downing et al., 2014).

When considering the mode of delivery, blended learning (combined in-person and online learning), online courses delivered in different languages (www.elearnicpcn.org), train the trainer approaches (Friedrichsdorf et al., 2019) and in-person courses can help widen access and participation. Within the limited pool of trainers/educators in the field, however, not all may feel equipped to teach all aspects (Liben et al., 2008).

The CPC Education Standard Framework (Neilson et al., 2021) supports the recommendation that each country should develop a bespoke interprofessional curriculum (Benini et al., 2022) through detailing levels of knowledge, skills and performance and guidance on the programme of learning content. Developed for use across learning settings and disciplines, the Framework extends across four levels: Public Health, Universal, Core and Specialist. The Framework ensures a standardised curriculum content but gives educators flexibility in both the delivery and assessment (Neilson et al., 2021, see Appendix A and Appendix B). This chapter provides examples of the design, delivery and evaluation of children's palliative care programmes of learning at Core level and Specialist level of the Framework and the CPCET Framework for Advance Care Planning (CPCET, 2020; 2023).

---

**LEARNING OBJECTIVES**

The reader will be able to do the following:

- Describe the principles of training and education design across settings.
- Describe and use different modes of delivering training and education.
- Evaluate the delivery and effectiveness of training and education.

---

## DESIGN

The educator's role is to facilitate a learning environment that enables identified learning outcomes to be met through activities. The environment may be in an educational, clinical or other setting. The setting will inform the education or training design, for example, through consideration of accessibility of the target audience such as the cost to attend in-person (such as fees, travel, etc.) or access to technology, if delivered online. *Constructive alignment* is the process of aligning identified learning outcomes with the learning activities and assessment of learning (Biggs and Tang, 2011, p. 97). This section covers the principles of designing education and training in different settings through constructive alignment.

## The principles of designing training and education across settings

The four levels within the CPCET Education Standard Framework (CPCET, 2020) and Standard Framework for Advance Care Planning for Children (CPCET, 2023) depict expected levels of developing knowledge and skills. Within the CPCET Education Standard Framework, these are mapped to academic levels, the Core level, for example, equating to diploma/degree level, whereas the CPCET Standard Framework for Advance Care Planning for Children was developed to encompass teaching and learning in both clinical and education settings. In both Frameworks the levels can be viewed as stand-alone or incremental (Neilson et al., 2021).

## Intended learning outcomes

Intended learning outcomes describe the knowledge, skills and/or competencies the learner should achieve by the end of the programme of learning. The elements of an intended learning outcome are what the learner should know/understand/achieve and an explanation of how achievement of the learning outcome will be evidenced (Table 10.1).

**TABLE 10.1** Standard Framework for Advance Care Planning (CPCET, 2023) extract, showing learning outcomes and suggested evidence

| Proficiency statement | Learning outcome | Suggested content exemplars; Skills, Understanding (knowledge) and Values (attitudes) | An explanation of how achievement of the learning outcome will be evidenced |
| --- | --- | --- | --- |
| CE1 Communicating effectively Demonstrate an understanding of the concept of advance care planning and set out the potential value and benefits to children and their carers, including understanding limitations | Discuss the context of advance care planning as well as potential barriers, limitations, and drivers to support advance care planning | *Skills* Able to demonstrate timely approaches to children and their carers *Understanding* Day-to-day demands of living with children with complex care needs *Values* Acceptance of avoidance as a legitimate coping practice | *Education* Written/verbal discussion on an advance care planning case study *Clinical* Verbal case discussion on an advance care planning case study |

**TABLE 10.2** SMART framework overview

| S | Specific | Outcomes need to be precise and not open to interpretation |
|---|---|---|
| M | Measurable | A means of assessing achievement of an outcome is required |
| A | Attainable | The outcomes need to be realistically achievable |
| R | Relevant | The outcomes need to be relevant to the learning and to the student |
| T | Time-bound | The timeframe for achievement needs to be realistic |

Learning outcomes should identify the important elements of learning, be achievable and clearly written. The SMART framework (Skrbic and Burrows, 2014) is a useful acronym for focusing intended outcomes (Table 10.2).

The defined Education Standard Framework levels enable practitioners to plan and develop their knowledge, understanding and skills, moving across levels, such as working at Core and moving to Specialist level (Table 10.3). For example, the intended learning outcome *"Discuss cultural, spiritual, and religious coping as related to children's palliative and end-of-life care"* is specific in being focused on cultural, spiritual and religious coping in a defined context (*palliative and end-of-life care*). It is relevant to those working with children and young people receiving

**TABLE 10.3** Extract from the CPCET Standard Framework for Advance Care Planning (CPCET, 2023) showing Core and Specialist level showing a learning outcome for the proficiency *Identifying and managing symptoms*

| Core | Specialist |
|---|---|
| This level would be focused on people who deliver care to children and their carers. It would include everyone who delivers care to children in education, social and health care who might encounter a child living with a life-limiting/-threatening condition and/or the child's carers (family and communities). The core programmes for sectors of health, education and social care might be different to address the needs of children accessing these types of care. In healthcare, this level should include care of the dying child and their carers, as well as supporting people with loss and bereavement following a child's death. | This level focuses on the leadership and management of palliative and end-of-life care for children. It would include clinical, research, education and management leadership. As well as addressing the needs of children and carers with complex and/or multiple palliative care needs, it would prepare practitioners to be a resource for those learning and delivering care at the other levels. This level would include learning to deliver end-of-life care in complex situations or where symptom management is challenging. |
| *Identifying and managing symptoms* | *Identifying and managing symptoms* |
| Demonstrate ability with support to plan advance care options inclusive of all settings, with children and their carers and record/communicate the plan | Demonstrate ability to independently plan advance care options with children and their carers and record/communicate the plan |

palliative care and measurable through a discussion where knowledge and understanding would be demonstrated. This outcome is attainable for a learner working at Core level within this field. The educator would ensure the outcome was time-bound in the setting.

SMART objectives can help educators identify their teaching focus and inform the mode of delivery and assessment. Bloom's Taxonomy (Bloom et al., 1956) is a framework that categorises complexity of intended learning objectives within six cognitive process categories: Knowledge, Comprehension, Application, Analysis, Synthesis and Evaluation (see Figure 10.1). The taxonomy was revised in 2001 (Anderson and Krathwohl, 2001). Four Knowledge Dimension levels were developed (Factual, Conceptual, Procedural and Meta-Cognitive) along with correlating action verbs. The noun-based category *Knowledge* in the original taxonomy became the verb-based category *Remember* in the revised taxonomy, and similarly *Evaluation* became *Create*.

While the cognitive process dimension categories (Remember–Create) in the Revised Taxonomy are seen as hierarchical, and areas of overlap have been described (Krathwohl, 2002, p. 215), Krathwohl (2002) highlights that the original taxonomy category *Comprehend* has been broadened in the Revised Taxonomy to *Understand* and notes a range in complexity of associated cognitive processes with the latter; *Explaining* being viewed as more cognitively complex than *Executing* which is located in the dimension *Apply*. Selecting verbs that have precise meanings aids the clarity of an intended learning outcome, for example, using the phrase 'to discuss' instead of 'to understand' provides a clear outcome that is measurable. For example, the wording in Learning Outcome 2, "Working with others in and across various settings" in the Core section of the Framework is "2.6 Discuss professional roles and

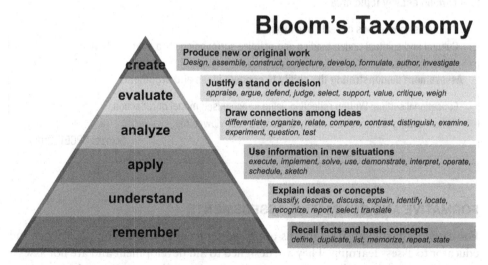

**FIGURE 10.1** Bloom's Revised Taxonomy

Source: Vanderbilt University Centre for Teaching. Available at: https://cft.vanderbilt.edu/guides-sub-pages/blooms-taxonomy/

responsibilities in a multi-disciplinary (or inter-professional) team delivering children's palliative and end-of-life care" (CPCET, 2020, see Appendix B).

## CONSTRUCTIVE ALIGNMENT

Constructive alignment is achieved through ensuring the verb informs the learning activity and the assessment (Biggs and Tang, 2011, p. 98). The activity within an intended learning outcome, for example, demonstrating understanding through discussion, highlights what is required to achieve the outcome and also informs the mode of assessment. Box 10.1 is an example of constructive alignment.

---

**BOX 10.1 CPCET STANDARD FRAMEWORK FOR ADVANCE CARE PLANNING: CORE LEVEL**

**Learning outcome**

Sustaining self-care and supporting the well-being of others

**Proficiency statement**

Can demonstrate the ability to reflect on own attitudes towards advance care planning and contributes to wider discussions.

**Intended learning outcome**

Analyse own attitudes to advance care planning, child death and bereavement.

**Learning activity topic area**

Children's conceptions of death and dying.
Cultural and spiritual understanding and practice surrounding child death and dying.

**Assessment demonstrating the ability to connect ideas and arguments**

Educational setting: Written reflection using a recognised model of reflection.
Clinical setting: Demonstrate ability to discuss their viewpoints.

Source: CPCET (2023).

---

## FORMATIVE AND SUMMATIVE ASSESSMENTS

Formative assessments are a means of providing feedback, enabling the learner and educator to assess learning. They are designed to aid development and are not assessments that are passed/failed. Formative feedback can be self-directed or peer- or educator-led. It needs to be timely so it can be used to develop the summative assessment. Feedforward comments are useful in providing direction for development of the work. Within clinical practice, reflecting on nursing practice can be a useful way to identify learning needs formatively, the summative assessment being the achievement of the identified competency, skill, etc. The summative assessment follows the completion of teaching. The mode of summative assessment will be determined by the learning outcome(s), teaching and learning activities and learning setting (e.g. educational/clinical). The assessment should be a means for learners to demonstrate achievement of the intended learning outcomes.

A constructively aligned assessment will help learners understand its relevance to the intended learning outcomes and teaching and learning activities. Assessment weighting also needs to be taken into consideration. This indicates how the mark for an assessment contributes to the overall course mark. In an academic setting, it is important that the assessment weighting also aligns with the level of study being undertaken, for example, certificate, diploma or degree level. Our learning in palliative care, informed through the unique experiences of each child, young person and their family, presents formative opportunities to reflect on our understanding, challenge our values and alter our behaviours.

It is suggested within the Education Standard Frameworks (CPCET, 2020, 2023), that programmes of learning should reflect the Pyramid Approach (Gabbay et al., 2014). This approach highlights the need for technical skills (theory and concepts that can be applied generally, such as symptom management), soft skills (personal and organisational skills, such as communicating effectively) and learning skills (learning together, such as multi-disciplinary holistic care delivered in any care setting), the premise being effective learning can improve the quality of care. The pyramid analogy reflects the need for a broad base (the organisational aspects such as the environment and resources) supporting the three sides (technical, soft and learning skills). Gabbay et al. (2014) also suggest that as well as a solid foundation (organisational support and action), each side of the pyramid must be developed in relation to the others; technical skills are developed simultaneously with soft and learning skills.

The principles for designing education and training are transferable across different settings. Time spent identifying the learning need is essential to ensure education and training are targeted at the correct level (Public Health, Universal, Core, Specialist) for the learner. Well-written learning outcomes and constructive alignment with the mode of delivery and assessment will ensure quality.

---

**LEARNING ACTIVITY**

Reflect on the learning objectives you have used to inform your palliative care knowledge, skills and competencies.

Consider:

- The level you are currently working at or aspire to be at, for example, Public Health, Universal, Core and Specialist, or if you are working across two levels.

- How to make your learning objectives SMART objectives.
- How you might use the Education Standard Framework to inform your next performance/ development review.
- Points to discuss with your assessor in your review.

## DIFFERENT MODES OF DELIVERING TRAINING AND EDUCATION

The format in which educational resources are delivered to those in need has evolved considerably, with the rapid advancement in technology and integration of information technology into society responsible for the transformation of learning broadly. Additional factors, with significant global influence, including the COVID-19 pandemic and the escalation of humanitarian crisis situations, have resulted in an urgent need to address care needs in challenging environments (Nouvet et al., 2018; Frenk et al., 2022). Innovative strategies and approaches applied to the delivery of educational resources serve to support healthcare providers across settings in their efforts to provide the best possible care to children living with palliative care needs and their families (Doherty et al., 2023).

Context-specific palliative care education influences the training content and how content is delivered to healthcare professionals. It requires careful consideration. It is important that the chosen mode of delivery is accessible, affordable and acceptable to target groups, including nurses. When delivering palliative care education globally, the range of diverse contexts/settings nurses operate in must be considered. For example, the lack of resources, such as essential medication, will impact on symptom management and local cultural practices around dying and death influence communication practices.

This section outlines various modes of delivery, highlights the importance of mentoring, and supervision and showcases the delivery of an international e-learning training course aimed at professionals working in a humanitarian setting.

## Modes of delivery

The need to equip healthcare professionals, especially in low- and middle-income countries, with adequate skills and knowledge to improve the quality of life (and death when appropriate) of children with palliative care needs and their families has been well documented (Connor et al., 2017; Knaul et al., 2018; Benini et al., 2022). In many regions, demand exceeds supply, and increasing access to children's palliative care education has been flagged as a priority (Downing and Ling, 2012). Nurses are central to the provision of quality children's palliative care, however, given the well-established global shortage of nurses, and out-migration of nurses to wealthier countries, further strain is placed on a reduced nursing workforce to provide complex specialised care to those in need (WHO, 2020b; Edwards et al., 2021).

Several modes may be used to communicate knowledge to learners, with each mode providing a range of opportunities and challenges. These include:

1. *Classroom based learning*: This traditional method of in-person training requires the learner to take time away from their clinical setting and travel to a dedicated venue to receive the training. While it allows for individual attention and group engagement, and is considered a useful method of augmenting professional's skills, it should ideally be reinforced by clinical practice to optimise benefits for the learner (Pulsford et al., 2013). In-person training is costly and accompanied by capacity constraints; it may be hard to replicate and achieve the level of consistency for each session. Classroom-based learning may exist as a stand-alone model or be combined with online learning formats and presented as blended learning.

2. *Distance learning*: This form of learning primarily involves the physical separation of educators and learners and uses a range of technologies to facilitate instruction and communication between them. Distance-based learning may take various forms including:

   a. Online or e-learning: These terms are used interchangeably and imply using digital devices and content for learning. Online learning may be described as asynchronous or synchronous. Synchronous learning happens in real time, i.e. learners meet regularly at a fixed time with a human facilitator, whereas asynchronous learning means the learner accesses learning materials at any time they choose and interaction is usually over a longer period without a human facilitator. An asynchronous approach to adult learning enables nurses and others to balance professional development with personal and professional obligations. However, online/e-learning may provide limited opportunities for group interactions and in palliative education, with an emphasis on skills for sensitive communication and interprofessional interaction, the learner's requirements may not be met (Rawlinson et al., 2014; Hughes et al., 2016; Cassum et al., 2020; Kimura et al., 2023).

   The e-learning industry has grown substantially in popularity and usage over the last decade with technology infiltrating every aspect of daily life in many parts of the world. E-learning enables learners to access educational content via computers, smartphones and tablets from the comfort of their homes, or any other desired location, thereby creating opportunities to fit learning around their lifestyle so that new skills and knowledge may be acquired at the learner's convenience.

   Since the COVID-19 pandemic, demand for online interactive engagement and learning has increased exponentially. Advances in technology that include the development and integration of Artificial Intelligence (AI) and e-learning apps using Augmented Reality (AR) and Virtual Reality (VR), have resulted in additional perks that serve to engage and improve the learners' experience. However, O'Connor et al. (2023) suggest that while new digital tools such as Chatbot ChatGPT are being used in nursing education, creating opportunities for nurse educators to enhance how they teach, nursing students are being cautioned to use AI tools responsibly, being mindful of the threats they may pose to academic integrity and professional practice. In addition, technology that includes the integration of video and audio files, images, Microsoft Word documents, pdfs, or infographic graphs into courses contributes to the creation of visually appealing, engaging, interactive courses that impact on the users' learning experience.

b. Blended or hybrid learning: This mode of delivery combines traditional classroom-style teaching with online learning. The face-to-face interaction lends itself to learner participation through role plays, group interaction and guidance from teachers, whereas with e-learning, with the focus on self-study, there is less opportunity for feedback from tutors and more time for the learner to select their own learning method. The EPEC-Pediatric Trainer programme uses a combination of online with in-person conference-style training, with the latter targeting modules that require the demonstration of interactional skills (Friedrichsdorf et al., 2019).

c. Videoconferencing: Videoconferencing can improve access to palliative care education for staff working across large geographic regions and is particularly helpful in resource-limited settings. Project ECHO (Extension for Community Healthcare Outcomes) combines videoconferencing with case-based discussions to connect specialist teams (the "Hub") with healthcare providers in communities (the "Spokes"). This tele-mentoring programme is used to deliver best practice education and guidance from specialists, in combination with case-based peer discussion, to address the increasing global demand for palliative care services in resource-limited settings (Ray et al., 2014: Doherty et al., 2021).

## INTERPROFESSIONAL COLLABORATION AND EDUCATION

Collaborative practice implies that healthcare workers from different professional backgrounds work collaboratively with patients, their families and local communities with a common goal of delivering the highest quality of patient care (WHO, 2010). Interprofessional education happens when mutual learning between two or more professionals takes place, resulting in effective collaboration and improved health outcome for the patient (Olenick et al., 2010).

This interprofessional approach to palliative care education and training presents a valuable opportunity for learning. The international expert panel that collaborated on the GO-PPaCS project reviewing children's palliative care standards, supports different disciplines learning interactively to improve interprofessional collaboration and ultimately the well-being of children and their families (Benini et al., 2022). Characteristics of interprofessional collaborative practice teams include strong patient and family focus, all team members are equal, there is no central leader, and leadership is shared among team members. Hence, responsibility and accountability are shared by team members and collectively by the team as a unit, input from other disciplines are deliberately sought and communication between team members is effective and seamless (Olenick et al., 2010: Golom and Schreck, 2018).

The benefits of interprofessional education are relevant to children's palliative care where an interprofessional team approach is required for exemplary care delivery. Examples of the benefits of interprofessional education in children's palliative care include:

- A greater understanding of other professionals' knowledge, skills and role.
- The prevention of isolation of each discipline.
- Enhanced communication and mutual respect of different point of views.
- The cultivation of interdisciplinary thinking.
- Increased understanding of the differences among multi-disciplinary, inter-disciplinary and trans-disciplinary levels of team collaboration.
- Increased collaboration on clinical and moral issues using a "shared language".
- Increased self-awareness, facilitated through group learning and mutual support among participants.

The gap between medical and nursing students appears to exist early on in their training programmes, and more opportunities for social interaction can address this and help them learn more about each other's role. Learning about the benefits of inter-professional education early on in their training can facilitate the successful integration of inter-disciplinary learning (Prentice et al., 2015).

## MENTORING AND SUPERVISING

It is important that the process of learning by integrating what has already been learnt is supported and the process of mentoring and supervision serves to affirm this (Downing et al., 2013). However, the traditional model of developing and nurturing a successful relationship between a less-experienced healthcare professional (mentee) and a more-experienced healthcare professional (mentor) has evolved with time. In the UK, national standards have been revised to reflect a shift in practice, with practice and academic assessors and practice supervisors being responsible for ensuring nursing students receive the necessary support and supervision to enhance learning in practice and simulated settings.

In a palliative care context, nurses have a professional responsibility to support less-experienced colleagues and mentoring is a powerful way of guiding new nurses through the core palliative care concepts and principles. This expands beyond nurturing skills and knowledge, extending to psychosocial support that nurses who may experience moral distress particularly need when caring for children living with serious illness and their families (Mazanec et al., 2016).

Professional support through the formal process of clinical supervision helps the individual to develop knowledge and competence in the field. Clinical supervision may take place individually or within a group context. Clinical supervision, in addition to supporting professional development, also nurtures well-being and optimises the quality of the work (Snowdon et al., 2017).

## DELIVERING EDUCATION AND TRAINING INTERNATIONALLY

The International Children's Palliative Care Network (ICPCN) is the only global organisation working towards improving access to palliative care for more than 21 million children who need it (Connor et al., 2017). The organisation's mission is to achieve the best quality of life for children and young people living with life-threatening or life-limiting conditions, their families, and carers worldwide and the acronym "CARES" describes the organisation's key areas of focus: Communication, Advocacy, Research, Education and Strategic Development. For more information about ICPCN, see https://icpcn.org/about-icpcn/.

The education and training of healthcare professionals are key considerations in response to the global need for children's palliative care. The ICPCN have developed two primary approaches to increase access to education on children's palliative care, namely face-to-face and e-learning training. In 2021, an evaluation of ICPCN's education programme was undertaken to assess the impact of face-to-face and online courses and to shape future improvements in both course content and presentation (eHospice, 2022). A questionnaire was distributed via Survey Monkey and nurses represented the largest number of respondents (>40%). The evaluation showed considerable knowledge gain in children's palliative care among 91% of respondents, skills gain at 88%, positive change in attitude at 86%, and improvement in clinical practice at 84%. The main outcome of both the online and face-to-face education initiatives was a positive impact in terms of developing further support services in children's palliative care.

The COVID-19 pandemic necessitated a shift in strategy with an increase in online opportunities for learning through webinars and other virtual platforms being created. These included:

1. The Global Palliative Care and COVID-19 series was created in collaboration with the Worldwide Hospice Palliative Care Alliance (WHPCA), the International Association for Hospice and Palliative Care (IAHPC) and Palliative Care in Humanitarian Aid Situations and Emergencies (PallCHASE). A set of briefing notes accompanied the series of webinars; these were developed by 127 subject experts representing 27 countries,

providing globally relevant palliative care information and guidance within the context of the COVID-19 pandemic (Worldwide Hospice Palliative Care Alliance, 2023).

2. The book, *Children's Palliative Care: An International Case-Based Manual*, edited by ICPCN (Downing, 2020), served as the catalyst for a series of webinars linked to the chapters in the book. This monthly webinar series, developed in collaboration with contributors to the book, drew together > 2800 attendees from > 110 countries over a period of 14 months.

3. Following the series of webinars linked to the book, regular monthly third-Thursday webinar meetings have continued with a range of topics being identified and a diverse panel of speakers invited to share their expertise with a global audience. All sessions are recorded and available on the ICPCN website (ICPCN, 2022).

4. Developing an online training course for healthcare providers in Iraq, as a key step to WHO's Global Initiative for Childhood Cancer (GICC), WHO Eastern Mediterranean Region (EMRO) entailed ICPCN developing a training package to be used for capacity-building of healthcare personnel in Baghdad and Basra. In consultation with WHO EMRO and colleagues on the ground in Iraq, a total of 20 hours of virtual training was designed and delivered via Zoom over a period of seven days, with the first session being two hours, followed by six sessions of three hours each, with two sessions per week.

## The ICPCN Education and Membership Hub

The purpose of ICPCN's Education and Membership Hub is to make children's palliative care education available and accessible to all those in need of training globally, including nurses. The Hub provides access to short courses, webinars and bespoke programmes. Several short children's palliative care courses have been developed covering a range of topics, some of which are available in 14 languages (Table 10.4). These taster courses serve as an introduction to the field and, upon completion, some participants may seek opportunities for intermediate or specialist training. Courses are endorsed by the University of South Wales and are freely available on the platform.

There are numerous issues to consider when delivering children's palliative care e-learning courses that target a global audience. These include varying needs, cultural differences, limited resources, and challenges with access to broadband. It is vital that collaboration with key stakeholders is initiated and nurtured to address the need for high-quality course content that may be adapted to meet both global and local needs.

**TABLE 10.4** List of courses and languages on ICPCN's Education and Membership Hub

| | English | Spanish | Portuguese | Dutch | French | Serbian | Czech | Russian | Mandarin | Malay | Farsi | Hindi | Vietnamese | Bengali |
|---|---|---|---|---|---|---|---|---|---|---|---|---|---|---|
| Introduction to CPC | ✓ | ✓ | ✓ | ✓ | ✓ | ✓ | ✓ | ✓ | ✓ | ✓ | ✓ | ✓ | ✓ | ✓ |
| Pain Assessment and Management | ✓ | ✓ | ✓ | X | ✓ | ✓ | ✓ | ✓ | ✓ | X | X | X | X | X |
| Communicating with children and emotional issues in CPC | ✓ | ✓ | ✓ | ✓ | ✓ | X | ✓ | ✓ | ✓ | X | X | X | X | ✓ |
| Child development and play in CPC | ✓ | ✓ | X | X | ✓ | X | ✓ | X | ✓ | X | X | X | X | ✓ |
| End of Life care in CPC | ✓ | ✓ | ✓ | ✓ | ✓ | X | ✓ | ✓ | ✓ | X | X | X | X | ✓ |
| Grief and Bereavement in CPC | ✓ | ✓ | ✓ | ✓ | ✓ | X | ✓ | X | ✓ | X | X | X | X | ✓ |
| Neonatal Palliative Care: An Introduction | ✓ | X | X | ✓ | ✓ | X | X | X | UR | X | X | X | X | X |
| Symptoms other than Pain in PPC | ✓ | X | X | X | X | X | X | X | UR | X | X | X | X | X |
| Adopting a CPC approach to the COVID-19 Pandemic | ✓ | X | X | X | X | X | X | X | X | X | ✓ | X | X | X |
| CPC in Humanitarian Settings | ✓ | X | X | X | X | X | X | X | X | X | X | X | X | X |
| Neonatal Palliative Care: An Enhanced Course | ✓ | X | X | X | X | X | X | X | X | X | X | X | X | X |

Key: UR = course Under Review.

## GLOBAL PALLIATIVE CARE COURSE CASE STUDY

The course on Children's Palliative Care in Humanitarian Settings was jointly developed by ICPCN and PallCHASE.

## Rationale for the course

A staggering 339 million people required humanitarian assistance in 2023, making the focus on care provision in humanitarian settings a priority. Although one of the most vulnerable groups, during a humanitarian crisis, children can be forgotten and face new threats to their health as well as exacerbations of existing health problems (Doherty, 2023).

The lack of skills and knowledge among healthcare workers has emerged as a significant barrier to children and families accessing much-needed palliative care services in humanitarian settings (Doherty et al., 2022). Motivation for this e-learning course stemmed from the need to explore ways to disseminate children's palliative care training resources to meet the needs of humanitarian health workers. Doherty et al. (2022) identified virtual training as a feasible model to support healthcare providers in a humanitarian health response and platforms such as Project ECHO had supported healthcare workers to provide essential palliative care in humanitarian settings.

---

**LEARNING OUTCOMES**

- It is expected that by the end of the course, the learner will be able to do the following:
- Understand key principles and philosophies in children's palliative care.
- Apply these principles and philosophies of care to a humanitarian setting.
- Apply practical communication techniques to children and families.
- Assess and prioritise palliative and end-of-life needs of children and their families.
- Understand and apply core principles of pain and symptom assessment and treatment options available in humanitarian settings.
- Describe the important self-care strategies which can be implemented when caring for children facing serious illness.

---

## Curriculum development/course outline

During the development phase, topics were identified by surveying humanitarian healthcare workers and the four modules serve to guide learners through the core palliative care topics (Figure 10.2).

Module 1: Discusses "What Is Children's Palliative Care" and learners are required to complete this module first, after which they are free to complete subsequent modules in their personal order of preference.

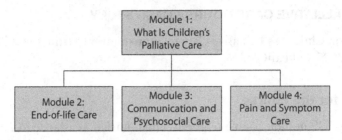

**FIGURE 10.2** Modules for the core palliative care topics

Module 2: Focuses on "End-of-life Care" for children in humanitarian settings, discussing locations of care, symptom management and communication challenges related to end-of-life situations.

Module 3: Provides clinicians with practice tools for communication and family-centred care, focusing on specific communication skills, such as active listening and responding with empathy.

Module 4: Outlines the core principles of pain and symptom assessment as well as management, focusing on treatments which are generally available and practical in humanitarian settings.

Table 10.5 provides an overview of the modules.

**TABLE 10.5** Overview of the modules

| Section | Module 1: What is Children's Palliative Care | Module 2: End of Life Care for Children | Module 3: Practical Approaches to Communicating with Children and Families in Palliative Care | Module 4: Pain and Symptom Care |
|---|---|---|---|---|
| 1 | Section 1: Define Children's Palliative Care and when it should be started | Defining the end life period and good death | Defining good communication | Pain Management |
| 2 | Describe why Children's Palliative Care is needed in humanitarian settings | Physiological Changes and Preparation | Practical Communication Techniques for Humanitarian Settings | GI Symptoms |
| 3 | Describe which children need palliative care | Discontinuing Artificial Hydration and Nutrition | Delivering Bad News using SPIKES Protocol | Respiratory Symptoms |

*(Continued)*

**TABLE 10.5** Overview of the modules *(Continued)*

| Section | Module 1: What is Children's Palliative Care | Module 2: End of Life Care for Children | Module 3: Practical Approaches to Communicating with Children and Families in Palliative Care | Module 4: Pain and Symptom Care |
|---|---|---|---|---|
| 4 | Describe how and where children's palliative care can be provided | Location of End-of-Life Care | Supporting Children facing Serious Illness and Death | |
| 5 | | Managing Symptoms at End-of-Life in Children | | |
| 6 | | Providing End-of-Life care for children | | |

## Course presentation/layout

One of the recommendations that arose from evaluating the ICPCN education pro-gramme in 2021 was to upgrade the online courses in an attempt to increase the quality of learner interaction and engagement (eHospice, 2022). The "Children's Palliative Care in Humanitarian Settings" course was the first ICPCN course that set out to address this upgrade. The course was developed in Rise 360 (Articulate, 2024), a web-based authoring tool, that allows for the creation of visually appeal-ing interactive courses. One Sharable Content Object Reference Model (SCORM) package per module was created in Rise 360 and exported onto the ICPCN Moodle platform for the learner to access.

Each module offers the learner opportunities for interactive learning experiences through the integration of graphics, audio and video clips, engagement through real-life case studies and opportunities to "test your knowledge" (Figure 10.3, Figure 10.4).

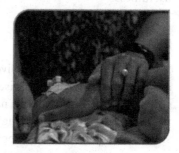

Empathy is the act of trying to imagine yourself in the other person's situation with the aim of trying to understand a person's thoughts and emotions.

'Responding with empathy' is when we convey this understanding back to the person to show we have understood.

**FIGURE 10.3** Two Worlds Cancer: responding with empathy

Source: Narendra Shrestha (2022).

Meet Leo.

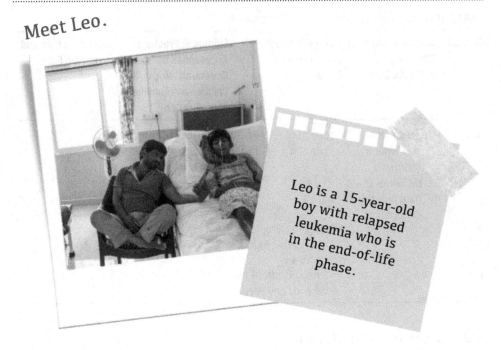

Leo is a 15-year-old boy with relapsed leukemia who is in the end-of-life phase.

**FIGURE 10.4** Two Worlds Cancer

Source: Harsha Vadlamani (2022). © 2022 Two Worlds Cancer/Harsha Vadlamani

## Course assessment

Each module is accompanied by a set of multiple-choice questions which are mandatory to complete and pass (80%) for a certification of completion to be issued.

## Course evaluation

An evaluation is available at the end of the course. This optional feedback form seeks to understand the learner's experience of the course, including ease of navigation and usefulness.

## EVALUATION

Innovative approaches to delivering children's palliative care education and training are required to meet recognised needs, especially those of low- and middle-income countries. International and national organisations have an important role to play in developing and supporting education and training models that are affordable, sustainable and culturally appropriate for the context. Consultation and collaboration, with strategic partners that support existing programmes are essential to optimise available resources and improve the quality of care provided. The evaluation of education and training will now be considered.

---

**LEARNING ACTIVITY**

Reflect on the delivery of the last training you completed:

- How well did the training meet your expectations?
- Were your personal/the training course learning outcomes met?
- How have you integrated/will you integrate learning from training into clinical practice?

---

It is good practice to evaluate teaching and learning to ensure it is fit for purpose and to inform future practice. The method and mode of evaluation should be decided during the development of the programme of learning. Identification of who should carry out the evaluation, for example, the healthcare practitioner, programme lead or external collaborator, and when and how findings will be actioned also need to be agreed.

Evaluation covers a number of elements, the experience of the learner and educator, the quality of the programme of learning, and the experience of any wider stakeholders. Where possible, learners should be involved in developing the evaluation tool and consideration of when it should be delivered. An evaluation may be carried out at the mid-point or the end of the programme of learning, either before or after the assessment. The timing can be crucial in informing the response rate. For example, completing at the end of a taught session may result in more students completing the evaluation. The ease of completion may also influence the completion rate and it is important to consider the number and type of questions in the planning stage. The type of question will be informed by what you want to know. For example, a true/false or yes/no question could be used to find out if the learning outcomes were clear, a Likert scale to find out how learning related to practice, and a free text answer to provide detail on these points.

Informal evaluation approaches include identifying what learners felt went well and what could be improved and how. This can be a useful check point as a verbal or written exercise at the end of a teaching session. It can also be a means of ascertaining the elements learners are struggling with, for example, directly asking what they found difficult or challenging in the session may inform changes to the mode or pace of delivery during the remainder of the programme. A means of gauging knowledge and understanding might be through students' spending 1 minute at the end of a session to note what they have learnt and any identified new knowledge deficits (Table 10.6). Identified knowledge deficits can then be incorporated into their personal development plan.

**TABLE 10.6** Examples of evaluation tools use

| Evaluation tool | Use |
| --- | --- |
| Online questionnaire/survey | Learner feedback on learning content, mode of delivery, for example, in-person lecture, online seminar, 1:1 peer learning, and assessment |
| Formative/summative assessments | Quality of programme of learning |
| Self-reflection | Educator reflection on performance, such as delivery of teaching, methods/language used, engagement of the learners, etc. can inform practice |

**BOX 10.2 THE CPCET EDUCATION STANDARD FRAMEWORK SELF-AUDIT TOOL**

Information page, extract, Core level (CPCET, 2020):

### CORE

In this level the focus will be on the learning for people who deliver care to children and their carers. It includes everyone who delivers care to children in education, social and health care who might encounter a child living with a life limiting/threatening condition and or the child's carers (family and communities). The core programmes for sectors of health, education and social care might be different to address the needs of children accessing these types of care. In healthcare this level should include care of the dying child and their carers as well as supporting people with loss and bereavement following a child's death.

| | |
|---|---|
| Course/Module name | |
| Organisation name | |
| Organisation's description of how this level Is used in their career pathways and workforce development, progression and assessment. | |
| Course/Module lead | |
| Email contact | |
| Date of self-audit | |
| Signature(s) | |

The CPCET Education Standard Framework Self-audit Tool programme of learning content, extract:

| Learning Outcome | Aligned course content | Method(s) of assessment | Changes made during last audit |
|---|---|---|---|
| **1. Communicating effectively**<br>1.3 Develop insight into positive cultures and patterns of communication when delivering "bad or unwanted" news/ information. | | | |

The CPCET Education Standard Framework Self-audit Tool action plan, extract:

### DEVELOPMENT ACTION PLAN

| Learning outcome identified for development | Audit improvement outcome | Actions | Lead name | Date | Outcome *Achieved Partially achieved Not achieved* |
|---|---|---|---|---|---|
| | | | | | |

It is important that learners are informed how their feedback has been used, for example, any changes made to the content or assessment of future course iterations. How this is communicated needs to be ascertained at the outset to ensure leaners who have completed the programme of learning are still informed.

An example of an evaluation through an online survey is ICPCN's recent Education Programme Evaluation (ehospice, 2022). Participants who had enrolled in one of their face-to-face or e-learning programmes over a 10-year period (2011–2021) were invited to complete the questionnaire via Survey Monkey. Alongside demographic data (such as participant age, geographical location, professional background), questions explored impact on knowledge base and skills, change in attitudes and clinical practice. Key findings included the need to enhance marketing within low- and middle-income countries and making e-learning courses more interactive.

The CPCET Education Standard Framework (CPCET, 2020) contains a self-audit tool for educators. The tool provides a template for reviewing pertinent information and developing an action plan (Box 10.2). It starts with an information page, a template for documenting the programme of learning content, assessment and changes in relation to learning outcome, and an action plan for each of the four levels.

The audit can be used by educators to reflect on and develop their own teaching/programmes of learning. An audit repository has been set up on the ICPCN webpage icpcn.org/resources/education-framework-self-audit-tool/.

---

**LEARNING ACTIVITY**

This activity is intended for learners and educators.

**Learner**

Reflect on your experience, knowledge, skills and competencies to date. Consider the level you are working at; this might be Public Health, Universal, Core or Specialist or a combination of levels for different proficiencies.

Review the CPCET Standard Framework and/or the CPCET Standard Framework for Advance Care Planning level you align with.

**Critical question to consider**

What strategies could you use to meet the identified competency learning objectives? For example, this might be through a validated training programme, local training course, peer observation in practice and/or self-directed study.

**Educator**

Reflect on your teaching to date and identify the level; this might be Public Health, Universal, Core or Specialist or a combination of levels for different proficiencies.

Review the levels of the CPCET Standard Framework CPCET (CPCET, 2020) and/or the CPCET Standard Framework for Advance Care Planning (CPCET, 2023) that align with your teaching.

---

**Critical questions to consider**

1.  What level(s) of the CPCET Standard Framework (CPCET, 2020) and/or the CPCET Standard Framework for Advance Care Planning (CPCET, 2023) does my programme of learning need to focus on?
2.  Are these the right levels for my target audience?

---

Evaluating education and training is an important step in quality control. Findings can help inform the design, delivery and evaluation of programmes of learning, ensuring they are fit for purpose, meeting the needs of the learner and wider stakeholders.

## SUMMARY

Developing effective education and training in any setting requires careful planning. Collaboration with stakeholders such as learners, children, young people and families will help educators identify the appropriate design, modes of delivery and evaluation tools for their programmes of learning. International interprofessional collaboration will help us work towards meeting the knowledge, skills and competency needs of those working with children and young people requiring palliative care globally across a range of diverse settings.

## KEY POINTS

*   Learners should be involved in developing the design, delivery and evaluation of education and training.
*   The CPCET Education Standard Frameworks and reflection on clinical practice can help identify knowledge, skills and competency deficits that inform SMART learning outcomes.
*   Innovative approaches to delivery and assessment should be considered.

## REFERENCES

Anderson, L. W., Krathwohl, D. R. (2001). *A taxonomy for learning, teaching, and assessing: A revision of Bloom's taxonomy of educational objectives: complete edition.* Addison-Wesley Longman.

Arias-Casais, N., Garralda, E., Rhee, J. Y., de Lima L., Pons J. J., Clark, D., Hasselaar, J., Ling, J., Mosoiu, D., Centeno, C. (2019). *EAPC atlas of palliative care in Europe 2019.* Available at: https://www.hospiz.at/wordpress/wp-content/uploads/2019/07/EAPC-Atlas-2019-final-web.pdf (accessed 14 May 2024).

Articulate (2024). Rise 360. Articulate.com. Available at: https://www.articulate.com/360/rise/ (accessed 14 May 2024).

Benini, F., Pappadatou, D., Bernada, M., Craig, F., De Zen, L., Downing, J., Drake, R., Friedrichsdorf, S., Garros, D., Giacomelli, L., Lacerda, A., Lazzarin, P., Marceglia, S., Marston, J., Mukaden, M. A., Papa, S., Parravicini, E., Pellegatta, F., Wolfe, J. (2022). International standards for pediatric palliative care: From IMPaCCT to GO-PPaCS. *Journal of Pain and Symptom Management,* 63(5), e529–e543. https://doi.org/10.1016/j.jpainsymman.2021.12.031

Biggs, J., Tang, C. (2011). *Teaching for quality learning at university* (4th edn). Open University Press/Society for Research into Higher Education.

Bloom, B. S., Engelhart, M. D., Furst, E. J., Hill, W. H., Krathwohl, D. R. (1956). *Handbook I: Cognitive domain*. David McKay.

Braun, M., Gordon, D., Uziely, B. (2010). Associations between oncology nurses' attitudes toward death and caring for dying patients. *Oncology Nursing Forum* 37(1), E43–E49. https://doi.org/10.1188/10.ONF.E43-E49

Cassum, S., Mansoor, K., Hirji, A., David, A., Aijaz, A. (2020). Challenges in teaching palliative care module virtually during COVID-19 era. *Asia-Pacific Journal of Oncology Nursing*, 7(4), 301–304. https://doi.org/10.4103/apjon.apjon_42_20

Connor, S. R., Downing, J., Marston, J. (2017). Estimating the global need for palliative care for children: A cross-sectional analysis. *Journal of Pain and Symptom Management*, 53(2), 171–177. https://doi.org/10.1016/j.jpainsymman.2016.08.020

CPCET (Children's Palliative Care Education and Training UK and Ireland Action Group). (2020). Education Standard Framework. ICPCN. Available at: https://icpcn.org/wp-content/uploads/2022/10/CPCET-Education-Standard-Framework.pdf (accessed 14 May 2024).

CPCET (Children's Palliative Care Education and Training UK and Ireland Action Group) and Child and Young Person's Advance Care Plan Collaborative (2023). ICPCN. Available at: https://icpcn.org/wp-content/uploads/2023/09/CPCET-Standard-Framework-for-Advance-Care-Planning-for-Children.pdf (accessed 14 May 2024).

Doherty, M. (2023). Children's palliative care in humanitarian settings. Available at: https://ehospice.com/inter_childrens_posts/childrens-palliative-care-in-humanitarian-settings-updated-e-learning-course/ (accessed 14 May 2024).

Doherty, M., Lynch-Godrei, A., Azad, T., Ladha, F., Ferdous, L., Ara, R., Groninger, H. (2022). Using virtual learning to develop palliative care skills among humanitarian health workers in the Rohingya refugee response in Bangladesh. *Journal of Medical Education and Curricular Development*, 9. https://doi.org/10.1177/23821205221096099

Doherty, M., Rayala, S., Evans, E., Rowe, J., Rapelli, V., Palat, G. (2021). Using virtual learning to build pediatric palliative care capacity in South Asia: Experiences of implementing a teleteaching and mentorship program (Project ECHO). *JCO Global Oncology*, 7(1), 210–222. https://doi.org/10.1200/GO.20.00481

Downing, J. (ed.) (2020). *Children's palliative care: An international case-based manual*. Springer.

Downing, J., Ling, J. (2012). Education in children's palliative care across Europe and internationally. *International Journal of Palliative Nursing*, 18(3), 115–120. https://doi.org/10.12968/ijpn.2012.18.3.115

Downing, J., Ling, J., Benini, F., Payne, S., Papadatou, D. (2013). *EAPC Core competencies for education in paediatric palliative care*; Report of the EAPC Children's Palliative Care Education Task Force; European Association for Palliative Care. Available at: https://www.ordemenfermeiros.pt/arquivo/colegios/Documents/2017/MCEESIP_PNAE_09_eapcnet_ppc_core_competencies.pdf

Downing, J., Ling, J., Benini, F., Payne, S., Papadatou, D. (2014). A summary of the EAPC White Paper on core competencies for education in paediatric palliative care. *European Journal of Palliative Care*, 21(5), 245–249.

Edwards, R. L., Patrician, P. A., Bakitas, M., Markaki, A. (2021). Palliative care integration: A critical review of nurse migration effect in Jamaica. *BMC Palliative Care*, 20, 155. https://doi.org/10.1186/s12904-021-00863-7

ehospice. (2022). Evaluation of ICPCN's Education programmes. Available at: https://ehospice.com/inter_childrens_posts/evaluation-of-icpcns-education-programme/ (accessed 14 May 2024).

Frenk, J., Chen, L. C., Chandran, L, Groff, E. O. H., King, R., Meleis, A., Fineberg, H. V. (2022). Challenges and opportunities for educating health professionals after the COVID-19 pandemic. *Lancet*, 400, 1539–1556. https://doi.org/10.10.1016/S0140-6736(22)02092-X

Friedrichsdorf, S. J., Remke, S., Hauser, J., Foster, L., Postier, A., Kolste, A., Wolfe, J. (2019). Development of a pediatric palliative care curriculum and dissemination model: Education in palliative and end-of-life care (EPEC) pediatrics. *Journal of Pain and Symptom Management*, 58(4), 707–720. https://doi.org/10.1016/j.jpainsymman.2019.06.008

Gabbay, J., le May, A., Connell, C., Klein, J. H. (2014). Skilled for improvement? Learning communities and the skills needed to improve care: An evaluative service development. The Health Foundation. Available at: https://www.health.org.uk/sites/default/files/SkilledForImprovement_fullreport.pdf (accessed 14 May 2024).

Gamondi, C., Larkin, P., Payne, S. (2013). Core competencies in palliative care: An EAPC White Paper on palliative care education: Part 2. *European Journal of Palliative Care*, 20(3), 140–145. https://www.sicp.it/wp-content/uploads/2018/12/6_EJPC203Gamondi_part2_0.PDF

Golom, F. D., Schreck, J. S. (2018). The journey to interprofessional collaborative practice: Are we there yet? *Pediatric Clinics of North America*, 65(1), 1–12. https://doi.org/10.1016/j.pcl.2017.08.017

Hain, R., Heckford, E., McCulloch, R. (2012). Paediatric palliative medicine in the UK: Past, present, future. *Archives of Disease in Childhood*, 97(4), 381–384. https://doi.org/10.1136/archdischild-2011-300432

Hughes, S., Preston, N. J., Payne, S. A. (2016). Online learning in palliative care: Does it improve practice? *European Journal of Palliative Care*, 23(5), 236–239.

ICPCN. (2022). ICPCN webinars. Available at: icpcn.org/resources/icpcn-webinars/ (accessed 14 May 2024).

Kimura, R., Matsunaga, M., Barroga, E., Hayashi, N. (2023). Asynchronous e-learning with technology-enabled and enhanced training for continuing education of nurses: A scoping review. *BMC Medical Education*, 23(1), 505. https://doi.org/10.1186/s12909-023-04477-w

Knaul, F. M., Farmer, P. E., Krakauer, E. L., De Lima, L., Bhadelia, A., Kwete, X. J., Arreola-Ornelas, H., Gómez-Dantés, O., Rodriguez, N. M., Alleyne, G. A. O., Connor, S. R., Hunter, D. J., Lohman, L., Radbruch, L., del Rocío, M. S. M., Atun, R., Foley, K. M., Frenk, J., Jamison, D.T., Rajagopal, M. R., & Lancet Commission on Palliative Care and Pain Relief Study Group. (2018). Alleviating the access abyss in palliative care and pain relief – an imperative of universal health coverage: The Lancet Commission report. *Lancet*, 391, 1391–1454. https://doi.org/10.1016/s0140-6736(17)32513-8

Krathwhol, D. R. (2002). A revision of Bloom's taxonomy: An overview. *Theory into Practice*, 41(4), 212–218. https://doi.org/10.1207/s15430421tip4104_2

Liben, S., Papadatou, D., Wolfe, J. (2008). Paediatric palliative care: Challenges and emerging ideas. *Lancet*, 371(9615), 852–864. https://doi.org/10.1016/S0140-6736(07)61203-3

Mancini, A., Kelly, P., Bluebond-Langner, M. (2013). Training neonatal staff for the future in neonatal palliative care. *Seminars in Fetal and Neonatal Medicine*, 18(2), 111–115. https://doi.org/10.1016/j.siny.2012.10.009

Martins Pereira, S., Hernández-Marrero, P., Pasman, H. R., Capelas, M. L., Larkin, P., Francke, A. L. (2021). Nursing education on palliative care across Europe: Results and recommendations from the EAPC Taskforce on preparation for practice in palliative care nursing across the EU based on an online-survey and country reports. *Palliative Medicine*, 35(1), 130–141. https://doi.org/10.1177/0269216320956817

Murakami, M., Yokoo, K., Ozawa, M., Fujimoto, S., Funaba, Y., Hattori, M. (2015). Development of a neonatal end-of-life care education program for NICU nurses in Japan. *Journal of Obstetric, Gynecologic & Neonatal Nursing*, 44(4), 481–491. https://doi.org/10.1111/1552-6909.12569

Mazanec, P., Aslakson, R. A., Bodurtha, J., Smith, T. J. (2016). Mentoring in palliative nursing. *Journal of Hospice & Palliative Nursing*, 18(6), 488–495. https://doi.org/10.1097/NJH.0000000000000297

Neilson, S., Randall, D., McNamara, K., Downing, J. (2021). Children's palliative care education and training: Developing an education standard framework and audit. *BMC Medical Education*, 21, 539. https://doi.org/10.1186/s12909-021-02982-4

Nouvet, E., Sivaram, M., Bezanson, K., Krishnaraj, G., Hunt, M., de Laat, S., Sanger, S., Banfeild, L., Rodriguez, P. F. E., Schwartz, L. J. (2018). Palliative care in humanitarian crises: A review of the literature. *Journal of International Humanitarian Action*, 3(5), 1–14. https://doi.org/10.1186/s41018-018-0033-8

O'Connor, S., Permana, A. F., Neville, S., Denis-Lalonde, D. (2023). Artificial intelligence in nursing education 2: Opportunities and threats. *Nursing Times*, 119(11), 28–32. Available at: https://s3-eu-west-1.amazonaws.com/emap-moon-prod/wp-content/uploads/sites/3/2023/10/231009-Artificial-intelligence-in-nursing-education-2-opportunities-and-threats.pdf (accessed 14 May 2024).

Olenick, M., Allen, L. R., Smego Jr, R. A. (2010). Interprofessional education: A concept analysis. *Advances in Medical Education and Practice*, 75–84. https://doi.org/10.2147/AMEP.S13207.

Parry, S. B. (1996). The quest for competencies: Competency studies can help you make HR decisions, but the results are only as good as the study. *Training*, 33, 48–56. https://www.proquest.com/docview/203398191/fulltextPDF/D71EC17C75274A8EPQ/1?accountid=8630&sourcetype=Trade%20Journals

Prentice, D., Engel, J., Taplay, K., Stobbe, K. (2015). Interprofessional collaboration: The experience of nursing and medical students' interprofessional education. *Global Qualitative Nursing Research*. https://doi.org/10.1177/2333393614560566

Pulsford, D., Jackson, G., O'Brien, T., Yates, S., Duxbury, J. (2013). Classroom-based and distance learning education and training courses in end-of-life care for health and social care staff: A systematic review. *Palliative Medicine*, 27(3), 221–235. https://doi.org/10.1177/0269216311429496

Rawlinson, F. M., Gwyther, L., Kiyange, F., Luyirika, E., Meiring, M., Downing, J. (2014). The current situation in education and training of health-care professionals across Africa to optimise the delivery of palliative care for cancer patients. *E Cancer Medical Science*, 8. https://doi.org/10.3332/ecancer.2014.492

Ray, R. A., Fried, O., Lindsay, D. (2014). Palliative care professional education via video conference builds confidence to deliver palliative care in rural and remote locations. *BMC Health Services Research*, 14, 272. https://doi.org/10.1186/1472-6963-14-272

Skrbic, N., Burrows, J. (2014). Specifying learning objective. In L. Ashmore, D. Robinson (eds), *Learning, teaching and development: Strategies for action* (pp. 54–87). Sage Publications.

Snowdon, D. A., Leggat, S. G., Taylor, N. F. (2017). Does clinical supervision of healthcare professionals improve effectiveness of care and patient experience? A systematic review. *BMC Health Services Research*. https://doi.org/10.1186/s12913-017-2739-5

Twamley, K., Kelly, P., Moss, R., Mancini, A., Craig, F., Koh, M., Polonsky, R., Bluebond-Langner, M. (2013). Palliative care education in neonatal units: Impact on knowledge and attitudes. *BMJ Supportive & Palliative Care*, 3(2), 213–220. https://doi.org/10.1136/bmjspcare-2012-000336

WHO (World Health Organization). (2010). Framework for action on interprofessional education and collaborative practice. Available at: https://www.who.int/publications/i/item/framework-for-action-on-interprofessional-education-collaborative-practice (accessed 14 May 2024).

WHO (World Health Organization). (2020a). Palliative care. Available at: https://www.who.int/news-room/fact-sheets/detail/palliative-care.

WHO (World Health Organization). (2020b). State of the world's nursing 2020: Investing in education, jobs and leadership. Available at: https://www.who.int/publications/i/item/9789240003279 (accessed 30 May 2024).

Worldwide Hospice Palliative Care Alliance. (2023). Global webinars and briefing notes. Available at: https://thewhpca.org/global-webinars-and-briefing-notes/?Itemid=368 (accessed 14 May 2024).

# CHAPTER 11

# Leadership for improvement

..................................................

*Julia Downing and Zodwa Sithole*

## INTRODUCTION

Children's palliative care nurses are in a key position to create change, to ensure quality of care and bring about improvement, not only in the lives of children and their families, but also in the provision of care, their self-development and the development of the team with which they work. They are leaders, not only in terms of nursing, but in the field of children's palliative care as a whole. Approximately 59% of the global health workforce are nurses (WHO, 2020a), and in many low- and middle-income countries this figure is a lot higher, e.g. in Uganda, nurses and midwives make up 72% of the public health workforce (Nursing Now, 2018), and in Brazil, it is 70% (de Oliveira et al., 2020), making them the first point of contact for most patients within the health system (Nursing Now, 2018), including in palliative care (Mwangi-Powell et al., 2015). In children's palliative care, many nurses are in leadership positions either within their team, the district, nationally or globally. However, often the leadership role of nurses is not recognised, particularly in low- and middle-income countries where nurses may have a low status and are not given the opportunity to be decision-makers, strategists, and professionals whose independent actions are based on education, evidence, and experience. Thus, they are not empowered to develop their leadership skills, to make change, bring about improvement and take a leading role. *"Leadership is about setting direction, opening up possibilities, helping people achieve, communication and delivering. It is also about behaviour, what we do as leaders is even more important than what we say* (Sir Nigel Crisp, NHS Institute for Innovation and Improvement, 2005).

Leadership is about setting direction, and about behaviour (NHS Institute for Innovation and Improvement, 2005) – as nurse leaders, we influence the behaviour of those around us, we bring about change and we address the big picture and show how regular duties affect the broader goals of the healthcare organisation.

DOI: 10.4324/9781003384861-15

In children's palliative care it is important to think about that change – what is it we need to change? How can we do it? How can we lead? Nurses working in children's palliative care need to be seen as full partners with other medical specialists and work in conjunction with leaders from other health professions. In order to prepare the nursing workforce to meet the needs of children's palliative care, nurses must take the lead in developing the curriculum and make improvements. They must also have positions on decision- and policy-making committees at institutional, national, regional, and international levels. Without good nursing leadership, and nurse leaders in decision-making positions, the healthcare system may not be able to meet the demands of children needing palliative care and their families.

Governments are responsible for including children's palliative care within the continuum of care (WHO, 2020b). The World Health Organization (WHO) cites "Leadership and Governance" as one of the six building blocks or core components of a health system (WHO, 2010). The WHO conceptual model for palliative care development (WHO, 2021a) identifies the core components for palliative care development, including children's palliative care, which helps to identify areas where nurses can lead improvement and on which global indicators for palliative care have been built. These components include: empowered people and communities; health policies related to palliative care; the use of essential medicines; education and training, research, and the provision of palliative care (WHO, 2021a). While all elements are essential, children's palliative care is provided within individual countries' legal frameworks and regulations, as is nursing, and so an understanding of policy issues is essential in bringing about improvement. Thus, in this chapter we will explore the policy landscape for children's palliative care and the politics of palliative care, the policy landscape for nursing, nurses working within the children's palliative care team, and finally nurses as leaders.

**LEARNING OBJECTIVES**

The reader will be able to do the following:

1. Describe the policy landscape for children's palliative care.
2. Critically discuss the policy landscape for nursing and how children's palliative care fits within this.
3. Critically discuss and evaluate the concept of the nurse as leading for improvement within children's palliative care, reflecting on their own setting.

## THE POLICY LANDSCAPE FOR CHILDREN'S PALLIATIVE CARE

It is important as nurses working in children's palliative care that we understand the global context in which we are seeking to bring about improvement. Which global policies, strategies and frameworks are influencing the development of children's palliative care, both by us as nurses, but also by global, regional and national policy- and decision-makers? What have governments, as member states of the World Health Organization, signed up to with regards to children's palliative care development? Have they made any commitments that we can support them with? That we can hold them accountable for? How do we make sure that improvements in children's palliative care that we are trying to introduce fit within any global or national frameworks, and include essential components of care, e.g. hospital or home-based care or both? Policy and legal frameworks exist to help us strengthen and promote the development of palliative care globally for all ages, including neonates, children, adolescents and young adults. The WHO conceptual model sets out what they mean by health polices, including policy and legal frameworks and regulations that help shape services but also guarantee the rights of children and their families (WHO, 2021a):

> This component refers to the political commitment and leadership expressed in governance and policy frameworks (strategies, standards, guidelines). It includes the development of a legal framework and regulations that guarantee the rights of patients, access to palliative care services and essential medicines and the financing and inclusion of palliative care in the national health service and benefits package. It also includes health system design and health care organisation, in addition to stewardship and multi-stakeholder action.
>
> *(WHO, 2021a, p. 15)*

Over the past 10–15 years, there has been a growing recognition at the global policy level for the need for palliative care for all ages, and key milestones including: the World Health Assembly Resolution on Palliative Care (WHO, 2014); defining Universal Health Coverage (WHO, 2023a) and Primary Health care (WHO and UNICEF, 2018); the publication of the Lancet Commission Report on "Alleviating the access abyss to pain control and palliative care" (Knaul et al., 2018); the publication of WHO documents including those for healthcare planners, implementers and managers (WHO, 2018a), assessing the development of palliative care worldwide (WHO, 2021a) and more recently the report "Left behind in pain" (WHO, 2023b); and, importantly, the inclusion of palliative care in the WHO COVID-19 guidelines (WHO, 2021b). While many of these high-level policies and frameworks highlight the importance of access to all in need of palliative care – for all children – and the need for equity of access around the world, they also recognise that access to palliative care and pain management is a human right – a right for every child who needs it, and their families, wherever they live around the world (Open Society Institute, 2015). Underpinning all of this are the UN Sustainable Development Goals (United Nations, 2023) with children's palliative care contributing not only to Sustainable Development Goal, No. 3 on "Good Health and Well-being", but also to others, including Sustainable Development Goal, No. 1 "No poverty", Sustainable Development Goal, No. 5, "Gender equality" and Sustainable Development Goal, No. 10, "Reduced inequalities".

The World Health Assembly resolution on palliative care (WHO, 2014) focuses on strengthening palliative care throughout the life course, with the World Health Organization keen in recent years to highlight a life-course approach, ensuring that no one is missed. The life-course approach provides evidence-based and human rights-based strategies to understand health (and palliative care) in today's context and is an important lens from which to review policies, programmes and interventions (Pan American Health Organization, WHO Americas, 2023), thus ensuring that children's palliative care is not left behind. The World Health Assembly resolution emphasises the need for palliative care for children as well as adults, and across a range of conditions, recognising that palliative care is fundamental to improving quality of life for children and their families, improving well-being, comfort and human dignity (see Chapter 1). It confirms that palliative care is an ethical responsibility of health systems and an ethical duty for all health professionals – including nurses. However, it also recognises the lack of integration and access to palliative care and recommendations are made to all member states, highlighting implementation, policy, access to medicines, and the importance of collaborations. 2024 is the tenth anniversary of this ground-breaking resolution, with a report having been published that evaluates progress as well as providing ongoing recommendations (Harding et al., 2024).

Palliative care has been included in both the definitions of Universal Health Coverage (WHO, 2023a) and Primary Health care (WHO and UNICEF, 2018), ensuring that if there is no access to children's palliative care, then governments are not providing Universal Health Coverage or adequate primary healthcare. This gives us as nurses, an advocacy tool, as focus is often on more general issues, rather than on specifics such as children's palliative care, particularly where the numbers needing such services are low, and where priorities are focused on cure. The Lancet Commission report, "Alleviating the access abyss to pain and palliative care" (Knaul et al., 2018) highlighted some key issues related to children's suffering and the need for palliative care, noting that while children and their families have specific palliative care needs, these can easily be overlooked as the absolute number of children needing palliative care is low compared with adults (only about 7% of those needing palliative care globally are < 20 years of age (Knaul et al., 2020)), yet a third of all children who died in 2015 experienced Serious Health-related Suffering associated with life-limiting or life-threatening conditions, and 98% were from low- and middle-income countries (Knaul et al., 2018). They also make a case that the provision of essential opioid analgesics for all children in low- and middle-income countries would cost just over US$1 million a year, which should be affordable.

Since the World Health Assembly resolution on palliative care (WHO, 2014), the World Health Organization have also strengthened their commitment to the development of children's palliative care, publishing a range of handbooks to support the development of palliative care across the age range, including for paediatrics (WHO, 2018a) along with in humanitarian aid settings (WHO, 2018b) and have recently set up a WHO working group for palliative care, comprising of WHO focal staff from the regional offices as well as headquarters, representatives of organisations in official relations with the WHO, WHO Collaborating centres, and those with Memorandums of Understanding with the WHO, which includes paediatric-focused organisations such as St Jude Global Children's Hospital, and the International Children's Palliative Care Network (ICPCN).

Thus, the global policy environment for children's palliative care continues to develop and strengthen, having an impact at the regional and national levels, as well as hopefully on service provision itself. Alongside this, at the service provision level, there are a range of useful frameworks and charters, including the ICPCN's Charter of Rights for Life-Limited and Life-Threatened Children (ICPCN, 2008), and the recent European Charter on Palliative Care for Children and Young People (EAPC, 2022), among others. These charters set out what can be expected through the provision of children's palliative care and can help guide nurses in identifying areas for improvement. There are also a range of examples of standards for children's palliative care, including the 'Global Overview – Paediatric Palliative Care Standards (GO-PPaCS, see Appendix B), published in 2022 (Benini et al., 2022) or the regionally focused African Palliative Care Standards, which include a section on children's palliative care (APCA, 2011) and can be used to guide nurses not only in the improvement of service provision, but also education, research, policy, etc.

At a national level, there are a range of policies for children's palliative care around the world, with some countries having an overall policy for palliative care which includes, but is not limited to, children's palliative care, with other countries having specific children's palliative care policies, and some having none (see Box 11.1). One of the challenges for children's palliative care is that it does not "fit neatly" into a box when it comes to policy. Often palliative care is included in disease-specific policies, e.g. Human Immunodeficiency Virus or Cancer, or those for communicable disease, or non-communicable disease (NCDs). As children's palliative care encompasses children with a wide range of conditions, and ages including neonates, children, adolescents and young adults, it needs to be included in any policy that covers these different groups, e.g. neonatal care, mother and child health, cancer, nutrition, etc. We have our work cut out to ensure that children's palliative care is included in all policies, so having an

---

**BOX 11.1 CASE STUDY: THE INTERNATIONAL CHILDREN'S PALLIATIVE CARE NETWORK (ICPCN) GLOBAL MAPPING OF CPC POLICIES**

A survey was sent out by the ICPCN to targeted members from each country to gather information about national policies. This was part of a wider mapping survey. Where the network did not know anyone within a specific country, we approached the regional associations to see if they could put us in contact with someone who would have information about children's palliative care development in that country. Information was received from 130 countries, covering all of the WHO regions, i.e. Africa, the Americas, the Eastern Mediterranean, Europe, Southeast Asia and the Western Pacific Region.

Only 11% of respondents said that they had a national children's palliative care policy in their country, 52% had a general national palliative care policy, some of which specified children and others did not, and 37% had no palliative care policy in their country. Of those with a children's palliative care policy, >70% were from high-income countries with the rest from upper-middle-income countries. Of those with no policy on palliative care, 21% were from high-income countries, 24% from upper-middle-income countries, 36% from lower-middle-income countries and 19% from low-income countries. Thus, there is a great need for advocacy to develop and implement policy on children's palliative care around the world.

overarching palliative care policy across the life span can be helpful. Yet at the same time, without a specific policy on children's palliative care, children can be left out. Often where an overarching palliative care policy exists, these tend to be adult-focused policy documents which may include some consideration of children's needs. However, this is challenging as the policy is designed for the majority group, i.e. adults, with only a minor focus on meeting the needs of the minority group, i.e. children. Thus, there is a danger of tokenism in these policies. This is a challenge not just within policy, but across the board in palliative care – in service provision, education, policy, advocacy and research – when it is assumed that overarching services will adequately provide for children, the minority group. There is a need for national, regional and international organisations to focus specifically on children's palliative care to ensure that the voice of children and their families is heard and respected and not just accorded lip service. The challenge for us as children's palliative care nurses is to ensure that this does not happen and that policy at both the national and service levels recognises the unique needs of children requiring palliative care and their families.

Global, regional and national organisations also have a key role in advocating for children's palliative care. The ICPCN has a global remit for children's palliative care and has been led by nurses from the outset. The organisation has worked in global collaboration with the International Association for Hospice and Palliative Care (IAHPC), the Worldwide Hospice Palliative Care Alliance (WHPCA), Palliative Care in Humanitarian Aid Situations and Emergencies (PallCHASE) and the Global Palliative Nursing Network (GPNN) (Box 11.2). Together, these networks have been influential in the development of global policy, such as the World Health Assembly resolution, Universal Health Coverage, Primary Health care, as well as the development of charters, standards, guidelines and resources to strengthen children's palliative care. Regionally the African Palliative Care Association (APCA), the European Association for Palliative Care (EAPC), the Asia Pacific Hospice Palliative Care Network (APHN) and the Asociación Latinoamericana de Cuidados Palliativos (ALCP) also have a strong voice and are crucial in the ongoing development of policy for palliative care across the life span, working closely with national palliative care organisations, many of whom are either led by nurses or have nurses within their leadership teams.

---

**BOX 11.2 CASE STUDY: THE GLOBAL PALLIATIVE NURSING NETWORK (GPNN)**

The GPNN aims to promote palliative nursing globally and establish a worldwide network to provide peer support and professional development for all nurses (adult and paediatric) working in palliative care – wherever they are. The network was set up by St Christopher's Hospice and the ICPCN in 2022 following St Christopher's pioneering nurse programme, a palliative nursing conference and other training, which engaged with over 1,200 palliative nurses from around the world. It is designed to complement existing networks and members can share insights and innovations as well as experiencing the support of like-minded professionals. Members can also enjoy regular webinars, a wide range of tools and resources, an annual conference and access to thought-provoking blogs (St Christophers, 2023).

In terms of children's palliative care leadership, some countries have specific children's palliative care networks such as Patch South Africa, Together for Short Lives (UK) and Kenniscentrum Kinderpalliatieve Zorg (The Netherlands), while others have a national organisation for palliative care that includes children, and some have none. A recent survey undertaken by the International Children's Palliative Care Network identified 25 countries as having specific national organisations for children's palliative care, e.g. South Africa; Brazil, Canada, and France. The majority of countries reported having national organisations which included children, but others had no national palliative care organisations. However, it was also interesting to note that many countries had professional associations, or special interest groups for those working in children's palliative care.

---

**LEARNING ACTIVITY**

Reflect on the policy environment in your country for palliative care:

1.   Does it include children's palliative care?
2.   Is there a separate policy for children's palliative care?
3.   Are you aware of the policies?
4.   How are nurses and nursing represented in the children's palliative care policy landscape?

---

## THE POLICY LANDSCAPE FOR NURSING LEADERSHIP

Strengthening nursing leadership is a global priority, emphasised in a range of fora including the Triple Impact Report (All Party Parliamentary Group, 2016), Nursing Now Challenge (Burdett Trust for Nursing, 2021), the Year of the Nurse and the Midwife (WHO, 2019a) and the ongoing development of a range of nursing leadership programmes around the world, such as the International Council of Nurses (ICN) Global Nursing Leadership Initiative, and the Florence Nightingale Foundation (FNF) Global Leadership programme, to name but a few. The strengthening of nursing leadership is recognised as one of the priority areas that can be used to address the global shortage of nurses (Oulton, 2006) and the World Health Organization Global Strategic directions for strengthening nursing and midwifery 2016–2020 had "optimising policy development, effective leadership, management and governance" as one of its four themes (WHO, 2016). The 2021–2025 Global Strategic directions for nursing and midwifery (WHO, 2021c) continue the theme of leadership as they identify four strategic directions and policy priorities: education, jobs, leadership, and service delivery. The emphasis here is to "increase the proportion and authority of midwives and nurses in senior health and academic positions and continually develop the next generation of nursing and midwifery leaders" (p. 6) through establishing and strengthening senior leadership positions for nursing and midwifery and investing in leadership skills development (WHO, 2021c). Alongside this, reports such as the Triple Impact Report (All Party Parliamentary Group, 2016) from the UK, recommend not only investing in leadership development but also creating structures that place nurse leaders within positions of influence.

The WHO agenda for "Making Health Systems Work" (WHO, 2007) along with the World Health Organization Leadership Framework has put particular emphasis on strengthening leadership and management in the health system with an emphasis on nursing and midwifery leadership (WHO, 2016; 2021c). They recommend creating an enabling leadership environment (organisational context, relationship with others, clear roles and responsibilities, supervision and incentives); and establishing functional critical support systems (to manage staff, information, and other resources) (WHO, 2007). This development and nurturing of leadership skills in nurses need to be available at every stage of nurses' careers to enable them to be influential leaders, and create ways that they can be nurtured and recognised (Burdett Trust for Nursing, 2021).

> Nursing and Health Policy is at the centre of what we do. Ensuring that nurses have a voice in the development and implementation of health policy is fundamental to ensuring these policies are effective and meet the real needs of patients, families and communities around the world.
>
> *(International Council of Nurses, 2023)*

Nurses can drive and need to be driving and leading policy change if they are to contribute to improvement in children's palliative care provision and to achieve health equity. Nurses are powerful leaders of policy-related nursing, healthcare and children's palliative care and need to have a voice (International Council of Nurses, 2023). Nurses are at the forefront of the development and implementation of children's palliative care around the world, to ensure access to quality care for all. Nurses are in a unique position to show leadership, influence and shape policy, to drive better outcomes and improve care, as well as improve job satisfaction and staff well-being. The skills and character developed by nurses extend far beyond the ten characteristics described by Cagliostro (2020) as reasons why nurses are uniquely placed to shape the future of healthcare (Box 11.3). The bedside experience of nurses lays the foundation for nurses to lead, to advocate for the marginalised, and to give a voice to the voiceless. As they lead in healthcare, they also lead in issues of gender equality and women's empowerment, speaking up for the needs and rights of women, as the majority in the nursing workforce are women. They are uniquely positioned to help reduce power inequities, build respect, contribute to improved working conditions, as well as to speak up for the vulnerable in society, such as those children needing palliative care. With their gender-sensitive leadership, nurses are represented at all levels of decision-making and can bring a global voice, through networks for children's palliative care or palliative nursing or bodies such as the WHO or the International Council of Nurses. They can use their unique opportunities to lead and make a difference to the provision of children's palliative care globally, bridging the gap between need and provision, and enhancing quality of life.

---

**BOX 11.3 TEN REASONS WHY NURSES ARE UNIQUELY PLACED TO SHAPE THE FUTURE OF HEALTHCARE**

1. Nurses remain calm under pressure – job performance can be a matter of life and death for their patients.
2. Nurses know that attention to detail is key, keeping patients safe and optimising healing and recovery.
3. Nurses are called upon to use the skills of critical thinking on a day-to-day basis.
4. The flexibility and creativity of nurses have become the foundation for excellent care.
5. Effective nursing teamwork is crucial – if teamwork suffers, patient outcomes suffer.
6. Nurses must be excellent communicators and adaptable.
7. Nurses have learnt to perform their role while showing empathy and compassion, leading to improved trust and better outcomes.
8. Patients entrust their lives to the integrity of nurses. In 2019, in the US, nurses were voted the most trusted profession for the 18th year in a row (Reinhart, 2020).
9. As patient advocates, nurses speak up as necessary to ensure positive outcomes.
10. Through their work, nurses develop a thorough understanding of the health needs of the patient population.

Source: Cagliostro (2020).

---

With only 25% of leadership positions in health globally being held by nurses, men hold a disproportionately high number of senior nursing roles. Nurses have a crucial role in speaking up for women, and for gender empowerment. Over the years, it has been recognised that there is "power" within the nursing profession, and it is important that nurses use that power wisely. Collectively nurses have the power to bring about change, in the health system, in children's palliative care, and in the empowerment of women. However, it is essential that nurses are trained in the skills to use this power wisely, to develop political awareness and skills, to push against the traditional, paternalistic healthcare system and to use a feminist model of empowerment to do this. This involves three dimensions: (1) raising consciousness of the socio-political realties of the nurse's world; (2) having strong and positive self-esteem and belief in their roles and skills as nurses; and (3) having the political skills needed in order to bring about change in the health system, and for children's palliative care (Mason et al., 1991). This link between nursing and feminism goes back many years, with Chinn and Wheeler (1985) posing the question as to whether nursing can afford to remain aloof from the women's movement and they consider nursing and women's health from a feminist perspective. More recently, Syed (2021), in the context of the COVID-19 pandemic, has explored the feminist political economy of health which suggests that discrimination against girls and women is a primary factor that influences social conditions and health. They recognise that women are vulnerable to health inequities at a range of levels, including their healthcare needs, their caregiving role and their position in the healthcare system. Feminist epistemological perspectives have impacted how women are perceived in society, and how these perceptions can affect women's paid and unpaid roles. With nurses, the majority of whom are women, being the majority of members of the workforce within the health system globally, we cannot avoid the recognition of feminist epistemology. As nurse leaders, we need to stand up against such inequities, and seek to empower not only other nurses, but also the vulnerable in society, such as the children and their families that we care for within palliative care settings. It is therefore essential that we build institutional capacity and leadership skills in nursing (WHO, 2020a) and specifically in children's palliative care. *The State of the World's Nursing 2020 Report* (WHO, 2020a) states that nurse leadership must be developed at country, regional and global levels, and that national policy-making forums should consider the nursing perspective in health system decision-making.

In the context of children's palliative care, there is a challenge around empowering nurses as leaders, but also recognising that in many countries, particularly in low- and middle-income countries not enough nurses have been trained in children's palliative care. In many countries, specialist children's palliative care nurses are not recognised and there is no career structure for nurses working in the field, or government-funded posts. Many nurses provide children's palliative care in their spare time, or care is provided by retired nurses for minimal renumeration (Downing et al., 2023), neither of which are sustainable if we are to develop children's palliative care further and decrease the gap between need and service provision. A balance also needs to be struck between recognising the specialist skills needed by children's palliative care nurses and making these so specialist that they are unattainable. We need nurses to be trained and competent to provide care at the different levels defined by the World Health Assembly resolution on PC (WHO, 2014) and in the EAPC core competencies for children's palliative care (Downing et al., 2014):

1. the palliative care approach (basic training and continuing education on children's palliative care);
2. general children's palliative care (intermediate training to all nurses who routinely work with children with life-threatening illnesses);
3. specialist children's palliative care.

With the Children's Palliative Care Education and Training Standard Framework (Neilson et al., 2021), these are expanded to four levels (see Introduction of this book):

1. Public Health
2. Universal
3. Core
4. Specialist.

While we must not lose sight of our goals as children's palliative care nurses: to care for children and their families; to relieve their suffering and help them to achieve the best possible quality of life; to care for them with competence and compassion; and to respectfully accompany the child and family on their journey; we can only do that through our leadership – at the bedside, within the community, within the hospital, within the district/region, nationally, regionally and globally. In order for nurses to provide the best possible palliative care that they can for children and their families, they need an enabling environment. An environment supported by:

• Policy and legal frameworks that empower them to provide care, rather than restricting it.
• Recognition of their specialist skills in children's palliative care.
• A career pathway and government posts for children's palliative care.
• Access to the medicines that they need – to the WHO essential medicines list as a minimum (WHO, 2023c).
• Access to appropriate education and training so that they are competent and "fit for practice".
• Access to data and research that support the care being provided.
• Empowered communities that understand what palliative care is and how it can help them.
• The formation of communities of like-minded nurses to support each other and mentor each other as leaders within the field – to give them a voice, and empower them to use that voice.

While we are far from this in many countries, particularly in low- and middle-income countries, we are moving forward and are gaining the momentum to support children's palliative care nurses to develop their leadership skills and to have a voice. Yet as we do this, there remain many challenges to nurses taking up those leadership roles, to leadership roles being open to them, and to children's palliative care nurses being given "a seat at the table", and, yet, without that we will never reach all children globally who need palliative care.

While in many high-income countries, the role of the children's nurse is well defined, in many low- and middle-income countries specific children's nurses do not exist, and in many settings, particularly outside of the capital cities and specialist children's hospitals, nurses will provide care to both adults and children. *The State of the World's Nursing Report 2020* (WHO, 2020a) cites the example of developing children's nursing in the African region where there are a growing number of governments who are investing in the development of children's nurses and recognising their value. Such nurses tend to be registered nurses with post-basic training as a specialist children's nurse with a growing number of registered children's nurses in the region, although not nearly enough. There are very few registered children's nurses trained in palliative care. In terms of specialist training, there are a growing number of programmes on specialist or advanced practice nursing, and as these develop, more nursing councils are recognising these specialist/advanced roles, which is essential to ensure nurses are practising within their competence and code of practice. Yet, even in countries where such roles are well developed, such as in the United States, there is a paucity of literature on roles such as the paediatric palliative Advanced Practice Registered Nurse (APRNs) (Cormack and Dahlin, 2022). Nursing leadership is therefore crucial to the development of regulation and scopes of practice which are appropriate for country health systems and culture. However, the training of nurses varies significantly from country to country and nursing roles need to develop according to competence and level of training, with advanced roles and task shifting proving challenging to some professions, e.g. doctors, in some parts of the world, according to the perceived status of nurses within their settings.

*The State of the World's Nursing Report 2020* (WHO, 2020a) stated that out of 115 countries, only 71% had a Chief Country Nursing Officer, ranging from 54% in the Eastern Mediterranean Region to 86% in the European Region, with only 53% of responding countries having a leadership development programme, with only 40% in the Southeast Asia Region. This demonstrates the wide disparity in nursing governance and leadership globally, impacting on the development of children's palliative care nurse leaders. This needs to be seen within individual country contexts, although in all settings there is potential for nurses to lead for improvement.

Task shifting, including nurse prescribing, can be seen within high-income and low- and middle-income countries. For example, in the United Kingdom, "nurses, midwives, pharmacists and other allied health professionals who have completed an accredited prescribing course and registered their qualification with their regulatory body, are able to prescribe" (RCN, 2014) There are two kinds of prescribers, including Independent Prescribers who have successfully completed the training and they are able to prescribe any medicine within their competency, including all controlled medicines in schedules two to five, which includes opioids (RCN, 2014; 2023). Lear (2023) undertook an evaluation of nurse prescribing in palliative care and found that it increases rapid symptom control for patients, and was in line with other studies showing improved symptom control (Edwards et al., 2022) and prevention of unplanned admissions (Latter et al., 2022). However, it was also clear that strong clinical leadership needed to be established among nursing independent prescribers in palliative care (Lear, 2023).

An example from low- and middle-income countries is that of nurse prescribing in palliative care in Uganda. In Uganda, access to palliative care was hampered by a lack of prescribers as the doctor:patient ratio is not high enough to ensure access to medications for individuals. Palliative care trained nurses have been able to prescribe in Uganda since 2004 when the statute was changed to enable this (Ministry of Health, 2004). The country has since been seen as a model for nurse prescribing in palliative care globally, promoting access to palliative care, including morphine down to the village level. Specific training is provided for nurse prescribers, including the Clinical Palliative Care Course, which commenced at Hospice Africa Uganda and is now run by Mulago School of Nursing, with well over 200 nurses completing the course to date. An evaluation of nurse prescribing found that the nurses are competent in assessing and managing pain, prescribing morphine and associated medications appropriately. The evaluation showed the benefit and safety of nurse prescribing for palliative care in Uganda, despite significant challenges (Downing et al., 2018).

While none of these programmes and evaluations focus specifically on children's palliative care, but on palliative care generally, neither exclude children's palliative care, and this is clearly an area where children's palliative care nurses can demonstrate leadership.

---

**LEARNING ACTIVITY**

Reflect on how nursing is seen as a profession in your country.

- Does this impact on your role within children's palliative nursing?
- Do you have strong nursing leaders within your country who you can learn from?
- What about children's palliative care nursing leaders?

---

## THE NURSE AS LEADER

Developing nurses as leaders is essential if we are to bring about improvement and change in children's palliative care. It is important that as nurses working in the field, we are innovative, resourceful, able to "think outside the box" while recognising our diversities, strengths and weaknesses. As nurses working in children's palliative care, we have a wide range of roles, including advocate, practitioner, teacher, co-ordinator, researcher, and counsellor, all of which are strengthened through our roles as leaders. However, our role as leaders can be impacted by different factors, such as: the status of nursing in our country and whether there are sufficient nurses to work in palliative care; the availability of training; the nurses' qualification and level of experience, knowledge and skills in children's palliative care. Another factor is lack of access to other members of an interdisciplinary team, which can lead to the nurse often fulfilling a variety of additional roles when other team members are not available, thus requiring them to have extra knowledge and skills. This is particularly the case in many low- and middle-income countries where nurses may be working in relative isolation.

Gender is another key factor impacting on the nurse's role as leaders, as discussed earlier. While making recommendations for policy-makers and implementers to strengthen nursing and midwifery leadership, Nursing Now (Newman et al., 2019) recognised that gender discrimination, bias and stereotyping were key inhibitors for nurses and midwives to develop appropriate leadership skills. Issues involved included societal and cultural perceptions about specific roles of women and men, female nurses and midwives having to juggle paid and unpaid work, their perceived limited decision-making authority, regardless of gender, along with a lack of self-confidence. Therefore, it is important to change the perception of the nursing profession and elevate the status and profile of nursing in the health sector, while building nurses' self-confidence and sense of preparedness to assume leadership positions (Newman et al., 2019). Women make up nearly 70% of the global health workforce, including 89% of the nursing workforce, yet, as highlighted earlier they only hold 25% of senior roles within healthcare (WHO, 2019b). However, there is evidence that shows that input from women leaders results in policies that are more supportive of women and children, which impacts on nurse retention and service provision (Ngabonzima et al., 2020), and strengthens progress towards Universal Health Coverage and the UN Sustainable Development Goals (Downs et al., 2016).

Every nurse is a leader, and we develop our leadership skills as we progress through our nursing career. Fundamental to all that we do is providing leadership in the care of our patients – of the children that we care for within palliative care, and their families, co-ordinating care, enabling access to treatment, medicines, resources, counselling, etc. Examples can be seen, such as at Rachel House in Indonesia, a pioneering children's palliative care programme, where the nurses have an essential role in co-ordinating care and helping families navigate through the care system (Rachel House, 2024). It is these skills that we develop in our clinical work, that we build on and develop throughout our careers.

Leaders come in all shapes and sizes, and lead in a range of different ways, some being more autocratic and others more democratic, some may be focused on the big picture and others on the small details. There are a range of leadership theories that are discussed in the literature. It has often been assumed that one is born with leadership skills or not, that some people were simply "born leaders". However, more recently, there is a view that some attributes that people have may make them more natural leaders, but that experience, education and skills development also have an important role to play. This resonates with the fact that many people develop and grow into leadership as they mature, or as they develop in their nursing careers. Also, from experience in conducting leadership training, it is clear that we can develop and learn new skills that are helpful in our leadership journey, and that reflection on our self as leaders is crucial as we try to lead for improvement in children's palliative care around the world.

While there are different leadership theories, the majority can be classified into one of the eight major types listed in Table 11.1. Having an understanding of the

**TABLE 11.1** Different leadership theories (Cherry, 2022; Indeed, 2023)

| Type | Description |
| --- | --- |
| 1. "Great Man" Theories | These theories assume the capacity for leadership is inherent – that great leaders are born and not made |
| 2. Trait Theories | These assume that people inherit certain qualities or traits that make them better suited to leadership |
| 3. Contingency Theories | These focus on variables related to the environment that might determine a particular style of leadership is best suited for a given situation |
| 4. Situational Theories | These propose that leaders choose the best course of action based upon situational variables, with different styles being more appropriate for certain types of decision-making |
| 5. Behavioural Theories | Based upon the belief that great leaders are made, not born, and focuses on the actions of leaders and not their qualities |
| 6. Participative Theories | Suggests the ideal leadership style is one that takes the input of others into account – encouraging participation from others in decision-making |
| 7. Management/Transactional Theories | These focus on the role of supervision, organisation and group performance – there is a system of rewards and punishments |
| 8. Relationship/Transformational Theories | These focus on the connections formed between leaders and followers through which they want every person to fulfil their potential |

different leadership theories not only can help as you reflect on your own leadership style, but also as you try and understand the leaders around you, those you see on the television, those you work with, those you aspire to be like and even those you don't want to be like.

It is also important to think about the differences between a leader and a manager – they can be, but are not necessarily, the same. Leaders and managers may share some similar attributes but generally a manager is someone placed in a position of authority who people have no choice but to follow. For example, we may be put into a position of authority in the post of ward manager and if those who work under us don't follow our instructions, then this can have repercussions for them. However, a leader is someone who attracts followers through charisma, success and other characteristics – we want to follow a leader and we have a choice as to whether we decide to do so or not (Indeed, 2023).

Alongside leadership theories there are also a range of leadership styles, each with its own distinct qualities, and these may include an aspect of how decisions are made. Common leadership styles include (Indeed, 2023):

- *The visionary* – they lead through inspiration and confidence – team morale is high which helps improve results.
- *Transformative* – they inspire people to strive beyond expectations towards a shared vision.
- *The coach* – they recognise individuals' strengths and weaknesses, help people set goals and provide feedback.
- *Autocratic* – they make decisions without input from others – a particularly important style of leadership where responding without question is literally a matter of life or death, e.g. in battle.
- *Bureaucratic* – they follow a strict hierarchy and expect their team members to follow procedures. This is often common within the healthcare setting, with nurses often being low down in the hierarchy.
- *Democratic* – they consider the opinions of others before making a decision.
- *Laissez-faire* – they delegate tasks and provide little supervision.

Different situations will require different leadership styles and not all will be appropriate in a children's palliative care context. In settings where children's palliative care is relatively new and may not be recognised within the health context, a visionary and transformative leader will be needed, however, at times, they will need to use a bureaucratic style, following strict hierarchy in order to bring about the change that is required. The development of children's palliative care globally has often been spearheaded by pioneers – they are known for their perseverance, for being headstrong and transforming challenges into opportunities. They recognise that change is constant, will take calculated risks, encourage creativity and maintain resilience (Miller, 2023). While important in the initial development of children's palliative care, pioneering leaders may not be the best people to move the field, or a service forward, when different skills are required. Generally, within children's palliative care the autocratic and laissez-faire styles of leadership are not appropriate, although as within any healthcare context, in times of emergency, an autocratic style may be required in order to ensure the safety of the child, their family and the healthcare staff. Supervision, mentorship, guidance and vision are key, although it is important to remember that we are all different, and each of us is unique, along with the situations in which we are working. However, if we are to lead for improvement, to bring about change for the best in children's palliative care, then transformational leadership is important as it provides inspiration, shows integrity, is based on relationships, encourages everyone to reach their potential, and focuses on the positive – it helps to bring about improvement. This is vital at a time when there is a shortage of nurses generally, insufficient children's palliative care nurses, increasing complexity in the children that we care for and rapid changes in health services around the world.

Another way of viewing leadership is through VUCA thinking (Volatile, Uncertain, Complex and Ambiguous). This is a mindset adopted by leaders around the world to function and lead in an ever-changing environment, with the VUCA framework providing a tool to help us to thrive in such a situation (Schulze et al., 2021; Cernega et al., 2024). As children's palliative care nurses we are used to working in such an environment, with the ever-changing needs of the children and families we care for, thus, we use a VUCA framework in all that we do. It is therefore important that not only are we technically sound but also that we enhance our leadership capabilities, build resilience and effectiveness in meeting the challenges of a rapidly changing and evolving health system (Campbell et al., 2020).

---

**LEARNING ACTIVITY**

Reflect on your own leadership styles.

- Which do you use and when?
- In what ways do you think you need to develop your leadership styles?

---

If we are to grow and develop in our leadership skills, then it is important that we reflect on how we lead, or prefer to lead. What are our strengths? What about our weaknesses? How can we become a better leader? What skills do we need in our present situation in children's palliative care? What help do we need to do this? As nurses, many of us have been taught about reflective practice and we have been encouraged to reflect on our practice as a routine part of what it means to be a nurse.

Campbell et al. (2020) identified four dimensions where nurses experience challenges as leaders: (1) leading others; (2) leading an organisation; (3) leading change; and (4) leading self (Figure 11.1). It is important for us to reflect on these four areas, to think about the challenges we experience as leaders in children's palliative care in these different areas, to think about the leadership styles that we use, and how we can help bring transformation and improvement in the settings and areas where we work. It can also help us identify areas where we need support and training in order to improve our skills. This will help us to think about how we

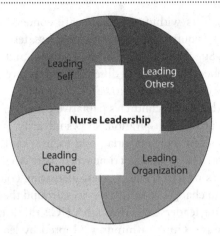

**FIGURE 11.1** The four dimensions where nurses experience challenges in leadership

Source: adapted from Campbell et al. (2020).

can develop and enhance our leadership skills, bringing together the depth of skill and technical expertise in children's palliative care alongside broader knowledge, including the "business" of healthcare and the relational skills needed to engage and lead teams.

Another example of a model that helps us to reflect on our leadership skills is the Five Practices of Exemplary Leadership developed in the early 1980s by Kouzes and Posner (2002). The five practices approach leadership as a measurable, learnable and teachable set of behaviours. The five practices that contribute to transformative leadership can be found in Table 11.2. They can help us look at contributors to transformative leadership, and review our strengths and weakness through the use of the Leadership Practices Inventory (LPI). They focus on growth rather than looking at what an individual does as good or bad, encourage self-reflection and allow individuals to commit to growing and developing. The LPI is an example of a

**TABLE 11.2** Exemplary leadership practices (Kouzes and Posner, 2002)

| Five exemplary practices | Ten commitments | Examples in children's palliative care |
|---|---|---|
| 1. Modelling the way | • Clarify values<br>• Set an example | Nurses working in children's palliative care all over the world are modelling the way in the provision of care in a range of settings, cultures and across a range of ages. We hope that this book, aimed at nurses working in children's palliative care, written and edited by nurses from around the world, will help model the way for the provision of children's palliative care globally, clarify values and give examples of how this can be done. |

*(Continued)*

**TABLE 11.2** Exemplary leadership practices (Kouzes and Posner, 2002) *(Continued)*

| Five exemplary practices | Ten commitments | Examples in children's palliative care |
|---|---|---|
| 2. Inspiring a shared vision | • Envisioning the future<br>• Enlisting others | There are many examples within children's palliative care where nurses have been in leadership positions, have been pioneers and have inspired others to follow a shared vision. For example, from the initial roots of palliative care Dame Cicely Saunders, who was a nurse as well as a doctor and social worker, Professor Ida Martinson from the University of Minnesota, Joan Marston, who set up the International Children's Palliative Care Network, to name but a few (ICPCN, 2024a). |
| 3. Challenging the process | • Searching for opportunities<br>• Experimenting and taking risks | Ruth Sims is a nurse who searched for opportunities and took risks. Setting up the Mildmay Centre in Uganda in 1998, along with colleagues, to provide palliative care for both children and adults with HIV. It was the first specialist palliative care centre for children in Uganda and the surrounding region (ICPCN, 2024a). |
| 4. Enabling others to act | • Fostering collaboration<br>• Strengthening others | Education and training are key in the development of children's palliative care, along with mentoring in order to enable others to act. Nurses worldwide are involved in enabling others to provide children's palliative care. Alex Mancini is one such nurse as she provides education and mentorship on neonatal palliative care, fostering collaboration between services, not just in the UK but globally (ICPCN, 2024b). |
| 5. Encouraging the heart | • Recognising contributions<br>• Celebrating the values and victories | In 2021, in recognition of the International Year of the Nurse, a report was launched on World Health Day to highlight the work of 27 nurses in palliative care. It was a celebration of the pivotal role of nurses in palliative care across the globe. It also aimed to act as an inspiration to policy-makers and managers, to support nurses so they could have a more prominent voice. While covering palliative nursing generally, there was a section specifically highlighting the role of nurses in children's palliative care (Downing, 2021). |

tool that has been used in many different parts of the world, including in low- and middle-income countries, for example, in Uganda (Nanyonga, 2015).

In the UK, the NHS has published a guide for leading improvement (NHS Institute for Innovation and Improvement, 2005) with the vision that every individual working in the NHS is enabled, encouraged and capable of working with others to bring about improvement. They developed the NHS Leadership Qualities framework (Figure 11.2) that describes 15 qualities in three areas: (1) Setting direction; (2) Delivering the service; and (3) Personal Qualities. They suggest the framework can be used to reflect on your own leadership abilities, to reflect on your team's leadership abilities in order to identify areas for improvement and develop and strengthen leadership capacity. They go on to discuss a leading modernisation framework developed by Plsek (NHS Institute for Innovation and Improvement, 2005), which says a leader of improvement needs to be a good leader, to shine in delivering excellent care or enabling us to do so, and to promote and support improvement. As we lead for improvement within children's palliative care, we need to strengthen the intersection of these three domains. The leader with the mindset for improvement focuses on process and systems, aims to improve the

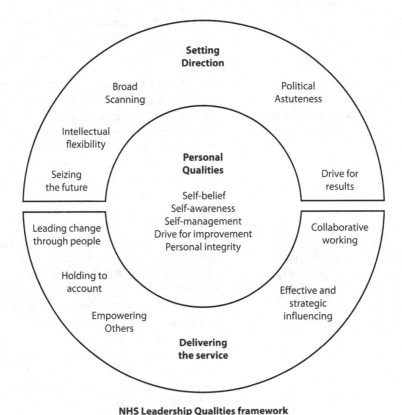

**NHS Leadership Qualities framework**

**FIGURE 11.2** NHS Leadership Qualities framework

Source: NHS Institute for Innovation and Improvement (2005), p. 4.

performance of the overall system; manages the variability in the system and deals with the chronic problems that underpin poor performance, i.e. treating the disease. It is about the leader having a mindset change from one of firefighting to one of continuous improvement (NHS Institute for Innovation and Improvement, 2005). While this is appropriate in the healthcare setting, it is also an interesting way to think about improvement in all areas of the WHO conceptual model (WHO, 2021a) if we are to improve the provision of children's palliative care in our service, our country, or globally.

So, for example, if we think about access to medicines, it is not about "treating the symptoms, but treating the disease" – understanding the underlying issue that means that palliative care medicines are not available and how we can deal with that underlying issue rather than "just the symptoms". We therefore need to try and develop a culture of improvement, encouraging learning and creating support mechanisms, collaborating together to ensure that the needs of children requiring palliative care and their families are at the centre of our planning. We need to make sure that all we do is aligned around improving the way children and their families are being cared for (NHS Institute for Innovation and Improvement, 2005). Box 11.4 and Box 11.5 present examples of leadership training in different areas.

---

**BOX 11.4 LEADERSHIP TRAINING FOR PALLIATIVE NURSES**

The Kenyan Hospice and Palliative Care Association (KEHPCA) ran a two-year nurse leadership programme for palliative nurses in Kenya. The programme aimed to equip nurse leaders and mentors working within palliative care with the skills and knowledge to enable them to grow in their leadership and take up leadership positions within palliative care in Kenya. Nurse leaders attended a mixture of face-to-face and virtual training over the two-year programme, which was funded by Hospice Care Kenya. Eight nurse leaders undertook the course, some being heads of community-based non-governmental organisations, some working in oncology and other palliative care settings.

---

**BOX 11.5 LEADERSHIP TRAINING FOR CHILDREN'S PALLIATIVE CARE**

Two Worlds Cancer Collaboration and the MNJ Institute at Hyderabad are running a multi-professional leadership institute for individuals working in children's palliative care. The programme involves a mix of self-directed learning, face-to-face training, virtual sessions, site visits, the development of leadership plans, a situational analysis of children's palliative care in their country and the implementation of a leadership project linked to the development of children's palliative care. The initial face-to-face session was held in Hyderabad prior to the Indian Association of Palliative Care Conference in February 2024, with ongoing virtual sessions and the implementation of their projects (ICPCN, 2024c).

## SUMMARY

Nurses are in a key position within children's palliative care to lead for improvement – to think outside of the box, to "treat the disease rather than the symptoms", to improve the overall system as well as the care that they provide in order to improve the quality of life of children needing palliative care and their families around the world. However, in order to do this, it is essential that they have a knowledge of the wider context for the provision of children's palliative care, of the policy landscape for both children's palliative care and nursing. As nurses develop as leaders, and step into positions of influence, a knowledge of leadership theories and skills is important, not only as they develop their own leadership skills but also in supporting others to do the same. Leadership for improvement is not an optional extra, but something that all of us as children's palliative nurses need to be committed to, to strive towards and to move forward together.

## KEY POINTS

- Children's palliative care nurses are in a key position to create change, however, often the leadership role of nurses is not recognised, and nurses are not given the opportunity to lead.
- There is a growing recognition of the need for children's palliative care at the global policy level, which has an impact at the regional, national and local levels.
- Strengthening nursing leadership is a global priority and is outlined in the WHO's Global Strategic Directions for Strengthening Nursing and Midwifery, and nurses have a crucial role in gender empowerment.
- There are a range of different leadership theories and styles and having an understanding of these can help nurses reflect on their own leadership styles and of those around them.
- Access to training is important as we seek to develop and empower the children's palliative care nurses of the future.

## REFERENCES

All Party Parliamentary Group on Global Health. (2016). *Triple Impact: How developing nursing will improve health, promote gender equality and support economic growth.* House of Commons.

APCA (African Palliative Care Association). (2011). APCA Standards for providing quality palliative care across Africa. Available at: https://www.africanpalliativecare.org/sites/default/files/2023-10/APCA_StandardsStandards-for-Providing-Quality-Palliative-Care-Across-Africa.pdf

Benini, F., Pappadatou, D., Bernada, M., Craig, F., De Zen, L., Downing, J., Drake, R., Friedrichsdorf, S., Garros, D., Giacomelli, L., Lacerda, A., Lazzarin, P., Marceglia, S., Marston, J., Mukaden, M. A., Papa, S., Parravicini, E., Pellegatta, F., Wolfe, J. (2022). International standards for pediatric palliative care: From IMPaCCT to GO-PPaCS. *Journal of Pain and Symptom Management*, 63(5), e529–e543. https://doi.org/10.1016/j.jpainsymman.2021.12.031

Burdett Trust for Nursing. (2021). Nursing now challenge. Available at: https://www.nursingnow. org

Cagliostro, J. (2020). 10 reasons why nurses are uniquely situated to shape the future of healthcare. Available at: https://www.linkedin.com/pulse/10-reasons-why-nurses-uniquely-situated-shape-future-jim-cagliostro

Campbell, C., Canning, M., Green, M. (2020). Nurse leadership in the 2020s. Duke Corporate Education. Available at: https://www.dukece.com/insights/nurse-leadership-in-the-2020s/

Cernega, A., Nicolescu, D. N., Imre, M. M., Totan, R. A., Arsene, A. L., Serban, R. S., Perpelea, A-C., Nedea, M-L., Pituru, S-M. (2024). Volatility, Uncertainty, Complexity and Ambiguity (VUCA) in healthcare. *Healthcare (Basel)*, 12(7), 773. https://doi.org/10.3390/healthcare12070773

Cherry, K. (2022). The major leadership theories. Available at: https://www.verywellmind.com/leadership-theories-2795323

Chinn, P. L., Wheeler, C. E. (1985). Feminism and nursing: Can nursing afford to remain aloof from the women's movement? *Nursing Outlook*, 33(2), 74–77.

Cormack, C. L., Dahlin, C. (2022). The Pediatric Palliative APRN: Leading the future. *Journal of Pediatric Health Care*, 36, 381–387. https://doi.org/10.1016/j.pedhc.2022.01.005

de Oliveira, A. P. C., Ventura, C. A. A., da Silva, F. V., Neto, H. A., Mendes, I. A. C., de Souza, K. V., Pinerio, M. I. C., da Silva, M. C. N., Padilla, M., Ramalho, N. M, de Souza, W. V. B. (2020). The state of nursing in Brazil. *Revista Latino-Americana de Enfermagem*, 28, e3404. https://doi.org/10.1590/1518-8345.0000.3404

Downing, J. (ed.) (2021). *Palliative care celebrating nurses' contributions*. Report by ICPCN, WHPCA, IAHPC. ICPCN.

Downing, J., Adongo, E. A., Kuma-Aboagye, P., Renner, L. A., Salifu, N., Paintsil, V., Odiko-Ollenu, W. A., Ossei Sekyere, B. (2023). Needs assessment and situational analysis for children's palliative care in Ghana. Unpublished report for the Ministry of Health.

Downing, J., Kivumbi, G., Nabirye, E., Ojera, A., Namwanga, R., Katusabe, R., Dusabimana, M., Kalema, K., Yayeri, B., Apollo, A., Batuli, M., Komunda, C., Nabukalu, R., Mwesige, J., Sekyondwa,: M., Kasirye, M., Amoris J. O., Nandutu, E., Acuda W., Adong, D., ... Leng, M. (2018). An evaluation of palliative care nurse prescribing: A mixed methods study in Uganda. *BMJ Supportive and Palliative Care*, 8(Suppl. 1), A6. https://doi.org/10.1136/bmjspcare-2018-ASPabstracts.15

Downing, J., Ling, J., Benini, F., Payne, S., Papadatou, D. (2014). A summary of the EAPC White Paper on core competencies for education in paediatric palliative care. *European Journal of Palliative Care*, 21(5), 245–249.

Downs, J. A., Mathad, J. S., Reif, L. K., McNairy, M. L., Celum, C., Boutin-Foster, C., Deschamps, M. M., Gupta, A., Hokororo, A., Katz, I. T., Konopasek, L., Nelson, R., Riviere, C., Gimcher, L. H., Fitzgerald, D. W. (2016). The ripple effect: Why promoting female leadership in global health matters. *Public Health Action*, 6, 210–211. https://doi.org/10.5588/pha.16.0072

EAPC (European Association for Palliative Care). (2022). The European Charter on Palliative Care for Children and Young People. EAPC. Available at: https://icpcn.org/wp-content/uploads/2023/01/FINAL-EAPC-CYP-Charter-1.pdf

Edwards, J., Coward, M., Carey, N. (2022). Barriers and facilitators to implementation of non-medical prescribing in primary care in the UK: A qualitative systematic review. *BMJ Open*, 12(1), 1–17. https://doi.org/10.1136/bmjopen-2021-052227

Harding, R., Hammerich, A., Peeler, A., Afolabi, O., Sleeman, K., Thompson, D., El Akoum, Gafer N. (2024). Palliative Care: How can we respond to 10 years of limited progress? WISH Report. Available at: https://wish.org.qa/research-report/palliative-care-how-can-we-respond-to-ten-10-years-of-limited-progress/

ICPCN. (2008). *The ICPCN Charter of Rights for Life Limited and Life Threatened Children*. Available at: https://icpcn.org/resources/publications-resources/ [English version].

ICPCN. (2024a). *A global history of children's palliative care.* Available at: https://icpcn. org/a-global-history-of-childrens-palliative-care/

ICPCN. (2024b). A new virtual course: Neonatal Palliative Care: An enhanced course. Available at: https://icpcn.org/news/a-new-virtual-course-neonatal-palliative-care-an-enhanced-course/

ICPCN. (2024c). Launch of the children's palliative care leadership initiative. Available at: https://icpcn.org/news/launch-of-the-childrens-palliative-care-leadership-institute/

Indeed. (2023). What are the main leadership theories and leadership styles? Available at: https://uk.indeed.com/career-advice/career-development/leadership-theories

International Council of Nurses. (2023). Nursing policy. Available at: https://www.icn.ch/ membership/specialist-affiliates/nursing-policy#:~:text=Nursing%20and%20Health% 20Policy%20is,and%20communities%20around%20the%20world

Knaul, F. M., Farmer, P. E., Krakauer, E. L., De Lima, L., Bhadelia, A., Kwete, X. J., Arreola-Ornelas, H., Gómez-Dantés, O., Rodriguez, N. M., Alleyne, G. A. O., Connor, S. R., Hunter, D. J., Lohman, L., Radbruch, L., del Rocío, M. S. M., Atun, R., Foley, K. M., Frenk, J., Jamison, D.T., Rajagopal, M. R., Lancet Commission on Palliative Care and Pain Relief Study Group. (2018). Alleviating the access abyss in palliative care and pain relief – an imperative of universal health coverage: The Lancet Commission report. *Lancet,* 391, 1391–1454. https://doi.org/10.1016/s0140-6736(17)32513-8

Knaul, F., Radbruch, L., Connor, S., de Lima, L., Arreola-Ornelas, H., Mendez Carniado, O., Jiang Kwete, X., Bhadelia, A., Downing, J., Krakauer, E. L. (2020). How many adults and children are in need of palliative care worldwide? In S. Connor (ed.), *Global atlas of palliative Care* (2nd edn, pp. 17–32). WHPCA.

Kouzes, J. M., Posner, B. Z. (2002). The leadership practices inventory: Theory and evidence behind the five practices of exemplary leaders. Available at: https://people.uncw.edu/ kozloffm/kouzesandposertheoryandevidence.pdf

Latter, S., Campling, N., Birtwistle, J., Richardson A., Bennett, M. I., Ewings, S., Meads, D., Santer, M. (2022). Supporting patient access to medicines in community palliative care: On-line survey of health professionals' practice, perceived effectiveness and influencing factors. *BMC Palliative Care,* 19(148), 1–9. https://doi.org/10.1186/s12904-020-00649-3

Lear, V. (2023). A review of nurse independent prescribers: Experiences, barriers and facilitators in palliative care. *International Journal for Advancing Practice,* 1(1), 18–22. https://doi.org/10.12968/ijap.2023.1.1.18

Mason, D. J., Backer, B. A., Georges, C. A. (1991). Toward a feminist model for the political empowerment of nurses. *Image: The Journal of Nursing Scholarship,* 23(2), 72–77. https:// doi.org/10.1111/j.1547-5069.1991.tb00646.x

Miller, J. (2023). Pioneering leadership: Transforming challenges into opportunities. Available at: https://www.linkedin.com/pulse/pioneering-leadership-transforming-challenges-jason-miller-qdvic/

Ministry of Health. (2004). *Statutory Instruments Supplement No 13. 23rd April 2004.* UPPC.

Mwangi-Powell, F. N., Downing, J., Powell, R. A., Kiyange, F., Ddungu, H. (2015). Palliative care in Africa. In B. R. Ferrell, N. Coyle, J. A. Paice (eds), *Oxford textbook of palliative nursing* (4th edn). Oxford University Press.

Nanyonga, R. C. (2015). *Leadership, followership, and the context: An integrative examination of nursing leadership in Uganda.* PhD thesis, Yale University, USA.

Neilson, S., Randall, D., McNamara, K., Downing, J. (2021). Children's palliative care education and training: Developing an education standard framework and audit. *BMC Medical Education,* 21, 539. https://doi.org/10.1186/s12909-021-02982-4

Newman, C., Stilwell, B., Rick, S., Peterson, K. (2019). Investing in the power of nurse leadership: What will it take? *IntraHealth.* 28(1).

Ngabonzima, A., Asingizwe, D., Kouveliotis, K. (2020). Influence of nurse and midwife managerial leadership styles on job satisfaction, intention to stay, and services provision in selected hospitals of Rwanda. *BMC Nursing*, 19(35). https://doi.org/10.1186/s12912-020-00428-8

NHS Institute for Innovation and Improvement. (2005). *Improvement Leaders' Guide. Leading Improvement: Personal and organisational development*. NHS.

Nursing Now (2018). Transforming nursing and midwifery in Uganda. Available at: https://archive.nursingnow.org/case-studies-uganda/

Open Society Institute. (2015). Public Health Fact Sheet: Children's Palliative Care and Human Rights. Available at: www.opensocietyfoundations.org

Oulton, J. A. (2006). *The global nursing shortage: An overview of issues and actions*. ICN.

Pan American Health Organization, WHO Americas. (2023). *Healthy life course*. Healthy Life Course - PAHO/WHO I Pan American Health Organization

Rachel House (2024). Bringing palliative care to children with life-limiting conditions in Indonesia. Available at: https://rachel-house.org

RCN (Royal College of Nursing). (2014). *RCN Fact Sheet on nurse prescribing in the UK*. Available at: www.rcn.org.uk/about-us/our-influencing-work/.

RCN (Royal College of Nursing). (2023). Non-medical prescribers. Available at: https://www.rcn.org.uk/Get-Help/RCN-advice/non-medical-prescribers

Reinhart, R. J. (2020). Nurses continue to rate highest in honesty, ethics. Available at: https://news.gallup.com/poll/274673/nurses-continue-rate-highest-honesty-ethics.aspx?fbclid=IwAR1Bz28gnxqAGQiRHzp5rH-HbTn4qksMkXmY33NAul1BpGTz0oH6CZMvuc8

Schulze, C., Welker, A., Kühn, A., Schwertz, R., Otto, B., Moraldo, L., Dentz, U., Arends, A., Welk, E., Wendorff, J-J., Koller, H., Kuss, D., Ries, M. (2021). Public health leadership in a VUCA world environment: Lessons learned during the regional emergency rollout of SARS-CoV-2 vaccinations in Heidelberg, Germany, during the COVID-19 pandemic. *Vaccines (Basel)*, 9(8), 887. www.ncbi.nlm.nih.gov/pmc/articles/PMC8402600

St Christophers. (2023). The Global Palliative Nursing Network. Available at: https://www.stchristophers.org.uk/gpnn/

Syed, I. U. (2021). Feminist political economy of health: Current perspectives and future directions. *Healthcare*, 9, 233. https://doi.org/10.3390/healthcare9020233

United Nations. (2023). Sustainable Development: The 17 Goals. Available at: https://sdgs.un.org/goals

WHO (World Health Organization). (2007). Making health systems work. Available at: https://www.who.int/management/mhswork/en/ (accessed December 2023).

WHO (World Health Organization). (2010). National health planning tools – health system building blocks. Available at: https://extranet.who.int/nhptool/BuildingBlock.aspx

WHO (World Health Organization). (2014). WHA67.19. Strengthening of palliative care as a component of comprehensive care throughout the life course. Available at: https://apps.who.int/gb/ebwha/pdf_files/wha67/a67_r19-en.pdf (accessed 19 June 2024).

WHO (World Health Organization). (2016). Global strategic directions for strengthening nursing and midwifery 2016–2020. Available at: https://www.who.int/publications/i/item/9789241510455

WHO (World Health Organization). (2018a). *Integrating palliative care and symptom relief into paediatrics: A WHO guide for health care planners, implementers and managers*. World Health Organization.

WHO (World Health Organization). (2018b). *Integrating palliative care and symptom relief into responses to humanitarian emergencies and crises: A WHO guide*. World Health Organization.

WHO (World Health Organization). (2019a). Executive Board designates 2020 as the "Year of the Nurse and Midwife". Available at: https://www.who.int/

WHO (World Health Organization). (2019b). Delivered by women, led by men: A gender and equity analysis of the global health and social workforce. Available at: https://www.who.int/

WHO (World Health Organization). (2020a). *State of the world's nursing 2020: Investing in education, jobs and leadership.* World Health Organization.

WHO (World Health Organization). (2020b). Palliative care. Available at: https://www.who.int/news-room/fact-sheets/detail/palliative-care (accessed 14 May 2024).

WHO (World Health Organization). (2021a). *Assessing the development of palliative care worldwide: A set of actionable indicators.* World Health Organization.

WHO (World Health Organization). (2021b). *Living guidance for clinical management of COVID-19.* World Health Organization.

WHO (World Health Organization). (2021c). Global strategic directions for strengthening nursing and midwifery 2021–2025. Available at: https://www.who.int/publications/i/item/9789240033863

WHO (World Health Organization). (2023a). What is Universal Health Coverage? Available at: https://www.who.int/health-topics/universal-health-coverage#tab=tab_1 (accessed 18 June 2024).

WHO (World Health Organization). (2023b). *Left behind in pain: Extent and causes of global variations in access to morphine for medical use and actions to improve safe access.* World Health Organization.

WHO (World Health Organization). (2023c). *WHO model list of essential medicines for children. 9th List.* World Health Organization.

World Health Organization and the United Nations Children Fund. (2018). *Declaration of Astana.* World Health Organization. Available at: https://iris.who.int/bitstream/handle/10665/328123/WHO-HIS-SDS-2018.61-eng.pdf?sequence=1 (accessed 18 June 2024).

# CHAPTER 12

# Evaluation and quality of care issues

..............................................

*Marie Friedel and Lucy Coombes*

## INTRODUCTION

The aim of palliative care is to improve the quality of life of patients, their families, and their caregivers by addressing their physical, psychosocial and spiritual needs through the prevention and relief of suffering. This is achieved through early identification and assessment, and treatment of pain and other symptoms (WHO, 1998). The Lancet Commission on Palliative Care and Pain relief study group affirms that: "Alleviation of the burden of pain, suffering and severe distress associated with life-threatening and life-limiting health conditions and with end-of-life is a global health and equity imperative" (Knaul et al., 2018; WHO, 2015).

There are the same pressures on palliative care services for children as there are for other healthcare provision. Integration of palliative care into existing healthcare systems can be achieved, according to the WHO, through its implementation in universal health coverage, financing it by public funds and integrating it into national insurance and social security programmes. With this social contract to resource children's palliative care comes a social contract to be accountable for the quality of the services, and to justify the resourcing in terms of outcomes and delivery.

Furthermore, palliative care must be anchored in clinical guidelines and referral systems at all levels of care. This requires monitoring and evaluation of legislative provisions, policies, interventions and programmes. However, we should be mindful that palliative care extends beyond financial accounting and regulatory requirements. "Progress on health and on human rights can be monitored with explicit outcome scales and benchmarks, using an appropriate set of metrics that extend beyond mortality and morbidity" (Knaul et al., 2018).

Children facing life-limiting and life-threatening conditions can be suffering from illnesses of all medical specialties (e.g. cardiology, pneumology, neonatology, genetics, oncology) and be aged from 0–18 years (Arias-Casais et al., 2020; Fraser et al.,

DOI: 10.4324/9781003384861-16

2012; Hain et al., 2013). They can be cared for in hospital, in a hospice, at home, or in respite healthcare settings. This heterogeneity in medical conditions, ages and care settings makes it difficult to reach consensus on, and consequently standards for, quality indicators used for evaluating the outcomes of children's palliative care (Kaye et al., 2017; Downing et al., 2018; Friedel et al., 2019).

While evaluating the quality of children's palliative care is challenging, in fulfilling the social contract and moral/ethical duty to care for seriously ill children, we also have to fulfil a duty to monitor resources, use them wisely and be able to demonstrate the effectiveness of care.

---

**LEARNING OBJECTIVES**

The reader will be able to do the following:

1. Critically discuss insights into the importance and needs to implement quality processes in children's palliative care.
2. Debate critically the conceptual, methodological and ethical complexity of evaluating palliative care and its outcomes.
3. Analyse the principles of evaluating quality in children's palliative care.

---

## WHY DO WE NEED TO EVALUATE QUALITY?

The overall goal of evaluating the quality of children's palliative care is to improve child and family outcomes, such as quality of life and care experience (Boyden et al., 2023). The care received at end of life, and the circumstances surrounding this, can have a significant effect on the bereavement outcomes of parents and siblings in terms of subsequent relationships, roles, friendships and ability to carry on with their lives (Mayland et al., 2022), as well as on the quality of life of the unwell child or young person. Therefore, there is a need to ensure that the care received by a child or young person is of high quality.

Globally, there is significant variability and inconsistency in models of children's palliative care service provision. Quality improvement activities make it possible for children's palliative care programmes to continuously monitor their care delivery and outcomes, while also methodologically organising efforts to interactively adjust care practices to better meet the needs of patients and families (Bogetz et al., 2022). They also enable teams to integrate across hospital systems and benchmark with other providers, enabling inequities in services to be identified and addressed (Bogetz et al., 2022).

Evaluating the quality of care serves four main purposes (adapted from Boyden et al., 2023):

- Ensure accountability of services
- Guide quality improvement initiatives
- Develop/produce new knowledge
- Aid clinical decision-making.

The Institute of Medicine (2001) lists six issues of quality, which we might slightly rephrase to apply to children's nursing care to include evaluating care as being:

1. Child- and childhood-centred
2. Safe
3. Effective
4. Timely
5. Sustainable
6. Just and equitable.

By identifying these issues of quality, we are in effect saying that a good quality children's palliative nursing care service would be child- and childhood-centred where children's specific childhoods within their communities are recognised (Randall, 2016a). This would include the essential aspects of childhoods, which are relational, generational and occur in a time and space socially. This means that parents and other carers, whose relationships with children are integral to the child's childhood, are also considered in terms of these relationships and the child's experience of a lived childhood. This allows us to value childhoods as both a process of learning to facilitate adulthoods, and as a process in and of itself. That a child being a child is sufficient with or without the prospect of a future adulthood. Evaluating this issue allows nurses to evaluate how well they can help children to be children, like their peers in their communities, irrespective of their life expectancy or prognosis (Randall, 2016a; 2016b).

The issues of safe, effective and timely care are perhaps better understood. It is easy to see how delayed care, ineffective care or care that people did not feel was safe, or which did perhaps cause unintentional harm to participants, would all constitute unsatisfactory care. In an increasingly fragile and uncertain world we might also agree that good care needs to be sustainable. This might include the environmental impact of care as well as sustainability in terms of resourcing, which would include people and their education and life-work balance as well as physical resourcing, spaces and time as a resource.

This brings us to how we might evaluate the quality issues of justice and equity. Can we judge nursing provision to be good if it only provides care for certain sections of a population, or if it underserves some people? In Western/Northern liberal democracies the answer may be clear, where work on inequality such as Wilkinson and Picket's (2010) spirit level or Michael Marmot's reports (Marmot, 2010; Marmot et al., 2020) have been largely accepted. The influence of this work can be seen in the prevalence of work showing inequalities in incidence and the prevalence of life-limiting and life-threatening conditions in childhood (Fraser et al., 2020) and in inequalities of access to place of death (Gibson-Smith et al., 2021). However, in other political contexts, such liberal arguments may not be valued or supported. While advocacy for children and carers might be seen as an essential function of children's nursing, and required by nursing regulators' evaluation of quality in terms of justice and equity, it remains a political nursing action.

We could use these quality issues to produce a self-assessment radar plot, much like that used in Normalisation theory tool kit (May et al., 2015), where one asks

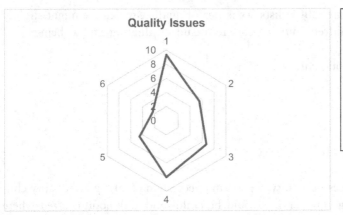

**FIGURE 12.1** Example of radar plot for children's palliative care nursing quality, using Institute of Medicine (2001) issues

the palliative care team to rate the nursing care using a visual line scale nominally from 0 to 10 for all six issues, using Disagree (= 0) or Agree (= 10) statements such as:

> The nurses help me (my child) to be a child living my (their) childhood.
>
> Disagree                                                                    Agree
>
> _____

It may be helpful to identify the evaluations of children, their carers and various professional team members separately to see if the overall assessment is in accordance with certain groups' views, i.e. that children agree with their parents' (carers') views (Figure 12.1).

What this sort of visualisation allows us to do is to see where there might be areas to develop. In the example, we can see that, while child-centred, the service could improve safety, sustainability as well as just and equitable access. As May et al. (2015) remind us, such an evaluation is not quantitative, the numbers give instead a sense of the feeling and conceptions people have about the issues. The numbers could be replaced with faces expressing emotions or words. It is also worth noting that in a radar plot there is no relationship between the issues, just an expression of the participants' conception of how well the nursing provided deals with each issue separately. Thus, while we may infer overall quality evaluation from the plot, it does not tell us how, for instance, safety relates to timely care, or sustainability of care.

## WHY IS IT CHALLENGING AND COMPLEX TO EVALUATE THE QUALITY OF CHILDREN'S PALLIATIVE CARE?

Understanding and measuring quality in children's nursing care, in general, have received little attention. Hargreaves et al. (2019) have noted that children's health services can lag behind the equivalent service for adults. They also remind us that states, which are signatories to the United Nations Convention on the Rights of the Child, have both a duty to provide the best possible healthcare for children and to listen to children's views on matters which affect them (Articles 24 and 12). Hargreaves et al. (2019) set out many of the measures taken in the UK to address quality in the children's services, while also discussing a lack of agreement about how quality should be measured. The indicators gleaned by national consultations focus on outcome measures of medical issues, with little opportunity to include quality measures focused on children's or their carers' views of care. Hargreaves et al. conclude that there is a lack of agreement on how quality should be measured and there are no frameworks or structures to involve all the stakeholders in agreeing on validated quality measures.

There is significant challenge and complexity in evaluating quality of life in children's palliative care:

- Children's palliative care research is quite recent (see Chapter 13).
- Ethical barriers to include children with life-limiting conditions in research (children are vulnerable, but social and moral agents).
- Variety of chronological ages and cognitive ability, diseases, care pathways, etc.
- Child-/family-centred care: research in children's care is marked by triangulation: child/parents/healthcare professionals. Research methods are therefore complex because they involve many stakeholders/actors.

---

**LEARNING ACTIVITY**

Using the National Institute of Clinical Excellence (UK) (NICE) audit form for guidance (NG61) (NICE, 2019), evaluate your own children's palliative care service. The form can be retrieved from https://www.nice.org.uk/guidance/ng61/resources/baseline-assessment-tool-excel-2729613133

There are columns with titles:

- Is the recommendation relevant?
- Current activity evidence
- Recommendation met?
- Actions needed to implement recommendations
- Is there a risk associated with not implementing this recommendation?
- Is there a cost saving?
- Deadline
- Lead

Remember, NICE is a government-funded and government-sponsored organisation.

1. What issues of quality are present, which are absent?
2. Are there voices that might not be heard?
3. Share your audit with colleagues you work with, can you identify areas for celebration and improvement?

## WHAT HAVE BEEN USED AS THE INDICATORS OF QUALITY IN CHILDREN'S PALLIATIVE CARE?

Despite the challenges, many researchers and clinicians have attempted to evaluate the quality of children's palliative care. However, what emerges from the literature is a range of strategies with little common conception or methodology of quality evaluation.

There are also the challenges of identifying nursing's unique contribution. Often the evaluation studies quite rightly evaluate the entirety of the palliative care team input, but this does make understanding nurses' input and the interaction of nursing with other professions in palliative care difficult (Friedel et al., 2019). The effect we are seeing may not be due to nurses or their work, but to other professions, or a combination of the effects of nurses' work and that of carers, other professional groups (both in health but also in other sectors such as education and social care).

With these caveats in mind, we might group the studies into four broad themes: (1) quality of life/symptom management; (2) parental perspectives; (3) identification of need and unmet needs; and (4) nursing services' productivity and efficiency.

### Quality of life/symptom management

Quality of life, or more accurately health-related quality of life measures, have been used in child palliative care populations (Huang et al., 2010). However, what Huang et al. (2010) found was that health-related quality of life measures were not reliably valid for use with children receiving palliative care. This was supported by Coombes et al.'s (2016) literature review which concluded that there was no ideal measure using quality of life. However, Friedel et al. (2021) found that adapting a short form individual quality of life measure (SEIQoL-DW; Hickey et al., 1996) could be helpful in children's palliative care. Thus, while the evidence is not conclusive, researchers have continued to use quality of life measures (Wolfe et al., 2014; Chong et al., 2018).

A health outcome has been defined as a "change in health status as a consequence of preceding healthcare or interventions" (Donabedian, 1980). The term "health status" should be understood from the broad perspective of well-being or quality of life. If we refer to Donabedian's model for evaluating quality of care, we must look at the structure, the process and the outcomes of a care programme. High-quality children's palliative care is presumed to improve quality of life. Quality of life, however, is a subjective, multi-dimensional construct and most probably not only influenced by children's palliative care interventions. Such conceptions do not conceptualise quality of dying, death and bereavement, as they are quality of life and health and well-being-related measures of quality of life. Thus, that they are not applicable to children who are dying is perhaps understandable.

Another definition of an outcome is related to patient-reported outcomes (PROMs), which are not directly the effect of interventions. Witt et al. (2015) have drawn the inference that the experience of care is not the same as outcome of care. Albeit that experience is likely to be positive if outcomes are those desired, but the reported outcomes of experiencing care are also closely related to being respected, listened to and heard. This does pose a challenge to children's nurses as few studies involve listening to or hearing children's voices. More often, the views of parents or adult carers are sought. However, we know that these parental views seen as a proxy for children cannot be relied upon as children's views often differ from those of their parents (Friedel et al., 2019; Coombes, Harðardóttir, Braybrook, Scott et al., 2023, see Table 12.1).

Friedel et al. (2019) have reviewed the use of patient-reported (child) measures in the research literature. They found only five such outcome measures were used in 19 studies alongside 10 other psychometric measures. They also note that often parental proxy views are sought on past events rather than prospective care. Namisango et al. (2019) also support this finding, i.e. that children themselves did not contribute to 30% of the studies about their needs. However, research teams are moving to address the gap in child-reported outcome measures, with ongoing work in Africa on the African Palliative Care Association Children's Palliative Outcome Scale (APCA c-POS) (Downing et al., 2012; Namisango et al., 2022), which has influenced the recent development of the C-POS:UK (Children's Palliative Outcome Scale) (Coombes et al., 2022; Coombes, Harðardóttir, Braybrook, Scott et al., 2023; Coombes, Harðardóttir, Braybrook, Roach et al., 2023; Coombes et al., 2024). The C-POS:UK team have conducted a multiphase, mixed method study following accepted methodological practice on outcome measure development. Validation studies are ongoing in the UK, Australia and New Zealand. The hope is that, once validated, this will provide a child-centred outcome measure, based on the priorities of children and their carers which can be routinely used in clinical children's palliative practice.

**TABLE 12.1** Comparison of interview data from children and Delphi results from parents (adapted from Coombes, Harðardóttir, Braybrook, Scott et al., 2023)

| Domain | Child report | Parental report |
| --- | --- | --- |
| Physical | Pain<br>Other symptoms | Getting enough sleep |
| Social practical | Being able to ask questions<br>Being able to undertake usual activities | Access to information about child's condition<br>Support needs of the child<br>Support to plan for future care |
| Emotional and psychological | Worry<br>Sharing feelings | Impact of child's condition on the family |
| Spiritual/existential | Being able to do things you enjoy<br>Living life to the fullest | Support to plan future care |

## Parental perspectives

While it may be accepted that parental views are not always an accurate proxy for those of their children, they are sought more often in evaluation studies. These studies have tended to report parental perspectives and satisfaction. For example, Hansson et al. (2022) interviewed parents about their satisfaction with a palliative home care model of provision, and Chocarro-González et al. (2021) studied satisfaction with an educational programme for parents to help them acquire care skills.

While much of the focus has been on the location of care with a clear preference by parents for home care, Wolff et al. (2010) have shown that, with support, more families choose home care, although satisfaction with care was high in both hospital and home settings.

## Identification of need and unmet needs

Several studies have been conducted attempting to identify the specific palliative care needs for children and some have tried to uncover where need may be unmet. Obviously, the identification of need in the population a service is providing care to is vital in evaluating whether a service is meeting the identified need. However, also vital is to understand where there may be unmet need and where the provision of nursing services might fall short.

Chong et al. (2020) found that the Paediatric Palliative Screening scale (PaPas) was congruent with clinician assessment and could be used to accurately identify those with additional need, resulting in longer treatment profiles. In addition, Song et al. (2021) showed the PaPas score could be used to set a referral score for primary care physicians to refer to hospital provision. A team led by Constantinou (Constantinou et al., 2019) found that a lack of respite and psychological supportive care, poor co-ordination, lack of organisation and poor communication by professionals contributed to unmet needs. Again, the focus here is very much on parental or carer perspectives rather than on children's perceived unmet needs.

## Nursing services' productivity and efficiency

As well as identifying needs, some studies have focused on the ability of providers of nursing services to deliver care. This is a broad theme including educational programmes and service efficiency, economic evaluation and the emergent use of technologies.

The focus of Bogetz et al.'s (2022) paper was quality improvement training and participation in children's palliative care. A majority of the 95 respondents reported involvement in quality improvement (66%) but 37% also reported not having any staff dedicated to this work. Barriers to engaging in quality work included lack of staffing, time, education, funding support and poor recognition of the importance of quality improvement work. Nilsson et al. (2020) also report on the use of the i-PARiHS framework (integrated-Promoting Action on Research Implementation in the Health Services) in knowledge translation in children's palliative care, suggesting this framework can guide nurses' establishment of evidence-based care. In Nilsson et al.'s study, this was most often applied to symptom relief in hospital contexts with a variety of educational strategies employed. The symptom of pain management was the focus of Thienprayoon et al.'s (2022) work in which they studied the establishment of a Paediatric Palliative Improvement Network. This collaborative approach was used to increase pain assessments over a year.

The organisation of care provision has received some attention. With Kernebeck et al. (2022) looking at improving nursing software to document care. Kaye et al. (2017) looked more directly at improving productivity in interdisciplinary palliative care teams, where they again found that productivity evaluation was challenging due to a lack of consensus on ways to define, measure and evaluate the work. However, Lo et al. (2022) found direct economic benefit from children's palliative care and an increase in frequency of death at home with associated improved care (Chong et al., 2018). It is noteworthy that their review of over 500 papers only yielded four that met their inclusion criteria on economic evaluation.

A key factor in children's palliative care can be the interface between what the CPCET (2020) group call Core nursing teams and Specialist teams. Nurses in the Core category deliver palliative care alongside curative/restorative care and those in Specialist category are those whose main occupation is to deliver and advise on palliative care. Streuli et al. (2019) undertook a systematic review of the impact of specialist children's palliative care which showed improvement in carer/professional communication which aided decision-making, although the data for children, siblings and other family members was limited and of poor quality.

Virdun et al. (2015) make the valid point in evaluating the optimal service provision that children and their carers wanted provision tailored to their needs. This might include receiving care in their location of choice, respite care, sibling support, psychological support and 24-hour access to specialist support.

Finally, we should consider the changing contexts of care. Holmen et al. (2020) reviewed the evidence on the acceptability of and satisfaction with the use of eHealth technologies in children's homecare. Holmen et al. (2020) found that children and carers held positive views of the technologies that enabled them to stay at home, but the views of professionals were less favourable (Box 12.1).

---

**BOX 12.1 HOW CAN WE EVALUATE QUALITY OF CHILDREN'S PALLIATIVE CARE?**

- Patient-centred outcomes measures (such as CPOS): Self and proxy report (child/parents/carers/healthcare professionals)
- Medical note review and administrative data (place of death and desired place of death, hospital admissions and length of stay)
- Observation studies
- Focus groups with healthcare professionals/parents/children/carers
- Specific apps integrated into the usual data registration system
- Audit, for example, benchmarking with peer review

## ALIGNMENT WITH INSTITUTE OF MEDICINE QUALITY ISSUES, AND THE UNSEEN QUALITIES

These studies detailed above are some of the current literature available that might show how children's palliative nursing care is currently being evaluated. It may not be an exhaustive review but it does give an indication of the current understanding of quality evaluation.

As mentioned above, the degree to which these papers reflect nursing's unique contribution is perhaps open to question. To identify children's nursing's unique contribution, we might need to have a clear conception of the features and functions of children's nursing. However, few attempts have been made to theorise what children's nursing is. The earlier work on family-centred care (Smith and Coleman, 2010) was not postulated as a theory, but as a philosophical approach. This approach has been questioned (Shields et al., 2007; 2012; Coyne et al., 2018) and later work by Randall (2016a) has not been widely adopted or developed. Thus, identifying the features and function of children's nurses in palliative care is difficult, with no real supportive consensus conceptions of what children's nursing actually is.

We can, however, see some elements of the Institute of Medicine's (2001) quality issues reflected in the analysis above. There are attempts to evaluate child-centred quality issues, albeit less frequently these are the focus of studies. Understanding of how children's childhoods are affected, or a framing of quality issues in terms of childhoods to be lived, is less often the focus of quality measures. However, we can see in the emergent work of the C-POS group that aspects of childhoods are being identified by children (see Table 12.1; Coombes, Braybrook, Harðardóttir, Scott et al., 2023).

Safety seems to be neglected with no studies considering safeguarding of children or the safety of carers. There is no discussion of how risks might be managed in relation to home care, for example. Effectiveness does seem to feature with economic aspects and productivity and service design to promote effectiveness considered. There is also consideration of outcomes, such as symptom management, which might equate to effectiveness of care, in some regards. However, sustainability does not seem to feature, and it is not clear if timeliness of care is evaluated systematically.

Although not included above, there is a study by Ananth et al. (2022) in which justice and equality are considered. They found that households with an income below $50,000 per annum were less likely to use the hospice and were more likely to be admitted to an intensive care unit and be ventilated, even when controlled for cancer diagnosis. They also point out that of 79 cancer decedents, only 17% used hospice services, which may have led to problems of unusual results from a small sub-sample (17% = 13 decedents).

It may, of course, be a legitimate response to ask if we *should* evaluate children's palliative care using the format of the Institute of Medicine quality issues. We do so here simply to give us a recognised framework for quality assessment, in lieu of agreed nursing measures.

That being said, there are a number of quality issues which are missing, and some voices unheard. Many would argue that children's palliative nursing must address children's spiritual and religious needs, including supporting children of no faith and those who are agnostic (Scott et al., 2023). The safety, effectiveness, timing and sustainability of spiritual care do not seem to have been considered, nor the issues of access and equity or how children's spiritual development might be affected. Yet, as Scott et al. (2023) identify in their qualitative study, these are issues that some children report are important.

Strangely for palliative care practitioners and researchers, evaluations of dying and death do not feature. We have some suggestions as to what a good death might look and feel like (Hendrickson and McCorkle, 2008; Chong et al., 2019) but no measures to evaluate if we are providing a good dying experience, nor if we achieve a good death for the child.

As we have seen above, the evaluation of quality issues in children's palliative care is moving forward at a pace, the African Palliative Care Association Children's Palliative Outcome Scale (APCA c-POS), the work of the C-POS group in the UK and the "what matters most" study in Canada (Widger, 2022) may well soon provide validated measures that give a set of agreed core indicators.

## SUMMARY

Although there has been a lack of consensus in evaluating the quality of children's palliative nursing care, there are now attempts to co-ordinate and agree on valid standardised measures. There has always been agreement on the importance of measuring and assuring the quality of nursing care and this is just as important in palliative care as in other aspects of children's nursing. Some of the nature of palliative work, and the complexities of delivering care to children in communities cared for by people, all of whom may hold differing views on many of the quality issues, make evaluating quality more challenging in children's palliative care.

Progress is being made, however, in agreeing a consensus, although we must be mindful of quality issues which may be overlooked, often considered too complex or controversial, but which are vital to delivering what most would agree are "good" children's nursing services to facilitate good dying, death and bereavement.

## KEY POINTS

- It is complex to evaluate outcomes in children's palliative care and the quality of children's palliative care activities and/or programmes due to the wide variety of health conditions, age range of children/adolescents and different care settings.
- Selecting the domain of children's palliative care that should be evaluated depends on the aim: what do we want to evaluate, why, and for whom?
- Different measurement instruments are available and should be selected wisely, depending on their validity and reliability.
- The evaluation must be culturally sensitive and context-appropriate.
- The measurement instruments or quality indicators should ideally be developed or used in a collaborative approach by children/parents/carers/healthcare professionals themselves (according to Patient Public Involvement standards).

## REFERENCES

Ananth, P., Lindsay, M., Nye, R., Mun. S., Feudtner, C., Wolfe, J. (2022). End-of-life care quality for children with cancer who receive palliative care. *Pediatric Blood & Cancer*, 69(9). https://doi.org/10.1002/pbc.29841.

Arias-Casais, N., Garralda, E., Pons, J. J., Marston, J., Chambers, L., Downing, J., Ling, J., Rhee, J. Y., de Lima, L., Centeno, C. (2020). Mapping paediatric palliative care development in the WHO European region: Children living in low-middle income countries are less likely to access it. *Journal of Pain and Symptom Management*. https://doi.org/10.1016/j.jpainsymman.2020.04.028

Bogetz, J. F., Johnston, E., Ananth, P., Patneaude, A., Cambia Advisory Workgroup, Thienprayoon, R., Rosenberg, A. R. (2022). Survey of pediatric palliative care quality improvement training, activities, and barriers. *Journal of Pain and Symptom Management*, 64(3), e123–e131. https://doi.org/10.1016/j.jpainsymman.2022.04.182

Boyden, J. Y., Bogetz, J. F., Johnston, E. E., Thienprayoon, R., Williams, C. S. P., McNeil, M. J., Patneaude, A., Widger, K. A., Rosenberg, A. R., Ananth, P. (2023). Measuring pediatric palliative care quality: Challenges and opportunities. *Journal of Pain and Symptom Management*, 65(5), e483–e495. https://doi.org/10.1016/j.jpainsymman.2023.01.021

Chocarro González, L., Rigal Andrés, M., de la Torre-Montero, J. C., Barceló Escario, M., Martino Alba, R. (2021). Effectiveness of a family-caregiver training program in home-based pediatric palliative care. *Children (Basel, Switzerland)*, 8(3), 178. https://doi.org/10.3390/children8030178

Chong, P. H., De Castro Molina, J. A., Teo, K., Tan, W. S. (2018). Paediatric palliative care improves patient outcomes and reduces healthcare costs: evaluation of a home-based program. *BMC Palliative Care*, 17(1), 11. https://doi.org/10.1186/s12904-017-0267-z

Chong, P. H., Soo, J., Yeo, Z. Z., Ang, R. Q., Ting, C. (2020). Who needs and continues to need paediatric palliative care? An evaluation of utility and feasibility of the Paediatric Palliative Screening scale (PaPaS). *BMC Palliative Care*, 19(1), 18. https://doi.org/10.1186/s12904-020-0524-4

Chong, P. H., Walshe, C., Hughes, S. (2019). Perceptions of a good death in children with life-shortening conditions: An integrative review. *Journal of Palliative Medicine*, 22(6): 714–723.

Constantinou, G., Garcia, R., Cook, E., Randhawa, G. (2019). Children's unmet palliative care needs: A scoping review of parents' perspectives. *BMJ Supportive & Palliative Care*, 9(4), 439–450. https://doi.org/10.1136/bmjspcare-2018-001705

Coombes, L., Braybrook, D., Roach, A., Scott, H., Harðardóttir, D., Bristowe, K., Ellis-Smith, C., Bluebond-Langner, M., Fraser, L. K., Downing, J., Farsides, B., Murtagh, F. E. M., Harding, R., C-POS. (2022). Achieving child-centered care for children and young people with life-limiting and life-threatening conditions: A qualitative interview study. *European Journal of Pediatrics*, 181(10), 3739–3752. https://doi.org/10.1007/s00431-022-04566-w

Coombes, L., Braybrook, D., Harðardóttir, D., Scott, H. M., Bristowe, K., Ellis-Smith, C., Fraser, L. K., Downing, J., Bluebond-Langner, M., Murtagh, F. E. M., Harding, R. (2024). Cognitive testing of the Children's Palliative Outcome Scale (C-POS) with children, young people and their parents/carers. *Palliative Medicine*. https://doi.org/10.1177/02692163241248735

Coombes, L., Harðardóttir, D., Braybrook, D., Roach, A., Scott, H., Bristowe, K., Ellis-Smith, C., Downing, J., Bluebond-Langner, M., Fraser, L. K., Murtagh, F. E. M., Harding, R. (2023). Design and administration of patient-centred outcome measures: the perspectives of children and young people with life-limiting or life-threatening conditions and their family members, *The Patient-Patient-Centered Outcomes Research*. https://doi.org/10.1007/s40271-023-00627-w

Coombes, L., Harðardóttir, D., Braybrook, D., Scott, H. M., Bristowe, K., Ellis-Smith, C., Fraser, L. K., Downing, J., Bluebond-Langner, M., Murtagh, F. E. M., Harding, R.

(2023). Achieving consensus on priority items for paediatric palliative care outcome measurement: Results from a modified Delphi survey, engagement with a children's research involvement group and expert item generation. *Palliative Medicine*. https://doi.org/10.1177/02692163231205126

Coombes, L., Wiseman, T., Lucas, G., Sangha, A., Murtagh, F. E. M. (2016). Health-related quality-of-life outcome measures in paediatric palliative care: A systematic review of psychometric properties and feasibility of use. *Palliative Medicine*, 30(10), 935–949. https://doi.org/10.1177/0269216316649155

Coyne, I., Holmström, I., Söderbäck, M. (2018). Centeredness in healthcare: A concept synthesis of family-centered care, person-centered care and child-centered care. *Journal of Pediatric Nursing*, 42, 45–56. https://doi.org/10.1016/j.pedn.2018.07.001

CPCET (Children's Palliative Care Education and Training UK and Ireland Action Group). (2020). Education Standard Framework. ICPCN. Available at: https://icpcn.org/wp-content/uploads/2022/10/CPCET-Education-Standard-Framework.pdf (accessed 14May 2024).

Donabedian, A. (1980). *Explorations in quality assessment and monitoring: The definition of quality and approaches to its assessment.* Vol. I. Health Administration Press.

Downing, J., Namisango, E., Harding, R. (2018). Outcome measurement in paediatric palliative care: Lessons from the past and future developments. *Annals of Palliative Medicine*, 7(Suppl. 3), S151–S163. https://doi.org/10.21037/apm.2018.04.02

Downing, J., Ojing, M., Powell, R. A., Ali, Z., Marston, J., Meiring, M., Ssengooba, J., Williams, S., Mwangi-Powell, F., Harding, R. (2012). A palliative care outcome measure for children in sub-Saharan Africa: Early development findings. *European Journal of Palliative Care*, 19(6), 292–294.

Fraser, L. K., Gibson-Smith, D., Jarvis, S., Norman, P., Parslow R. (2020). 'Make Every Child Count': Estimating current and future prevalence of children and young people with life-limiting conditions in the United Kingdom. Available at: https://www.york.ac.uk/media/healthsciences/documents/research/public-health/mhrc/Prevalence%20reportFinal.pdf (accessed 14 May 2024).

Fraser, L., Miller, M., Hain, R., Norman, P., Aldridge, J., McKinney, P. A., Parslow, R. C. (2012). Rising national prevalence of life-limiting conditions in children in England. *Paediatrics*, 129, 1–7. https://doi.org/10.1542/peds.2011-2846

Friedel, M., Aujoulat, I., Dubois, A. C., Degryse, J. M. (2019). Instruments to measure outcomes in pediatric palliative care: A systematic review. *Pediatrics*, 143(1), e20182379. https://doi.org/10.1542/peds.2018-2379

Friedel, M., Brichard, B., Boonen, S., Tonon, C., De Terwangne, B., Bellis, D., Mevisse, M., Fonteyne, C., Jaspard, M., Schruse, M., Harding, R., Downing, J., Namisango, E., Degryse, J. M., Aujoulat, I. (2021). Face and content validity, acceptability, and feasibility of the adapted version of the children's palliative outcome scale: A qualitative pilot study. *Journal of Palliative Medicine*, 24(2), 181–188. https://doi.org/10.1089/jpm.2019.0646

Gibson-Smith, D., Jarvis, S. W., Fraser, L. K. (2021). Place of death of children and young adults with a life-limiting condition in England: A retrospective cohort study. *Archives of Disease in Childhood*, 106, 780–785. https://doi.org/10.1136%2Farchdischild-2020-319700

Hain, R., Devins, M., Hastings, R., Noyes, J. (2013). Paediatric palliative care: development and pilot study of a 'Directory' of life-limiting conditions. *BMC Palliative Care*, 12(1), 43. doi: 10.1186/1472-684X-12-43

Hansson, H., Björk, M., Santacroce, S. J., Raunkiaer, M. (2022). End-of-life palliative home care for children with cancer: A qualitative study on parents' experiences. *Scandinavian Journal of Caring Sciences*, 10.1111/scs.13066. https://doi.org/10.1111/scs.13066

Hargreaves, D. S., Lemer, C., Ewing, C., Cornish, J., Baker, T., Toma, K., Saxena, S., McCulloch, B., McFarlane, L., Welch, J., Sparrow, E., Kossarova, L., Lumsden, D. E.,

Ronny, C., Cheung, L. H. (2019). Measuring and improving the quality of NHS care for children and young people. *Archives of Disease in Childhood*, 104, 618–621. https://doi.org/10.1136/archdischild-2017-314564

Hendrickson, K., McCorkle, R. (2008). A dimensional analysis of the concept: Good death of a child with cancer. *Journal of Pediatric Oncology Nursing*, 25(3), 127–138.

Hickey, A. M., Bury, G., O'Boyle, C. A., Bradley, F., O'Kelly, F. D., Shannon, W. (1996). A new short form individual quality of life measure (SEIQoL-DW): Application in a cohort of individuals with HIV/AIDS. *BMJ (Clinical Research edition)*, 313(7048), 29–33. https://doi.org/10.1136/bmj.313.7048.29

Holmen, H., Riiser, K., Winger, A. (2020). Home-based pediatric palliative care and electronic health: Systematic mixed methods review. *Journal of Medical Internet Research*, 22(2), e16248. https://doi.org/10.2196/16248

Huang, I. C., Shenkman, E. A., Madden, V. L., Vadaparampil, S., Quinn, G., Knapp, C. A. (2010). Measuring quality of life in pediatric palliative care: Challenges and potential solutions. *Palliative Medicine*, 24(2), 175–182. https://doi.org/10.1177/0269216309352418

Institute of Medicine, (IOM). (2001). *Crossing the quality chasm: A new health system for the 21st century*. National Academy Press.

Kaye, E. C., Abramson, Z. R., Snaman, J. M., Friebert, S. E., Baker, J. N. (2017). Productivity in pediatric palliative care: Measuring and monitoring an elusive metric. *Journal of Pain and Symptom Management*, 53(5), 952–961. https://doi.org/10.1016/j.jpainsymman.2016.12.326

Kernebeck, S., Busse, T. S., Jux, C., Dreier, L. A., Meyer, D., Zenz, D., Zernikow, B., Ehlers, J. P. (2022). Evaluation of an electronic medical record module for nursing documentation in paediatric palliative care: Involvement of nurses with a think-aloud approach. *International Journal of Environmental Research and Public Health*, 19(6), 3637. https://doi.org/10.3390/ijerph19063637

Knaul, F. M., Farmer, P. E., Krakauer, E. L., De Lima, L., Bhadelia, A., Kwete, X. J., Arreola-Ornelas, H., Gómez-Dantés, O., Rodriguez, N. M., Alleyne, G. A. O., Connor, S. R., Hunter, D. J., Lohman, L., Radbruch, L., del Rocío, M. S. M., Atun, R., Foley, K. M., Frenk, J., Jamison, D. T., Rajagopal, M. R., Lancet Commission on Palliative Care and Pain Relief Study Group. (2018). Alleviating the access abyss in palliative care and pain relief: An imperative of universal health coverage: the Lancet Commission report. *Lancet*, 391, 1391–1454. https://doi.org/10.1016/s0140-6736(17)32513-8

Lo, D. S., Hein, N., Bulgareli, J. V. (2022). Pediatric palliative care and end-of-life: A systematic review of economic health analyses. *Revista paulista de pediatria: Orgão oficial da Sociedade de Pediatria de São Paulo*, 40, e2021002. https://doi.org/10.1590/1984-0462/2022/40/2021002

Marmot, M. (2010). *Fair society, healthy lives: Marmot review*. University College London.

Marmot, M., Allen, J., Boyce, T., Goldblatt, P., Morrison, J. (2020). *Health equity in England: The Marmot review 10 years on*. Institute of Health Equity.

May, C., Rapley, T., Mair, F. S., Treweek, S., Murray, E., Ballini, L., Macfarlane, A. Girling, M., Finch, T. L. (2015). Normalization Process Theory On-line Users' Manual, Toolkit and NoMAD instrument. Available at: http://www.normalizationprocess.org (accessed 29 May 2024).

Mayland, C. R., Sunderland, K. A., Cooper, M., Taylor, P., Powell, P. A., Zeigler, L., Cox, V., Gilman, C., Turner, T., Flemming, K., Fraser, L. K. (2022). Measuring quality of dying, death and end-of-life care for children and young people: A scoping review of available tools. *Palliative Medicine*, 02692163221105599. https://doi.org/10.1177/02692163221105599

Namisango, E., Bristowe, K., Allsop, M. J., Murtagh, F. E. M., Abas, M., Higginson, I. J., Downing, J., Harding, R. (2019). Symptoms and concerns among children and young people with life-limiting and life-threatening conditions: A systematic review highlighting meaningful health outcomes. *The Patient: Patient-Centered Outcomes Research*, 12(1), 15–55. https://doi.org/10.1007/s40271-018-0333-5

Namisango, E., Bristowe, K., Murtagh, F. E. M., Downing, J., Powell, R. A., Atieno, M., Abas, M., Zipporah, A., Luyirika, E. B., Meiring, M., Mwangi-Powell, F. N., Higginson, I. J., Harding, R. (2022). Face and content validity, acceptability, feasibility, and implementability of a novel outcome measure for children with life-limiting or life-threatening illness in three sub-Saharan African countries. *Palliative Medicine*, 36(7), 1140–1153. https://doi.org/10.1177/02692163221099583

NICE. (2019). End-of-life care for infants, children and young people with life-limiting conditions: Planning and management. Available at: https://www.nice.org.uk/guidance/ng61 (accessed 29 May 2024).

Nilsson, S., Ohlen, J., Hessman, E., Brännström, M. (2020). Paediatric palliative care: A systematic review. *BMJ Supportive & Palliative Care*, 10(2), 157–163. https://doi.org/10.1136/bmjspcare-2019-001934

Randall, D. (2016a). *Pragmatic children's nursing: A theory for children and their childhoods*. Routledge.

Randall, D. (2016b). Pragmatics and bringing dying back into children's nursing. eHospice International children's edition published online 11 August 2016. Available at: https://ehospice.com/inter_childrens_posts/pragmatics-and-bringing-dying-back-into-childrens-nursing/ (accessed 28 May 2024).

Scott, H. M., Coombes, L., Braybrook, D., Roach, A., Harðardóttir, D., Bristowe, K., Ellis-Smith, C., Downing, J., Murtagh, F. E. M., Farsides, B., Fraser, L. K., Bluebond-Langner, M., Harding, R. (2023). Spiritual, religious, and existential concerns of children and young people with life-limiting and life-threatening conditions: A qualitative interview study. *Palliative Medicine*, 2692163231165101. Advance online publication. https://doi.org/10.1177/02692163231165101

Shields, L., Pratt, J., Davis, L., Hunter, J. (2007). Family-centred care for children in hospital. *Cochrane Database Systematic Review*, CD004811. https://doi.org/10.1002/14651858.CD004811.pub2

Shields, L., Zhou, H., Pratt, J., Taylor, M., Hunter, J., Pascoe, E. (2012). Family-centred care for hospitalised children aged 0–12 years. *Cochrane Database of Systematic Reviews*, Issue 10. Art. No. CD004811. https://doi.org/10.1002/14651858.CD004811.pub3.

Smith, L., Coleman, V. (2010). *Child and family-centred healthcare: Concept, theory and practice* (2nd edn). Palgrave Macmillan.

Song, I. G., Kwon, S. Y., Chang, Y. J., Kim, M. S., Jeong, S. H., Hahn, S. M., Han, K. T., Park, S. J., Choi, J. Y. (2021). Paediatric palliative screening scale as a useful tool for clinicians' assessment of palliative care needs of pediatric patients: A retrospective cohort study. *BMC Palliative Care*, 20(1), 73. https://doi.org/10.1186/s12904-021-00765-8

Streuli, J. C., Widger, K., Medeiros, C., Zuniga-Villanueva, G., Trenholm, M. (2019). Impact of specialized pediatric palliative care programs on communication and decision-making. *Patient Education and Counseling*, 102(8), 1404–1412. https://doi.org/10.1016/j.pec.2019.02.011

Thienprayoon, R., Jones, E., Humphrey, L., Ragsdale, L., Williams, C., Klick, J. C. (2022). The Pediatric Palliative Improvement Network: A national Healthcare Learning Collaborative. *Journal of Pain and Symptom Management*, 63(1), 131–139. https://doi.org/10.1016/j.jpainsymman.2021.06.020

Virdun, C., Brown, N., Phillips, J., Luckett, T., Agar, M., Green, A., Davidson, P. M. (2015). Elements of optimal paediatric palliative care for children and young people: An integrative review using a systematic approach. *Collegian (Royal College of Nursing, Australia)*, 22(4), 421–431. https://doi.org/10.1016/j.colegn.2014.07.001

WHO (World Health Organization). (1998). Definition of palliative care. Available at: https://www.who.int/cancer/palliative/definition/en/

WHO (World Health Organization). (2015). Fact sheet N°402, Palliative Care, July 2015. Available at: http://www.who.int/mediacentre/factsheets/fs402/en/

Widger, K. (2022). What matters most: Identifying a core indicator set for quality pediatric palliative care. Available at: https://kimwidger.ca/what-matters-most/ (accessed 4 June 2024).

Wilkinson, R., Picket, K. (2010). *The spirit level: Why equality is better for everyone.* Penguin Books.

Witt, J., Murtagh, F. E. M., de Wolf-Linder, S., Higginson, I. J., Daveson, B. A. (2015). Introducing the Outcome Assessment and Complexity Collaborative (OACC) Suite of Measures. Available at: https://www.kcl.ac.uk/cicelysaunders/attachments/Studies-OACC-Brief-Introduction-Booklet.pdf

Wolfe, J., Orellana, L., Cook, E. F., Ullrich, C., Kang, T., Geyer, J. R., Feudtner, C., Weeks, J. C., Dussel, V. (2014). Improving the care of children with advanced cancer by using an electronic patient-reported feedback intervention: Results from the PediQUEST randomized controlled trial. *Journal of Clinical Oncology*, 32(11), 1119–1126.

Wolff, J., Robert, R., Sommerer, A., Volz-Fleckenstein, M. (2010). Impact of a pediatric palliative care program. *Pediatric Blood & Cancer*, 54(2), 279–283. https://doi.org/10.1002/pbc.22272

## CHAPTER 13

# Research readiness and leadership

...............................................

*Jane Coad, Regina Szylit,*
*Maiara Rodrigues dos Santos and Julia Downing*

### INTRODUCTION

Previous chapters have illuminated that "palliative care" is reported to be a multi-disciplinary, multi-dimensional, active process aimed at improving the quality of life of babies, children and young people with any of the four categories of life-limiting or life-threatening conditions (Box 13.1). It is widely perceived as a total approach to care, from the point of diagnosis (or before when no diagnosis is made) or recognition of life-threatening and life-limiting conditions (Hawley, 2015).

---

**BOX 13.1 CATEGORIES OF LIFE-LIMITING CONDITIONS**

*Category 1*: Life-threatening conditions for which curative treatment may be feasible but can fail.

*Category 2*: Conditions where premature death is inevitable.

*Category 3*: Progressive conditions without curative treatment options.

*Category 4*: Irreversible but non-progressive conditions causing severe disability leading to susceptibility to health complications and likelihood of premature death.

Source: adapted from Together for Short Lives (2018), p. 11.

---

Research plays a fundamental role in advancing knowledge, addressing challenges, promoting innovation, and facilitating well-informed decision-making across diverse fields and disciplines. Research is therefore needed to develop the evidence base for children's palliative care and thus improve the decisions and interventions of care, treatment and outcomes.

DOI: 10.4324/9781003384861-17

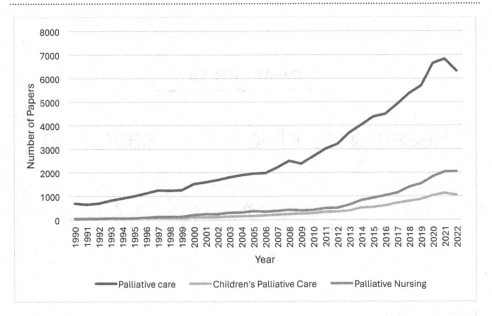

**FIGURE 13.1** Published papers in children's palliative care

Source: Reproduced with permission from Julia Downing.

Despite this recognition and awareness, there is a paucity of international research regarding improving services and holistic care for families who have a life-threatened or life-limited child. In many countries, research on babies, children and young adult's palliative care has significantly lagged behind research in adult palliative care (Downing et al., 2024) A preliminary search of the literature in PubMed from 1990–2022 (see Figure 13.1) showed that while the published literature on children's palliative care has grown, it is still way behind that of general palliative care, and the literature on palliative nursing is not much better.

While some researchers internationally systematically illuminated growing numbers of children needing palliative care (Fraser et al., 2012; Fraser et al., 2013; Connor and Sepulveda, 2014; Connor et al., 2017; Knaul et al., 2018; Fraser, Gibson-Smith et al., 2020; 2021; Connor, 2020), figures for the numbers of babies, children and young adults who have life-limiting or life-threatening conditions and health needs vary enormously. There is also a growing number of researchers who have undertaken small to medium-sized projects to understand the experience and the needs of children and their families, however, overall, the evidence base remains limited in generalisability in terms of international transformation. While in the field there is some consensus and policy development, there are still no best models of care based on international robust evidence.

Based on these deliberations, we aim in this chapter to set the scene with regards to research in children's palliative care and to draw together and critically discuss examples from international settings where palliative care research has taken place. We will draw out the need for research, the challenges and priorities for research in children's palliative care and will discuss a few areas of research within the field to highlight research that has been undertaken well and what could be done better. We will also then discuss some of the ethical issues raised by children's palliative care research.

---

**LEARNING OBJECTIVES**

The reader will be able to do the following:

1. Understand the current state of research in children's palliative care, including the global context, key challenges, and priorities that shape the research agenda.
2. Be able to use examples of palliative care research from international settings.
3. Recognise the need, challenges and priorities in children's palliative care research.
4. Explore and comprehend the ethical considerations associated with children's palliative care research.

---

## BACKGROUND

The environment for research in children's palliative care is developing and changing, with the importance seen in developing an evidence base within the field (Dombrecht et al., 2023). Over the years, this lack of an evidence base has been highlighted by many, including by the World Health Organization (WHO) in the development of their pain guidelines (Milani et al., 2011; WHO, 2012; 2020), by a team looking at children's palliative care in sub-Saharan Africa (Harding et al., 2010; 2014) and in many papers from around the world (e.g. Poles and Bousso, 2009; Rabello et al., 2010; Beecham et al., 2016; Downing, 2016; de Pinho et al., 2020; Passone et al., 2020; Dombrecht et al., 2023).

Drawing on evidence in Brazil, for example, the growing awareness of the importance of this specialty coexists with significant challenges in conducting research. The scarcity of resources, the lack of comprehensive studies, and the difficulties in communicating with families in this specific domain underscore substantial barriers to the advancement of children's palliative care in the country. Overcoming these obstacles requires not only a more robust investment in resources but also a renewed commitment to research, aiming to enhance not only clinical practice but also the sensitive and crucial interactions with involved families. National research in children's palliative care still relies on international data (integrative reviews) for progress in the field (Poles and Bousso, 2009; Rabello et al., 2010; de Pinho et al., 2020; Passone et al., 2020).

Therefore, the need for evidence in the field of children's palliative care is vital if we are to progress the evidence that underpins children's palliative care nursing. This is a global priority. Harding et al. (2013) emphasised the need for research into children's palliative care in sub-Saharan Africa and in doing so recommended that

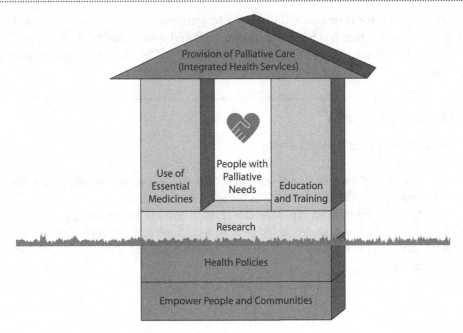

**FIGURE 13.2** The WHO conceptual model for palliative care development

Source: adapted from WHO (2021).

research be adopted as another pillar in the Public Health Strategy for developing palliative care (Stjernsward et al., 2007). More recently, the WHO published their conceptual model for palliative care development (Figure 13.2), highlighting the need for research which informs evidence-based improvements and improving the scientific evidence to guide the care of people and decisions about the organisation of health services (WHO, 2021), including palliative care for babies, children and young adults.

We are saying in this chapter that research is not an optional extra but essential for the provision and development of children's palliative care. Currently, much of children's palliative care practice is based on evidence from adult palliative care or expert opinion. It is therefore important that as nurses we contribute to the development of the evidence needed and ensure that this evidence does not just come from high-income countries, but from across the world (Downing, 2016).

In an attempt to strengthen the evidence-base for palliative care, Hospice UK published a report, "Research in palliative care: Can hospices afford not to be involved?" (Payne et al., 2013). While recognising the importance of academic institutions in research, the report also acknowledged the important role that hospices, and other palliative care providers, have in the development and utilisation of research. They recommended a "Research Framework for Hospices", which provided guidance for levels of research-focused participation within hospice care settings (Payne and Turner, 2012) identifying three levels of research active hospices (Box 13.2). These levels clearly show that research is *everyone's business* – whether we are at the level of research awareness – a "critical consumer of research" or whether we are leading and developing research, or most commonly somewhere in-between. While this framework was developed with UK hospices in mind, and across adult and children's hospices, it is a framework that has utility beyond UK hospices, to palliative care, and children's palliative care services around the world.

---

**BOX 13.2 LEVELS OF RESEARCH ACTIVE HOSPICES**

Level 1: Research awareness in all professionals.
Level 2: Engagement in research generated by others.
Level 3: Engagement in research activities and leadership in developing and undertaking research.

*Source*: Payne and Turner (2012).

---

As nurses providing palliative care to children and their families around the world, it is essential that we are committed to the utilisation and generation of evidence. The recently published international standards for children's palliative care (Benini et al., 2022, see Appendix B) highlight the need to improve research in the field and the World Health Assembly Resolution on palliative care (WHO, 2014) stressed the importance of research to ensure evidence-based care and service provision, encouraging research across low- and middle-income countries and encouraging collaboration. However, the literature and practice both suggest that there are challenges to this. For example, the team at the Louis Dundas Centre for Children's Palliative Care asked 76 delegates who had attended the 7th Paediatric Palliative Care Conference in Cardiff in 2016, what they had found to be the biggest barriers to palliative care research in children (Beecham et al., 2016). The delegates included individuals from a range of professions, working in a range of settings (e.g. hospital, community, hospice) and from a range of countries. Key barriers were identified as:

1. Time and other resources.
2. Clinicians' attitudes towards research.
3. Clinicians' perceptions of patients and their families.
4. Ethical approval processes.

Other challenges identified in the literature are: how to include children, young people and their families in research; patient diversity and small sample sizes; limited funding; the unpredictable nature of the illnesses; society's perceptions of the burden of research for children and their families; a lack of competence in research methods; the need to change attitudes; interdependencies and dynamic interactions; a lack of outcome and measurement tools; and the lack of the workforce and infrastructure available to undertake research (Harding et al., 2010; 2014; Beecham et al., 2016; Downing, 2016; Feudtner et al., 2019; Siden and Widger, 2021; Aldridge and Downing, 2020).

Yet despite these challenges we know that it is possible to do high-quality research into children's palliative care, involving all those concerned in the provision of care and children, young adults and their families. We also know that methods and studies will be refined and developed over time as we gain more information and skill within the development of evidence. Two closely linked examples of this, which also highlight the complexity of children's palliative care, can be seen in studies estimating the need for children's palliative care and those mapping the development of children's palliative care, both of which have implications for our research.

Estimating the number of children needing palliative care within countries, and globally, is an area where results differ, sometimes showing large differences from one study to another (see Introduction). Differences in results can be explained, such as the age range of those included, where the data is from, use of mortality and/or morbidity data, how need is calculated. However, it is also important to note that as methods change and improve, data also has become more accurate, and the need for palliative care for children is dynamic and changing, with access to life-sustaining care improving and many children living longer and needing care for longer periods of time. For example, the work done by Fraser and her colleagues (Fraser et al., 2012; Fraser et al., 2013, Fraser, Gibson-Smith et al., 2020; 2021) shows the change in need in the UK over a period of 10 years and illustrates not only the dynamic nature of children's palliative care, but also the refinement and development in estimation. Globally, the figures vary across a wide range from 3.96 million children (Connor, 2020) to the figure of 21.1 million (Connor et al., 2017).

However, over time, there has been a shift in how we calculate the numbers of children needing palliative care and the Lancet Commission introduced the concept of Serious Health-related Suffering (SHS), emphasising suffering for measuring the global burden associated with life-limiting or life-threatening conditions or the end of life (Knaul et al., 2018). As this method has developed, it has been recognised that the recent figure of 3.96 million children (Connor, 2020) is too low and is therefore under revision. Thus, there has been much discussion on how we identify the need, demonstrating the dynamic nature of research, and how studies build on each other and are refined over the years.

Over the past few years there have been a range of Atlases published, looking at palliative care development globally (Connor and Sepulveda, 2014; Connor, 2020) and regionally – Africa (Rhee et al., 2017), Europe (Arias-Casais et al., 2019), Latin America (Pastrana et al., 2012; 2021) and the Eastern Mediterranean Region (Osman et al., 2017). Some of these, though not all, include an overview of children's palliative care, such as the European Association of Palliative Care (EAPC) *Atlas on Palliative Care in Europe* (Arias-Casais et al., 2019; 2020). This was important data as it was the first time that data had been included specifically on children 's palliative care services (Fraser, Gibson-Smith et al., 2020; 2021). Taken as a snapshot in time, mapping of services can be useful to show developments, however, often they are out of date as soon as they are published. There can be challenges as to how you define a children's palliative care service, how you know its reach, and importantly how you collect the data. Since its inception in 2005, the ICPCN has been mapping service development, with the most recent map being published in 2024 (ICPCN, 2024). It is essential that data on children's palliative care services is gained through individuals working in the field in the country, and that methods of collecting data continue to be refined and developed in order to provide data that is as accurate as possible.

Fraser, Bluebond-Langner et al. (2020) in their paper, "Advances and Challenges in European Paediatric Palliative Care", discussed the data in the European Atlas (Arias-Casais et al., 2019; 2020). The data collection included two surveys and included 51 out of 54 countries across Europe. It highlighted that, in the main, children and young people's palliative care provision was flourishing across Europe in the five areas, but also showed that some countries in Europe did not have any palliative care provision. Arguably, if there is no provision, then the opportunities for collecting data are impacted and this highlights the need for further research that seeks to understand experiences and views of palliative care as well as collation of robust standardised data. It is worth noting that the scarcity of data does not mean that children do not exist, nor that children do not have palliative care needs, but it clearly impacts the funding and provision of palliative care services for children and families in these countries.

If we take a broader international view and look at Brazil, for example, the mapping of palliative care in Brazil has revealed a significant rise in children's palliative care services over the last decade, signifying recent advancement in the field. However, there remains an uneven distribution of these services across different regions of Brazil, mirroring the need for improvements in various aspects. This includes enhancing access to opioids, allocating dedicated time for children's palliative care, implementing continuous education programmes, and prioritising the well-being of professionals engaged in this line of work (Ferreira et al., 2022).

In 2023, a study entitled "Exploring the Brazilian Paediatric Palliative Care Network: A Quantitative Analysis of Survey Data" was published. This study aimed to identify characteristics of services comprising the Brazilian Paediatric Palliative Care (PPC) Network in Brazil (Ferreira et al., 2023). The study conducted an online survey with 90 Brazilian children's palliative care services participating. Results showed that the majority of services (88.9%) were established after 2010, with 57.9% located in the southeast region. Challenges included 36.7% of services expressing concern about healthcare professionals' well-being and 40% reporting difficult or no opioid access. The inequalities in access to health in Brazil extend to education and to research. Research and services are concentrated in the southeast region of the country, with few children's palliative care services linked to universities and only about a third of them developing research in the area (Ferreira et al., 2023).

With the dearth in the evidence base for children's palliative care, it can be a challenge knowing where to start – what our priorities should be and what we should look at first. Work has been undertaken globally, regionally, nationally, and locally to identify priorities for research. A Delphi study undertaken by the International

Children's Palliative Care Network (ICPCN) identified 26 priorities, with the top six being: (1) children's understanding of illness; (2) dying and death; (3) managing pain in children where there is no morphine; (4) funding; (5) training; and (6) assessment of the WHO two-step analgesic ladder for pain management in children (Downing et al., 2015). This study involved 153 participants (32% Europe, 28% sub-Saharan Africa, 12% North America, 11% Latin America, 10% Asia, 6% Oceania and 1% Middle East), 25% of whom were nurses. Likewise, Baker et al. (2015) used a Delphi study with both experts and family members to identify research priorities for children's palliative care within the US. They identified 20 research priorities which were grouped into the five themes: (1) decision making; (2) care co-ordination; (3) symptom management; (4) quality improvement; and (5) education. Feudtner et al. (2019) identified six priorities which covered similar themes to Baker et al. such as (1) training and development; (2) symptom management; (3) communication; (4) improving systems of care; (5) policy; (6) education. While these studies focused specifically on children, a consensus-building process for palliative care research in Africa (Powell et al., 2014) looked more generally at palliative care and highlighted three thematic priorities: (1) patient, family and volunteers; (2) health providers; and (3) health systems, and stressed the importance of research in children's palliative care, such as the palliative care needs for children. The results of these research papers have been summarised in the word cloud in Figure 13.3.

Figure 13.3 draws together a number of papers to show key issues from our background review. In this section, we have set the scene, identified the challenges and priorities, emphasised the need for research globally, shown that research is a dynamic process that builds on previous studies, and highlighted its importance within the field.

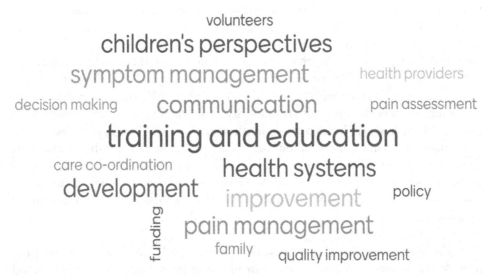

**FIGURE 13.3** Priorities for research in children's palliative care: Word cloud generated from research papers (Baker et al., 2015; Downing et al., 2015; Feudtner et al., 2019; Powell et al., 2014)

## APPROACHES TO CHILDREN'S PALLIATIVE CARE RESEARCH: WHAT WOULD THE IDEAL LOOK LIKE?

Having set the scene on research in children's palliative care, we wanted to reflect on what the ideal environment and team would be that would support this research. We know that children's palliative care requires a holistic approach which is grounded in the values that span the care and support needs of children and their family carers, including clinical, social, psychological, financial, educational and spiritual domains. Whether a study is quantitative (measuring objective data), or qualitative (exploring values and perceptions), at the core of that work must be participation and involvement of the children who are in receipt of palliative care services, or their family carers.

There are a number of research pieces that have sought to contribute to the evidence base of this group, including collating data from stakeholders which include babies, children, young adults, families and/or professionals. Here we share research approaches in two specific areas: (1) service provision; and (2) family bereavement. This made our focus very specific, but we felt this would be the most practical and useful approach.

### Research focusing on children's palliative care services including stakeholder views

Overall, there is limited evidence which uses research and robust evidence to recommend ways to assess the needs of children, families and caregivers. Many of the studies we identified detailed challenges with assessment and allocation of services, treatment and care, although more recent papers published as part of the development of outcome measures, identified the needs of children (Namisango et al., 2019; Scott et al., 2023).

Many researchers chose to use both qualitative (using words) and quantitative (using numbers) approaches to explore palliative care for children. In Australia, for example, a study by Monterosso et al. (2007) suggested that existing criteria for accessing services were perceived as narrow and inconsistent. This was an important study in that 497 families were identified as potential participants with 129 agreeing to take part in a two-phase study. Both qualitative and quantitative data were analysed to highlight the following related issues: the need for more co-ordination of care by families, better forward planning, decreased perceived bureaucratic processes, broader eligibility criteria, increased leadership to facilitate inter-agency collaboration, and the need for a case-management approach. A lack of funding and resources underpinned the key barriers discussed.

Some studies use qualitative approaches exclusively. For example, in a study conducted in Switzerland by Bergstraesser et al. (2013), the team included health professionals from different international countries based on the clinical leadership in their country, region, academic institution and/or organisations. They used qualitative methods in a two-part descriptive study to develop a tool to facilitate appropriate and timely involvement of specialist children's palliative care services. Semi-structured interviews were used in Part 1 with palliative care experts from the UK, France, the USA and Canada – paediatricians aged 45–49 years (n = 5) and nurses aged 47–58 years. In Part 2, focus groups were used with paediatric health professionals from Zurich, Switzerland (including four physicians, three nurses, two social workers, one psychologist, and one physiotherapist).

Studies by Mitchell et al. (2018), Coad et al. (2014), Coyne et al. (2014) and Carter et al. (2012) have been pivotal in their impact in this field in the UK. Each used qualitative voices in order to understand complex health and care needs, including access to or use of palliative care services. One example by Carter et al. (2012) undertook workshops and interviews with children, families and health professional stakeholders to examine UK community children's nursing services and what could be improved. Further barriers to appropriate decision-making about care were identified by Carter et al. (2012) who state, "services needed to be commissioned by people with an appreciation of what is needed". Commissioning did not always work well and was acknowledged as problematic even by the commissioners who contributed to the study. "Inconsistency" in decision-making and lack of prioritisation and appreciation of "what is needed',' meant that children's care at home could be compromised by ineffective commissioning. There was also evidence that where staffing allocation was inadequate, resources were reallocated to meet greatest need. In particular, Carter et al. (2012) refer to shifting resources from more routine aspects of caseload work to free up staffing hours to provide care to families whose child was dying.

More recently, Brenner et al. (2021) undertook a qualitative research project with 20 parents of children with complex health needs including palliative care needs and 23 stakeholders (including Health and Safety Executive, Senior Managers, Administrators, Case Managers, Nurses, and Home Care Service Workers) (n = 15). An open-ended survey and descriptive analysis were used to highlight a number of issues. One key issue they found was a continuous need to focus on standardised care assessment and reassessment of family needs, and communication of these processes and roles to families using the service. In cases where a service is not available, assessment of need may highlight where funding is required. Brenner et al. (2021) identified that to progress their service, better assessment of the need for additional funding for enhanced respite care was needed. Participants also suggested that a key contributing factor to this enhanced care was the specialist knowledge of the service manager, case managers and nurses leading and delivering care to this population. Integrating the views of the skilled workforce into an assessment instrument can support their self-determination, empowering them both in their role and in supporting participation from families and young people.

Study participants interviewed by Law et al. (2011) offered suggestions about how services could be improved through better integration of services. For example, a "one-stop clinic opportunity for families that offers an orthopaedic surgeon, spinal specialist if necessary, dietician, physiotherapist, paediatrician, wheelchairs, orthotics in one session" (Physiotherapist). The same study provided examples of partnership working focused on comprehensive Service Level Agreements, whereby allocation of resources across sectors and professional boundaries were agreed, aiming at facilitating improved service provision. The use of care pathways in the integration and coordination of services was perceived to be beneficial as soon as the child with complex needs was identified.

One of the areas identified as a challenge for research in children's palliative care has been the lack of outcome measures and tools (Downing et al., 2018). Following on from studies by Harding et al. on children's palliative care in sub-Saharan Africa (2010; 2014), work began to develop the first children's palliative outcome scale: "C-POS" (Downing et al., 2012). In refining and validating the tool, a cross-sectional qualitative study was undertaken in Kenya, Namibia, South Africa and Uganda in order to identify the symptoms, concerns and other outcomes that matter to children with life-limiting conditions and their families in sub-Saharan Africa (Namisango et al., 2020). Some 61 interviews were conducted with children with life-limiting conditions (7–17 years of age) and 59 with caregivers of children (0–17 years) unable to self-report. This study was important as it was one of the first in the region to interview the children themselves, or their caregivers, and to understand the symptoms' concerns and priority outcomes that were important to them. Outcomes were identified which included physical concerns, psycho-social concerns, existential concerns, and the quality of healthcare. This work provides the evidence on what matters to children living with palliative care needs in sub-Saharan Africa and feeds into the development of appropriate services as well as the development of an outcome measure. It also showed that using developmental and age-appropriate research methods, children can and should be engaged in research. Refining of the C-POS continues, and work carried out in sub-Saharan Africa fed into work being done in other countries, such as Belgium (Friedel et al., 2021) and the UK (Coombes et al., 2021; 2023). That work is now feeding back into the work in sub-Saharan Africa, and to work in other countries including India, Bangladesh, and Turkey – highlighting the ongoing developments within the science of paediatric palliative care research.

In a study conducted in Brazil, the primary aim was to investigate ethical and moral conflicts within the realm of paediatric oncology, specifically from the perspective of nursing professionals. The research employed a qualitative secondary analysis methodology, involving semi-structured interviews with ten nursing professionals working at a paediatric cancer hospital. Thematic data analysis was applied to the interview data, leading to the identification of two prominent themes. The first theme, "living with conflicts intrinsic to the relationships", encapsulates the diverse sources of conflict experienced by nursing professionals in their interactions with colleagues, families, and seriously ill children. This theme underscores the need to address sensitive topics to mediate these conflicts effectively. The second theme, "developing moral resilience", illuminates how nurses reframe conflicts and employ strategies to mitigate personal harm. The findings shed light on the intricate and demanding environment of paediatric oncology, acknowledging the multi-faceted nature of sensitive issues faced by nursing professionals during clinical decision-making. The study emphasises self-reflection and intuitive strategies as protective measures that can aid nurses when confronted with ethical and moral conflicts in their daily paediatric oncology practice. Moreover, due to the limited support services available for nursing professionals, there is a call for institutional policies to foster the development of moral resilience within this context (Dos Santos et al., 2023).

Box 13.3 presents research approaches utilised in children's palliative care.

---

**BOX 13.3 RESEARCH APPROACHES TO CHILDREN'S PALLIATIVE CARE**

Collectively, in children's palliative care, researchers have used a number of qualitative approaches, carrying out reviews and using exploratory and creative approaches to seek views. This is important groundwork, but robust quantitative studies are also needed to measure the change in outcomes and impact of interventions to fully understand the phenomena of children's palliative care in more depth.

Arguably a mix of both approaches would move the research and evidence forward to make the real differences that are needed.

---

## Research focusing on family bereavement

In the realm of bereavement research, there exists a continuous effort to explore experiences of grieving families and those at the end-of-life stage in children's palliative care. This endeavour involves innovative approaches, including intricate utilisation of theories, such as the Dual Process Model of Coping with Bereavement (Stroebe and Schut, 1999), which serves to enhance both research and clinical practice. Furthermore, the Family Management Style Framework (Knafl et al., 2008) has been adapted for palliative care, incorporating a novel conceptual aspect related to "Preparing for Death" (Bousso et al., 2012). This research yields valuable insights into the care of grieving family members, offering guidance on how to identify and harness unique family strengths with practical applications. There is a critical gap concerning recognition of anticipatory grief and the support offered to families during a child's end-of-life journey (Dos Santos et al., 2019). Anticipatory grief and emotional distress experienced before a child's death are common aspects of end-of-life care yet are often under-recognised and under-supported. Researchers and clinical practitioners in Brazil have worked together to bridge this gap by emphasising the importance of acknowledging and addressing anticipatory grief (Dos Santos et al., 2019; Dos Santos et al., 2020). This approach aims to raise awareness among healthcare professionals about the emotional complexities faced by families during this phase and the imperative need for tailored support.

Grasping the crucial role of bereavement research in addressing the unique challenges of children's palliative care ensures comprehensive and tailored support for families facing loss. This can be done through recognising and applying key theoretical models, and using innovative approaches in order to foster a more nuanced understanding of grief in children's palliative care.

Sustained efforts have revolved around integrating the Dual Process Model of Coping with Bereavement into the care of grieving families within palliative care settings. This model recognizes that individuals alternate between two primary coping processes: loss-oriented and restoration-oriented. Loss-oriented coping involves actively addressing emotional aspects of loss, whereas restoration-oriented coping entails tending to practical tasks and adapting to changes brought about by loss (Bousso et al., 2012). By applying this model, the aim has been to provide a comprehensive and individualised approach to support grieving families by acknowledging and validating diverse coping strategies employed by families which have been shown to facilitate their adjustment to loss. Furthermore, work has highlighted the importance of recognising the unique needs and strengths of each family member throughout the bereavement process.

In research, the Family Management Style Framework has also been adapted specifically for palliative care (Bousso et al., 2012). An innovative component, "Preparing for Death", has been incorporated into the framework to recognise anticipatory grief experienced by families as they navigate end-of-life care and prepare for impending loss (Bousso et al., 2012).

Through their research and clinical practice, the Brazilian team has identified strategies for recognising and mobilising family strengths, empowering families to effectively cope with grief and bereavement. They have developed interventions that facilitate open communication, promote shared decision-making, and provide psychosocial support to families throughout their child's end-of-life journey. Implementation of these approaches not only contributes to theoretical understanding of grief and bereavement in palliative care but also serves as a valuable resource for informing clinical practice. Healthcare professionals can thus better meet the complex and evolving needs of grieving families, nurturing resilience, and facilitating the healing process.

---

**LEARNING ACTIVITY**

1. Reflect on the examples given on bereavement research and research focusing on services and stakeholders views.
2. What have you learnt from this and how can you apply that to your own research?

---

## ETHICS

So far in this chapter we have discussed some background and examples drawn from research in the field of children's palliative care. However, whatever the approach taken, studies often raise a number of ethical concerns and challenges. These may encompass issues related to obtaining consent, ensuring confidentiality, addressing potentially challenging language and age-appropriate content, navigating sensitive subject matter, and effectively concluding the study.

---

**LEARNING ACTIVITY**

1.  Reflect on your own research in children's palliative care, or other research that you have read.
2.  What have been the main ethical issues that you have encountered?
3.  How have you overcome these?

---

In the field of children's palliative care research there is very little published literature to guide ethical principles and practice in this area although they are often raised as a challenge (Rahimzadeh et al., 2015; DeCamp et al., 2022). Ethical issues can arise at any time in the study and while researchers may have attempted to predict and even plan for ethical challenges, they can be difficult to navigate and require much reflexivity. To illustrate this, we have drawn some examples from the field.

## Power dynamics, participants and researchers' harms

Ethical considerations are of paramount importance when conducting research involving children in palliative care. Given the vulnerable nature of this population, it is crucial to ensure their rights, well-being, and protection throughout the research process, aiming to mitigate power dynamics, participants, and researchers' harms.

In one research study involving a bereaved population (Dos Santos et al., 2019; Dos Santos et al., 2020), a multi-disciplinary team was established to provide support to researchers during data collection and analysis. This team comprised nurses, psychologists, doctors, and social workers. We established the need to support members of the team according to their different backgrounds, roles in the hospital where data collection took place or their clinical or research expertise. Thus, we anticipated assisting in participant engagement within the clinical setting, of providing support in the analysis process, and in offering emotional support for both families and researchers.

By involving a diverse team with different areas of expertise, we aimed not only to ensure comprehensive support, but also to enhance the quality and trustworthiness of our research (Lincoln and Guba, 1985). It also helped to expand the horizon for the interpretative process through deepening reflexivity for data analysis, as well as ensuring reliability through multiple coders per data set. The collaborative approach during data collection allowed us to address ethical considerations effectively and provide the necessary support to participants and researchers throughout the study. Ongoing monitoring and support are essential throughout the research process.

Researchers should ensure that appropriate resources and support services are available for children and their families, providing access to counselling or other forms of assistance. Furthermore, it is essential to adhere to ethical guidelines and regulations in research, ensuring the protection of participants' rights, confidentiality and informed consent. These principles should guide our research practices and contribute to the overall ethical integrity of our studies.

Potential harms and damages must be considered in a broad perspective, beyond that for the assigned participant. Ethically, it is important to take into consideration that the research may produce data or arouse emotional issues in the whole family. For this reason, the researcher might want the participant to discuss their enrolment with their families, depending on the approach and theme of the research or the setting, such as interviews in bereaved families' homes (Dos Santos et al., 2020). There should also be discussion about the use of any piece of art, photo or video produced with the child for the research.

## Managing relationships

Ethics recommendations for authentic engagement have been delineated by DeCamp et al. (2022) and these are useful for end-of-life palliative care research with children and families, enabling adequate management of relationships as those individuals involved dive into sensitive topics. Researchers and participants can develop deep bonds over time as they discuss complex issues, which can evolve into a desire to take part in family rituals, or even a request from the family to keep data produced during research, as a memory after the child's death. The recommendations set out by DeCamp et al. (2022) involve considering time and preparation for an acceptable approach to including children and their families as research partners and managing "relationship ethics".

Interestingly, Rahimzadeh et al. (2015) discuss the need for a "more engagement-centred approach" in children's palliative care research, based on human rights and social tenets of childhood. Planning research with children and families in palliative care involves best practice for tailoring the approach and conduct to the child and family's needs, according to the child's development, physical or cognitive impairment, and the family's cultural background.

Due to cultural and policy-specific needs, some ethical issues may be country-specific, thus we need to tailor the nuances of ethical conduct for sensitive research. Without understanding the country's politics, cultures and ways of working, it could be damaging to the research reputation, and participants may not want to engage with future palliative care or other research. For example, in the UK, participants may be offered some of kind of reward for participation, usually offered after the data collection to prevent coercion and by way of a thank you. However, in Brazil, researchers are not allowed to offer any kind of compensation to research participants, apart from the costs of the research for food and transportation. Thus, what is acceptable and ethically permissible may vary from country to country, and this needs to be acknowledged in multi-country/multi-site research.

In this way, researchers need to manage the relationships between the healthcare team and the service, adapting the language and approach with potential participants. It is necessary to manage relationships well in research, so that reputational damage does not occur, discouraging institutions from receiving research, as well as participants from wanting to engage in palliative care. Most importantly, reducing risks involves caring for families beyond the assigned participant and ensuring that researchers have proper time available to manage distress along the research process.

## Minimising additional upset

Preventing additional upset is a vital consideration when undertaking research in the field of children's palliative care. An example of this is a research study that focused on models of interaction/relationships between children, parents and providers, with evidence about the development of positive and negative relationships during end-of-life care and its impact on family grief (Dos Santos et al., 2019; Dos Santos et al., 2020). The study used multiple data collection strategies (document review, interviews and participant observation), across all stages of the childhood and multiple illness trajectories. Different data sources can help the researcher to obtain more insights about the research phenomenon, with less burden on the participants. In addition, the integration of the interdisciplinary team into research teams can reduce upset to researchers and participants when carrying out research relating to grief, for example (Dos Santos et al., 2020). This type of research can overwhelm both vulnerable participants and researchers and ethical care must be taken throughout all phases of the research (Butler et al., 2019).

Palliative care, dying and death are all sensitive and upsetting areas to discuss, particularly when relating to one's self, a child or family member. This does not mean that we should not undertake research in children's palliative care, however, we need to be aware of the emotional nature of our research and make every effort to minimise or reduce any additional upset. Research conducted with children and families has highlighted the importance of research in the field, and family members have noted that although interviews can be hard and upsetting, that is natural, and it should not mean that they are not involved or asked difficult questions. While finding some questions upsetting, Coombes et al. (2023) found that despite getting upset and crying, parents still felt it was important that researchers asked them the questions, even if they did get emotional when answering. Box 13.4 summarises the ethical principles in researching children's palliative care.

---

**BOX 13.4 ETHICAL PRINCIPLES**

It is essential to consider the vulnerable nature of children's palliative care research, for participants, researchers and providers. Sound ethical principles must be adhered to, including rights, well-being and protection throughout the research process, aiming to mitigate power dynamics, participants' and researchers' harms. It is also important to provide adequate management of relationships in children's palliative research, as involved individuals dive into sensitive topics and researchers need to be considerate to cultural backgrounds and country-specific policies. The nature of research into children's palliative care is that it is sensitive, poses ethical challenges, and that it can be upsetting, but this doesn't mean that we shouldn't do it.

## SUPPORTING AND SUSTAINING THE CULTURE OF CHILDREN'S PALLIATIVE CARE RESEARCH

In this chapter, we have discussed several issues that arise when conducting research with children and their families as well as the professionals who care for them. Despite all the issues we have raised, supporting research from ideas to implementation is part of not only building a research career, but also transforming the landscape of the field. However, internationally there are huge variations when it comes to support, funding and infrastructures.

We have advocated that adopting a team and ideally an international, regional or national collaborative approach to research is increasingly important to address priorities if there is to be real change for this group of children. It is thus important that funding bodies around the world share lessons learned from successful funding examples and frameworks that support research focused on benefits, impact and improved health outcomes.

The CoPPAR (Collaborative Paediatric Palliative Care Research Network) is an example of a national collaboration and partnership between those delivering care and those with skills to deliver research. It was established in the UK in January 2022, funded by the National Institute for Health Research, and brought together academics and clinical teams to share experiences and expertise to improve research confidence (Fraser, 2023). Importantly it also involved parents of children with life-limiting or life-threatening conditions or whose child had died. Ultimately the success of the network in addressing the need for more high-quality research in children's palliative care was dependent on the collaborative ethos that was shared and developed across the network. A similar collaboration is planned for sub-Saharan Africa, linking in with UK and African academics alongside practitioners, in order to develop and strengthen the children's palliative care evidence in the region, but also to build capacity for research.

Other collaborations exist, such as the Palliakid project which includes partners from Spain, Finland, Romania, the Netherlands, Denmark, Latvia, Italy, Turkey, Belgium and the UK (ICPCN). Through the project, they aim to evaluate the feasibility, effectiveness, and cost-effectiveness of novel interventions for children with palliative and end-of-life care needs in different healthcare systems across Europe (ehospice, 2024). Global Health and Palliative Care (GHAP): Expanding Access is another collaboration, with a component on children's palliative care in Uganda, including King's College London, the African Palliative Care Association, ICPCN, Makerere University, Mulago Hospital, Mildmay Uganda and Kawempe Home Care (King's College London, 2024). This builds upon many regional and international collaborations for children's palliative care in sub-Saharan Africa. Both the GHAP project, and a project being led by the University of Coimbra (EoL in Place Project), which has collaborators in Portugal, The Netherlands, the USA, and Uganda (University of Coimbra, 2024), are providing opportunities to strengthen research capacity for children's palliative care research generally, but also offering opportunities to African clinicians for PhD study.

Another example of creating global collaborative networks is drawn from Brazil where the research team has been dedicated to creating global collaborative networks with the aim of supporting positive outcomes in children's palliative care and family-centred care. The network aims to sustain outcomes for family-centred palliative care through creative efforts to address the needs of individuals who are dying and their families; through developing a curriculum for families who have lost a child, provide opportunities for dissemination of research; and provide opportunities for doctoral and post-doctoral studies. For example, through the network's contribution to the post-graduate programme in Brazil, the quality and outcomes of children's palliative care have been enhanced, particularly in relation to: grief as a family experience; the skills of nurses caring for these families; the nurses' role in supporting end-of-life decision-making; and palliative care policies and programmes in Brazil and worldwide (Dos Santos et al., 2020; Downing et al., 2012; Downing et al., 2015). In the United Kingdom there is also a Research network led jointly by the Association of Paediatric Palliative Medicine (APPM) and Together for Short Lives (2024), which aims to advance the science of children's palliative care in order to: (1) make it easier to carry out children's palliative care research, specifically supporting children's hospices to become research-ready; (2) support research in all aspects of children's palliative care, in its holistic definition; (3) support translation of research into practice; and (4) have an ongoing commitment to research prioritisation.

The significance of networks, globally, regionally and nationally, in children's palliative care research cannot be overstated. Relationships serve as the connective tissues that link individual researchers with team members, participants, institutions, communities, and organisations. Healthy and supportive relationships, rooted in sensitivity and appreciation for diverse backgrounds and aspirations, provide protection and nurturing for everyone involved. As nurse researchers in children's palliative care, we assume various roles such as primary investigators, community partners, mentors, educators, and collaborators. Good relationships in children's palliative care enable us to fulfil our roles, ensuring the success of the projects but also the well-being of all involved. Ultimately, these relationships can help us to understand the research context, establish a foundation for success in research endeavors, nurture talent of other healthcare professionals and enhance the overall quality of our work (Mooney-Doyle and Deatrick, 2023). In this, we all have a key role to play.

---

**LEARNING ACTIVITY**

1. Reflect on your role as a nurse within research in children's palliative care. Are you a full-time nurse researcher? A clinical nurse involved in research? Leading research projects?

2. In your role do you have strong networks with other nurse researchers in children's palliative care? What about researchers from other disciplines? How can you strengthen your networks and how can you collaborate in research within children's palliative care?

## SUMMARY

What we have set out here is the complexity of undertaking research when children are living with a serious illness. While challenging, various strategies can be employed to engage with the complexities associated with data collection in children's palliative nursing care research. However, raising awareness of research of nurses delivering palliative care is vital, as is the investment in education for nurses, but also the public, other healthcare professionals and policy-makers, in order to develop a research-aware community, which is the foundation for research engagement and participation.

When working with a group of children where nursing needs might be related to long-term conditions, disability or end of life, it is important to define the population, their needs, challenges and priorities. Only once the definitions are clear can concise and meaningful research questions be formulated to address the research agendas of the various stakeholders.

As research adds to the picture of children's palliative nursing care needs, it is becoming increasingly important that researchers across the globe coordinate and collaborate to ensure that children's palliative care is understood in the context of geopolitical healthcare and defined population needs. Research leadership has a vital role to play in advocating for universal access to palliative nursing care for children and their carers.

## KEY POINTS

- While there is a developing research literature, research into children's palliative care lags behind palliative care research undertaken with adults.
- Research is not an optional extra but is essential for the provision and development of children's palliative care nursing.
- All levels of improving research in this field are needed from awareness and participation through to research leadership.
- Methods and the accuracy of data are refined and developed over time as we gain more information and skill in the development of evidence within children's palliative care.
- Ethical issues are complex but should not prevent us from undertaking this important work, in particular, making sure children's voices are represented and acted on.
- There are some solid examples of communities and cultures of researchers and case examples that can be accessed to spread positive research cultures and thus build global evidence-based knowledge and capacity in children's palliative care.

## REFERENCES

Aldridge, J., Downing, J. (2020). Integrating research into care. In J. Downing (ed.), *Children's palliative care: An international case-based manual* (pp. 273–284). Springer.

Arias-Casais, N., Garralda, E., Pons, J. J., Marston, J., Chambers, L., Downing, J., Ling, J., Rhee, J. Y., Lima, L. D., Centeno, C. (2020). Mapping paediatric palliative care development in the WHO European region: Children living in low-middle income countries are less likely to access it. *Journal of Pain and Symptom Management*, 60(4), 746–753. http//doi.org/10.1016/j.jpainsymman.2020.04.028

Arias-Casais, N., Garralda, E., Rhee, J. Y., Lima, L. D., Pons-Izquierdo, J. J., Clark, D., Hasselaar, J., Ling, J., Mosoiu, D., Centeno, C. (2019). *EAPC atlas of palliative care in Europe 2019*. Vilvoorde.

Baker, J. N., Levine D. R., Hinds, P. S., Weaver, M. S., Cunningham, M. J., Johnson, L., Anghelescu, D., Mandrell, B., Gibson, D. V., Jones, B., Wolfe, J., Feudtner, C., Friebert, S., Carter, B., Kane, J. R. (2015). Research priorities in pediatric palliative care. *The Journal of Pediatrics*, 167(2), 467–470.e3. http//doi.org/10.1016/j.jpeds.2015.05.002

Beecham, E., Hudson, B. F., Oostendorp, L., Candy, B., Jones, L., Vickerstaff, V., Lakhanpaul, M., Stone, P., Chambers, L., Hall, D., Hall, K., Ganeshamoorthy, T., Comac, M., Bluebond-Langner, M. (2016). A call for increased paediatric palliative care research: Identifying barriers. *Palliative Medicine*, 30(10), 979–980. http//doi.org/10.1177/0269216316648087

Benini, F., Papadatou, D., Bernadá, M., Craig, F., De Zen, L., Downing, J., Drake, R., Friedrichsdorf, S., Garros, D., Giacomelli, L., Lacerda, A., Lazzarin, P., Marceglia, S., Marston, J., Muckaden, M. A., Papa, S., Parravicini, E., Pellegatta, F., Wolfe, J. (2022). International Standards for Pediatric Palliative Care: From IMPaCCT to GO-PPaCS. *Journal of Pain and Symptom Management*, 63(5), e529–e543. http//doi.org/10.1016/j.jpainsymman.2021.12.031

Bergstraesser, E., Hain, R. D., Pereira, J. L. (2013). The development of an instrument that can identify children with palliative care needs: The Paediatric Palliative Screening Scale (PaPaS Scale): A qualitative study approach. *BMC Palliative Care*, 12(1), 20. http//doi.org/10.1186/1472-684X-12-20

Bousso, R. S., Misko, M. D., Mendes-Castillo, A. M., Rossato, L. M. (2012). Family management style framework and its use with families who have a child undergoing palliative care at home. *Journal of Family Nursing*, 18(1), 91–122. http//doi.org/10.1177/1074840711427038

Brenner, M., Doyle, A., Begley, T., Doyle, C., Hill, K., Murphy, M. (2021). Enhancing care of children with complex healthcare needs: An improvement project in a community health organisation in Ireland. *BMJ Open Quality*, 10(1), e001025. http//doi.org/10.1136/bmjoq-2020-001025

Butler, A. E., Copnell, B., Hall, H. (2019). Researching people who are bereaved: Managing risks to participants and researchers. *Nursing Ethics*, 26(1), 224–234. http//doi.org/10.1177/0969733017695656

Carter, B., Coad, J., Bray, L., Goodenough, T., Moore, A., Anderson, C., Clinchant, A., Widdas, D. (2012). Home-based care for special healthcare needs: Community children's nursing services. *Nursing Research*, 61(4), 260–268. http//doi.org/10.1097/NNR.0b013e31825b6848

Coad, J., Gibson, F., Horstman, M., Milnes, L., Randall, D. C., Carter, B. (2014). Be my guest! Challenges and practical solutions of undertaking interviews with children in the home setting. *Journal of Child Health Care*, 19(4). http//doi.org/10.1177/1367493514527653

Connor, S. R. (ed.). (2020). *Global atlas of palliative care* (2nd edn). Worldwide Hospice Palliative Care Alliance.

Connor, S. R., Downing, J., Marston, J. (2017). Estimating the global need for palliative care for children: A cross-sectional analysis. *Journal of Pain and Symptom Management*, 53(2), 171–177. http//doi.org/10.1016/j.jpainsymman.2016.08.020

Connor, S. R., Sepulveda, C. (eds) (2014). *Global atlas of palliative care at the end-of-life*. World Health Organization/Worldwide Hospice Palliative Care Alliance.

Coombes, L., Bristowe, K., Ellis-Smith, C., Aworinde, J., Fraser, L. K., Bluebond-Langner, M., Chambers, L., Murtagh, F. E. M., Harding, R. (2021). Enhancing validity, reliability and participation in self-reported health outcome measurement for children and young people: A systematic review of recall period, response scale format, and administration modality. *Quality of Life Research*, 30(7), 1830–1832. http//doi.org/10.1007/s11136-021-02814-4

Coombes, L., Hardardóttir, S., Braybrook, D., Roach, A., Scott, H., Bristowe, K., Ellis-Smith, C., Downing, J., Bluebond-Langner, M., Fraser, L. K., Murtagh, F. E. M., Harding, R. (2023). Design and administration of Patient-Centered Outcome Measures: The perspectives of children and young people with life-limiting or life threatening conditions and their family members. *The Patient-Patient-Centered Outcomes Research*, 16, 473–483. http//doi.org/10.1007/s40271-023-00627-w

Coyne, I., Amory, A., Kiernan, G., Gibson, F. (2014). Children's participation in shared decision-making: Children, adolescents, parents and healthcare professionals' perspectives and experiences. *European Journal of Oncology Nursing*, 18, 273–280. http://dx.doi.org/10.1016/j.ejon.2014.01.006

DeCamp, M., Alasmar, A., Fischer, S., Kutner, J. S. (2022). Meeting ethical challenges with authenticity when engaging patients and families in end-of-life and palliative care research: A qualitative study. *BMC Palliative Care*, 21(1), 74. http//doi.org/10.1186/s12904-022-00964-x

de Pinho, A. A. A., do Nascimento, I. R. C., do Ramos, I. W. da S., Alencar, V. O. (2020). Repercussões dos cuidados paliativos pediátricos: Revisão integrativa. *Revista Bioética*, 28(4), 710–717. http//doi.org/10.1590/1983-80422020284435

Dombrecht, L., Lacerda, A., Wolfe, J., Snaman, J. (2023). A call to improve paediatric palliative care quality through research. *BMC Palliative Care*, 22, 141. http//doi.org/10.1186/s12904-023-01262-w

Dos Santos, M. R., da Silva, L. T. P., de Araújo, M. M., Ferro, T. A., Silva, I. N., Szylit, R. (2023). Ethical and moral conflicts in the nursing care of pediatric patients with cancer and their families. *Cancer Nursing*, 46(4), 314–320. http//doi.org/10.1097/NCC.0000000000001113

Dos Santos, M. R., Szylit, R., Deatrick, J. A., Mooney-Doyle, K., Wiegand, D. L. (2020). The evolutionary nature of parent-provider relationships at child's end-of-life with cancer. *Journal of Family Nursing*, 26(3), 254–268. http//doi.org/10.1177/1074840720938314

Dos Santos, M. R., Wiegand, D. L., Sá, N. N., Misko, M. D., Szylit, R. (2019). From hospitalization to grief: Meanings parents assign to their relationships with pediatric oncology professional. *Revista da Escola de Enfermagem da USP*, 53, e03521. http//doi.org/10.1590/S1980-220X2018049603521

Downing, J. (2016). Editorial: To research or not to research – An important question in paediatric palliative care. *Palliative Medicine*, 30(10), 902–903. doi:10.1177/0269216316675570

Downing, J., Atieno, M., Powell, R. A., Ali, Z., Marston, J., Meiring, M., Ssengooba, J., Williams, S., Mwangi-Powell, F. N., Harding, R., APCA AIDSTAR Project Advisory Group. (2012). Development of a palliative care outcome measure for children in sub-Saharan Africa: Findings from early phase instrument development. *European Journal of Palliative Care*, 19(6), 292–295.

Downing, J., Knapp, C., Muckaden, M. A., Fowler-Kerry, S., Marston, J., ICPCN Scientific Committee. (2015). Priorities for global research into children's palliative care: Results of an international Delphi Study. *BMC Palliative Care*, 14, 36. http//doi.org/10.1186/s12904-015-0031-1

Downing, J., Namisango, E., Harding, R. (2018). Outcome measurement in paediatric palliative care: Lessons from the past and future developments. *Annals of Palliative Medicine*, 7(Suppl. 3), S151–S163. http//doi.org/10.21037/apm.2018.04.02

Downing, J., Namukwaya, E., Nakawesi, J., Mwesiga, M. (2024). Shared-decision-making and communication in paediatric palliative care within Uganda. *Current Problems in Pediatric and Adolescent Health Care*, 54(1), 101556. https://doi.org/10.1016/j.cppeds.2024.101556

ehospice. (2024). Press release: SJD Barcelona Children's Hospital coordinates a European project to improve paediatric palliative care. Available at: https://ehospice.com/inter_childrens_posts/press-release/

Ferreira, E. A. L., Barbosa, S. M. M., Costa, G. A. (2022). *Mapeamento dos cuidados paliativos pediátricos no Brasil*. Rede Brasileira de Cuidados Paliativos Pediátricos (RBCPPed).

Ferreira, E. A. L., Valete, C. O. S., Barbosa, S. M. D. M., Costa, G. D. A., Molinari, P. C. C., Iglesias, S. B. D. O., Castro, A. C. P. D. (2023). Exploring the Brazilian pediatric palliative care network: A quantitative analysis of a survey data. *Revista Paulista de Pediatria*, 41, e2022020. http//doi.org/10.1590/1984-0462/2023/41/2022020

Feudtner, C., Rosenberg, A. R., Boss, R. D., Wiener, L., Lyon, M. E., Hinds, P. S., Bluebond-Langner, M., Wolfe, J. (2019). Challenges and priorities for pediatric palliative care research in the U.S. and similar practice settings: Report from a pediatric palliative care research network workshop. *Journal of Pain and Symptom Management*, 58(5), 909–917.e3. http//doi.org/10.1016/j.jpainsymman.2019.08.011

Fraser, L. K. (2023). Introducing the CoPPAR Toolkit. International Children's edition of ehospice. Available at: https://ehospice.com/inter_childrens_posts/introducing-the-coppar-toolkit/

Fraser, L. K., Bluebond-Langner, M., Ling, J. (2020). Advances and challenges in European Paediatric Palliative Care. *Medical Sciences (Basel, Switzerland)*, 8(2), 20. http//doi.org/10.3390/medsci8020020

Fraser, L. K., Gibson-Smith, D., Jarvis, S., Norman, P., Parslow, R. (2020). 'Making Every Child Count': Estimating current and future prevalence of children and young people with life-limiting conditions in the United Kingdom. Final Report. UK. Available at: https://www.togetherforshortlives.org.uk/app/uploads/2020/04/Prevalence-reportFinal_28_04_2020.pdf.

Fraser, L. K., Gibson-Smith, D., Jarvis, S., Norman, P., Parslow, R. (2021). Estimating the current and future prevalence of life-limiting conditions in children in England. *Palliative Medicine*, 35(9), 1641–1651. http//doi.org/10.1177/0269216320975308

Fraser, L. K., Miller, M., Aldridge, J., McKinney, P. A., Parslow, R.C. (2013). Prevalence of life-limiting and life-threatening conditions in young adults in England 2000–2010: Final report for Together for Short Lives. York University. Available at: www.togetherforshortlives.org.uk/app/uploads/.

Fraser, L. K., Miller, M., Aldridge J., McKinney P. A., Parslow R. C., Hain, R. (2012). Life-limiting and life-threatening conditions in children and young people in the United Kingdom; national and regional prevalence in relation to socioeconomic status and ethnicity: Final report for Together for Short Lives. Leeds University and Together for Short Lives. Available a: https://www.togetherforshortlives.org.uk/app/uploads/2018/01/ExRes-Childrens-Hospices-Ethnicity-Report-Leeds-Uni.pdf

Friedel, M., Brichard, B., Boonen, S., Tonon, C., De Terwangne, B., Bellis, D., Mevisse, M., Fonteyne, C., Jaspard, M., Schruse, M., Harding, R., Downing, J., Namisango, E., Degryse, J-M., Aujoulat, I. (2021). Face and content validity, acceptability, and feasibility of the adapted version of the Children's Palliative Outcome Scale: A qualitative pilot study. *Journal of Palliative Medicine*, 24(2), 181–188. http//doi.org/10.1089/jpm.2019.0646

Harding, R., Albertyn, R., Sherr, L., Gwyther, L. (2014). Pediatric palliative care in sub-Saharan Africa: A systematic review of the evidence for care models, interventions, and outcomes. *Journal of Pain and Symptom Management*, 47(3), 642–651. http//doi.org/10.1016/j.jpainsymman.2013.04.010

Harding, R., Selman, L., Powell, R. A., Namisango, E., Downing, J., Merriman, A., Ali, Z., Gikaara, N., Gwyther, L., Higginson, I. (2013). Research into palliative care in sub-Saharan Africa. *The Lancet, Oncology*, 14(4), e183–e188. http//doi.org/10.1016/S1470-2045(12)70396-0

Harding, R., Sherr, L., Albertyn, R. (2010). *The status of paediatric palliative care in sub-Saharan Africa: An appraisal.* The Diana Princess of Wales Memorial Fund and King's College London. Available at: https://icpcn.org/wp-content/uploads/2022/11/The-Status-of-Paediatric-Palliative-Care-in-sub-Saharan-Africa_July-2010.pdf

Hawley, P. H. (2015). The bow tie model of 21st century palliative care. *Journal of Pain and Symptom Management*, 47(1), e2–e5. http//doi.org/10.1016/j.jpainsymman.2013.10.009

ICPCN. (2024). International children's palliative care services locator. Available at: https://icpcn.org/map-of-services.

King's College London. (2024). Global health and palliative care. Available at: https://www.kcl.ac.uk/research/global-health-and-palliative-care

Knafl, K., Deatrick, J. A., Gallo, A. M. (2008). The interplay of concepts, data, and methods in the development of the Family Management Style Framework. *Journal of Family Nursing*, 14(4), 412–428. http//doi.org/10.1177/1074840708327138

Knaul, F. M., Farmer, P. E., Krakauer, E. L., De Lima, L., Bhadelia, A., Kwete, X. J., Arreola-Ornelas, H., Gómez-Dantés, O., Rodriguez, N. M., Alleyne, G. A. O., Connor, S. R., Hunter, D. J., Lohman, L., Radbruch, L., del Rocío, M.S.M., Atun, R., Foley, K. M., Frenk, J., Jamison, D. T., Rajagopal, M. R., Lancet Commission on Palliative Care and Pain Relief Study Group. (2018). Alleviating the access abyss in palliative care and pain relief – an imperative of universal health coverage: The Lancet Commission report. *Lancet*, 391, 1391–1454. http//doi.org/10.1016/s0140-6736(17)32513-8

Law, J., McCann, D., O'May, F. (2011). Managing change in the care of children with complex needs: healthcare providers' perspectives. *Journal of Advanced Nursing*, 67(12), 2551–2560. https://doi.org/10.1111/j.1365-2648.2011.05761.x

Lincoln, Y. S., Guba, E. G. (1985). *Naturalistic inquiry*. Sage.

Milani, B. A., Magrini, N., Gray, A., Wiffen, P., Scholten, W. (2011). WHO calls for targeted research on the pharmacological treatment of persisting pain in children with medical illnesses. *Evidence-Based Child Health: A Cochrane Review Journal*, 6(3), 1017–1020. http//doi.org/10.1002/ebch.777

Mitchell, S. J., Slowther, A. M., Coad, J., Dale, J. (2018). The journey through care: Study protocol for a longitudinal qualitative interview study to investigate the healthcare experiences and preferences of children and young people with life-limiting and life-threatening conditions and their families in the West Midlands, UK. *BMJ Open*, 8. http//doi.org/10.1136/bmjopen-2017-018266

Mooney-Doyle, K., Deatrick, J. A. (2023). Relationships make research – and researchers – whole. *Revista da Escola de Enfermagem da USP*, 57, e2023E001. https://doi.org/10.1590/1980-220X-REEUSP-2023-E001en

Monterosso, L., Kristjanson, L. J., Aoun, S., Phillips, M. B. (2007). Supportive and palliative care needs of families of children with life-threatening illnesses in Western Australia: Evidence to guide the development of a palliative care service. *Palliative Medicine*, 21(8), 689–696. http//doi.org/10.1177/0269216307083032

Namisango, E., Bristowe, K., Allsop, M. J., Murtagh, F. E. M., Abas, M., Higginson, I. J., Downing, J., Harding, R. (2019). Symptoms and concerns among children and young people with life-limiting and life-threatening conditions: A systematic review highlighting meaningful health outcomes. *The Patient: Patient Centered Outcomes Research*, 12, 15–55. http//doi.org/10.1007/s40271-018-0333-5

Namisango, E., Bristowe, K., Murtagh, F. E., Downing, J., Powell, R. A., Abas, M., Lohfeld, L., Ali, Z., Atieno, M., Haufiku, D., Guma, S., Luyirika, E. B., Mwangi-Powell, F. N.,

Higginson, I. J., Harding, R. (2020). Towards person-centred quality care for children with life-limiting and life-threatening illness: Self-reported symptoms, concerns and priority outcomes from a multi-country qualitative study. *Palliative Medicine*, 34(3), 319–335. http//doi.org/10.1177/0269216319900137

Osman, H., Rihan, A., Garralda, E., Rhee, J. Y., Pons, J. J., de Lima, L., Tfayli, A., Centeno, C. (2017). *Atlas of palliative care in the Eastern Mediterranean region*. IAHPC Press.

Passone, C. G. B., Grisi, S. J., Farhat, S. C., Manna, T. D., Pastorino, A. C., Alveno, R. A., Miranda, C. V. S., Waetge, A. R., Cordon, M. N., Odone-Filho, V., Tannuri, U., Carvalho, W. B., Carneiro-Sampaio, M., Silva, C. A. (2020). Complexity of pediatric chronic disease: Cross sectional study with 16,237 patients followed by multiple medical specialities. *Revista Paulista de Pediatria*, 38, e2018101. http//doi.org/10.1590/1984-0462/2020/38/201810

Pastrana, T., De Lima, L., Sánchez-Cárdenas, M., VanSteijn, D., Garralda, E., Pons, J. J., Centeno, C. (2021). *Atlas de cuidados paliativos en Latinoamérica 2020*. IAHPC Press.

Pastrana, T., De Lima, L., Wenk, R., Eisenchlas, J., Monti, C., Rocafort, J., Centeno, C. (2012). *Atlas of palliative care in Latin America ALCP* (1st edn). IAHPC Press.

Payne, S., Preston, N., Turner, M., Rolls, L. (2013). *Research in palliative care: Can hospices afford not to be involved?* A report for the Commission into the Future of Hospice Care. Help the Hospices. https://hospiceuk-files-prod.s3.eu-west-2.amazonaws.com/s3fs-public/2022-11/Research%20in%20palliative%20care.pdf

Payne, S., Turner, M. (2012). Methods of building and improving the research capacity of hospices. *European Journal of Palliative Care*, 19(1), 34–37.

Poles, K., Bousso, R. S. (2009). Morte digna da criança: Análise de conceito [Dignified death for children: Concept analysis]. *Revista da Escola de Enfermagem da U S P*, 43(1), 215–222. http//doi.org/10.1590/s0080-62342009000100028

Powell, R. A., Harding, R., Namisango, E., Katabira, E., Gwyther, L., Radbruch, L., Murray, S. A., El-Ansary, M., Leng, M., Ajayi, I. O., Blanchard, C., Kariuki, H., Kasirye, I., Namukwaya, E., Gafer, N., Casarett, D., Atieno, M., Mwangi-Powell, F. N. (2014). Palliative care research in Africa: Consensus building for a prioritized agenda. *Journal of Pain and Symptom Management*, 47(2), 315–324. http//doi.org/10.1016/j.jpainsymman.2013.03.022

Rabello, C. A. F. G., Rodrigues P. H. de A. (2010). Saúde da família e cuidados paliativos infantis: Ouvindo os familiares de crianças dependentes de tecnologia. [Family health programme and children palliative care: Listening to the relatives of technology-dependent children]. *Ciênc & Saúde Coletiva*, 15(2), 379–388. http//doi.org/10.1590/S1413-81232010000200013

Rahimzadeh, V., Bartlett, G., Longo, C., Crimi, L., Macdonald, M. E., Jabado, N., Ells, C. (2015). Promoting an ethic of engagement in pediatric palliative care research. *BMC Palliative Care*, 14, 50. http//doi.org/10.1186/s12904-015-0048-5

Rhee, J. Y., Luyirika, E., Namisango, E., Powell, R. A., Garralda, E., Pons, J. J., de Lima, L., Centeno, C. (2017). *APCA atlas of palliative care in Africa*. IAHPC Press.

Scott, J. M., Coombes, L., Braybrook, D., Roach, A., Hardardóttir, D., Bristow, K., Ellis-Smith, C., Downing, J., Murtagh, F. E. M., Farsides, B., Fraser, L.K., Bluebond-Langner M., Harding, R., on behalf of C-POS. (2023). Spiritual, religious and existential concerns of children and young people with life-limiting and life-threatening conditions: A qualitative interview study. *Palliative Medicine*. http//doi.org/10.1177/026921632316501

Siden, H., Widger, K. (2021). Research in children's palliative care. In R. Hain, A. Goldman, A. Rapoport, M. Meiring (eds), *Oxford textbook of palliative care for children* (pp. 410–148). Oxford University Press.

Stjernswärd, J., Foley, K. M., Ferris, F. D. (2007). The public health strategy for palliative care. *Journal of Pain and Symptom Management*, 33(5), 486–493. http//doi.org/10.1016/j.jpainsymman.2007.02.016

Stroebe, M., Schut, H. (1999). The dual process model of coping with bereavement: Rationale and description. *Death Studies*, 23(3), 197–224. http//doi.org/10.1080/074811899201046

Together for Short Lives (2018). *A guide to children's palliative care: Supporting babies, children and young people with life-limiting and life-threatening conditions and their families* (4th edn). Together for Short Lives. Available at: https://www.togetherforshortlives.org.uk/app/uploads/2018/03/TfSL-A-Guide-to-Children%E2%80%99s-Palliative-Care-Fourth-Edition-5.pdf (accessed 27 June 2024).

Together for Short Lives (2024). Research in the children's palliative care sector. Available at: https://www.togetherforshortlives.org.uk/changing-lives/supporting-care-professionals/research/ (accessed 27 June 2024).

University of Coimbra. (2024). EoL in place. Available at: https://www.uc.pt/en/eolinplace/ (accessed 27 June 2024).

WHO (World Health Organization). (2012). Guidelines on the pharmacological treatment of persisting pain in children with medical illnesses. Available at: https://iris.who.int/handle/10665/44540 (accessed 27 June 2024).

WHO (World Health Organization). (2014). Strengthening of palliative care as a component of integrated treatment throughout the life course. *Journal of Pain & Palliative Care Pharmacotherapy*, 28(2), 130–134. http//doi.org/0.3109/15360288.2014.911801

WHO (World Health Organization). (2020). Guidelines on the management of chronic pain in children. Available at: https://iris.who.int/bitstream/handle/10665/337999/9789240017870-eng.pdf?sequence=1 (accessed 27 June 2024).

WHO (World Health Organization). (2021). Assessing the development of palliative care worldwide: A set of actionable indicators. Available at: https://iris.who.int/bitstream/handle/10665/345532/9789240033351-eng.pdf?sequence=1 (accessed 27 June 2024).

# Appendix A: CPCET UK and Ireland Education Standard Framework (2020) mapped to chapters

| | Public Health | Universal | Core | Specialist |
|---|---|---|---|---|
| 1. Communicating effectively | 1.1 Gain an appreciation of both "helpful" and "unhelpful" patterns of communication with children and their carers who are living with life-limiting/life-threatening conditions, and those who have experienced a bereavement. **[Chapters 2 and 3]** | 1.2 Identify positive cultures of communication and -approaches to use when communicating with people who are distressed or grieving. **[Chapters 2 and 3]** | 1.3 Develop insight into positive cultures and patterns of communication when delivering "bad or unwanted" news/information. **[Chapter 4]** <br> 1.4 Discuss the design, delivery and evaluation of play for children living with life-limiting/life-threatening conditions. **[Chapter 6]** | 1.5 Analyse cultures and patterns of communication in managing complex issues in children's palliative and end-of-life care. **[Chapter 9]** |
| 2. Working with others in and across various settings | 2.1 Discuss how to build and sustain compassionate communities and how all children can be included to experience a childhood alongside their peers. **[Chapter 1]** | 2.2 Discuss principles of safeguarding children with palliative care needs. **[Chapter 1]** <br> 2.3 Identify own organisation's policies and practices which support, facilitate and sustain palliative and end-of-life care for children and their carers. **[Chapter 1]** | 2.4 Analyse the practice and approaches to identifying palliative and end-of-life care needs of children and their carers. **[Chapters 4 and 6]** <br> 2.5 Identify and reflect on your own role within the team delivering palliative and end-of-life care. **[Chapter 5]** <br> 2.6 Discuss professional roles and responsibilities in a multi-disciplinary (or inter-professional) team delivering children's palliative and end of life care. **[Chapter 5]** <br> 2.7 Explain the legal and practical requirements related to the care of a child's body after death. **[Chapter 8]** | 2.8 Critically evaluate policy and practices of team working and suggest ways forward to improve team cohesion and performance. **[Chapter 11]** <br> 2.9 Engage in critical dialogue of leadership for quality improvement and for equality of access in children's palliative and end-of-life care. **[Chapters 11 and 13]** |

*(Continued)*

| | Public Health | Universal | Core | Specialist |
|---|---|---|---|---|
| 3. Identifying and managing symptoms | 3.1 Describe common reactions to health and wellness, stress and grieving and set out potential interventions/ strategies. **[Chapters 1 and 3]**<br><br>3.2 Reflect on own beliefs, attitudes and understanding of personal and community responses to death in childhood. **[Chapter 1]** | 3.3 Describe common reactions and mental health issues and strategies to support well-being for children and their carers who are living with life-limiting/life-threatening conditions and the bereaved. **[Chapter 3]**<br><br>3.4 Recognise and list common symptoms that children and their carers who are living with life-limiting/life-threatening conditions and the bereaved might experience, and set out potential interventions. **[Chapter 3]** | 3.5 Assess, plan and implement effective symptom management approaches for a number of common symptoms encountered in children's palliative and end-of-life care. **[Chapter 7]**<br><br>3.6 Analyse and evaluate the assessment of care and the evidence base of symptom management to include a number of common symptoms encountered in children's palliative and end-of-life care. **[Chapter 7]**<br><br>3.7 Discuss the principles and practice of caring for a child's body after death, and supporting those who are bereaved. **[Chapter 8]** | 3.8 Assess, plan and implement for complex symptom management, including the management of different interacting symptoms encountered in children's palliative and end-of-life care. **[Chapter 9]**<br><br>3.9 Analyse and evaluate complex symptom management, including the management of different interacting symptoms. **[Chapter 12]**<br><br>3.10 Critically evaluate the evidence base for the management of complex/inter acting symptoms. **[Chapters 7 and 13]** |

| 4. Sustaining self-care and supporting the well-being of others | 4.1 Develop an awareness of, and reflect on, their own beliefs, attitudes, values relating to child death in their communities. **[Chapters 2 and 3]** | 4.4 Examine children's understanding and reactions to living with life-limiting/life-threatening conditions and dying and death in childhood. **[Chapter 4]** | 4.6 Analyse and evaluate your role, both as an individual and a professional, in self-care and supporting others to manage reactions to complex and/or multiple interacting issues contexts. **[Chapter 9]** |
| | 4.2 Explore strategies designed to manage stress and promote coping and well-being for self. **[Chapter 2]** | 4.5 Reflect on and discuss own experiences of delivering and interactions with those receiving care and the team delivering care. **[Chapter 5]** | 4.7 Demonstrate the understanding, skills and attitudes to design, deliver and evaluate learning opportunities for others. **[Chapter 10]** |
| | 4.3 Identify how own behaviour and practices influence others who are distressed and/or grieving. **[Chapter 2]** | | |

*Source*: CPCET (Children's Palliative Care Education and Training UK and Ireland Action Group) (2020). Education Standard Framework. ICPCN. Available at: https://icpcn.org/wp-content/uploads/2022/10/CPCET-Education-Standard-Framework.pdf (accessed 14 May 2024).

# Appendix B: Global Overview: Paediatric Palliative Care Standards (adapted from Benini et al. 2021)

## 1. THE DEFINITION OF PAEDIATRIC PALLIATIVE CARE AND ELIGIBILITY CRITERIA

### Standards

- Paediatric palliative care is a right for all children with a life-threatening or life-limiting illness and their families.
- All children with a life-limiting, life-threatening or terminal disease are eligible for paediatric palliative care.
- Paediatric palliative care should improve Quality-of-Life and address the needs, choices and wishes of children and their families.
- Paediatric palliative care should not be limited to end-of-life care but introduced at the time of the diagnosis of a life-limiting or life-threatening condition or, in some instances, prior to diagnosis when it may become challenging, for example, cost of tests, a rare condition, advanced disease.
- The level of care provided should be defined according to the specific needs of the child and family and may change over time.
- There are distinct levels of palliative care (palliative approach by all healthcare providers, generalised paediatric palliative care, specialised paediatric palliative care), which should be offered by professionals with appropriate levels of training in paediatric palliative care.
- All definitions are general and should represent the ultimate goal of practice in paediatric palliative care. Local conditions and resources should be taken into account.

## 2. THE MAGNITUDE OF THE NEED FOR PAEDIATRIC PALLIATIVE CARE

### Standards

- It is necessary to define the approaches used for the collection of data on the epidemiology of paediatric palliative care.
- Healthcare providers and policymakers should design care models and allocate resources according to the number and needs of children and families eligible for paediatric palliative care.

## 3. NEEDS

### Standards

- Healthcare providers should evaluate the specific needs of the child and their family and define a care plan and priorities accordingly.
- The evaluation of needs should be global, taking into account clinical, psychological, social, organisational, educational, spiritual, cultural and ethical needs of the child and family.
- The evaluation of needs must take into account the situation of the child and family, but also the foreseeable needs, wishes and desires, and those 'hidden' (i.e. those covered or unaddressed by the child and family during consultations).
- "Hidden" needs can be unmasked by actively listening to the child and their family.

## 3.1 THE CHILD'S NEEDS

### Standards

- Paediatric palliative care should address the physical, psychosocial, spiritual and developmental needs of a child.
- Distress caused by the disease should be minimised in order to improve the quality of life for the child and family.
- Symptom control should be adapted to the child's age, setting and culture.
- All interventions, pharmacological or non-pharmacological, should be continuously monitored.
- Evaluation, treatment, monitoring of symptoms and all other needs should be performed by qualified healthcare providers within an interdisciplinary team.
- All paediatric palliative care plans should be shared with the child, if possible, and their family.

### 3.1.1 CLINICAL NEEDS

## Standards

- Preventing, alleviating or eradicating distressing symptoms are one of the main goals of paediatric palliative care.
- Evaluation, treatment and monitoring of physical symptoms should be performed according to the specific response of each child.
- The perceived impact of each symptom on the child's functioning and daily life should be regularly evaluated.

### 3.1.2 DEVELOPMENTAL NEEDS

## Standards

- Paediatric palliative care plans must take into account infants', children's and adolescents' developmental needs which are affected by their life-threatening and life-limiting condition.
- Paediatric palliative care providers should be aware of how children's and adolescents' developmental stages affect how they cope with illness, dying, and death.
- Members of the paediatric palliative care team must have the competence to relate with infants, children and adolescents according to their cognitive, emotional, social, and physical stages of development.
- Comprehensive transition procedures for adequate referral of adolescents from PPC teams to adult teams should be planned.

### 3.1.3 PSYCHOLOGICAL AND SOCIAL NEEDS

## Standards

- Children with serious illness or facing the dying process should be helped to cope with a range of feelings, thoughts and behaviours reflective of their anxiety and distress.
- Psychological concerns and needs should be evaluated where possible by trained specialists within the multidisciplinary team, or if these are not available, by individuals trained in psychological care.
- Suitable psychosocial tools should help identify children's difficulties and plan appropriate interventions (verbal, symbolic, play or art therapy).
- Approaches that foster the child's resilience should enhance self-esteem and promote autonomy.
- PPC providers should actively listen and decode non-verbal language when communicating with children
- Parents should be helped to function effectively in their parenting role.
- The child's social abilities (right to play and have fun, to attend school, to maintain relations with friends) should be promoted and adapted to their developmental age and physical condition.

#### 3.1.4 SPIRITUAL NEEDS

#### Standards

- Spiritual support should be provided to every child who wishes to discuss spiritual issues and concerns.
- It is essential to maintain a respectful attitude towards the child's and family's cultural and spiritual/religious background.

### 3.2 FAMILY NEEDS

#### Standards

- Parents and other family members who have a close bond with the child should be involved in all care steps.
- The assessment of family needs should begin at the initiation of paediatric palliative care and be extended up to bereavement after the child's death.
- The needs of the family members (parents, siblings, grandparents, other persons if necessary) should be evaluated throughout the child's illness trajectory.
- The family's needs should be included in the development of the paediatric palliative care plan and addressed, when possible, by interdisciplinary team members skilled in active listening and communication and respectful of each family member's dignity.

#### 3.2.1 COMMUNICATION NEEDS

#### Standards

- Honest, continued and open communication with the family is crucial.
- Communication and discussions about the child's diagnosis and prognosis should take place in an appropriate and safe setting, taking into account the culture of the child and the family.
- Parents should be assisted in maintaining their parental role and effectively address children's distressing behaviours.

#### 3.2.2 PSYCHOLOGICAL NEEDS

#### Standards

- Family members should be offered the opportunity to share and discuss their personal feelings and thoughts and receive appropriate support from compassionate professionals with advanced communication skills.
- Potential situations of conflict should be identified early, prevented, and managed.
- Trained members of the interdisciplinary team should offer psychological support to family members, and when possible, by specialised mental health

professionals, especially when distress is very high, abuse occurs, and dysfunctional family dynamics perpetuate over time.

- Psychological support should be available to all family members after the death of the child and, when possible, for as long as needed.

### 3.2.3 NEED FOR HOME CARE AND ORGANISATIONAL SUPPORT

**Standards**

- Parents and other family members should be trained and supported 24/7 in caring for their child at home, when possible.
- They should be assisted in maintaining their social roles (e.g., work, future perspectives).
- Economic issues should be investigated and addressed, if possible.

### 3.2.4 SIBLINGS' AND GRANDPARENTS' NEEDS

**Standards**

- Siblings' and grandparents' concerns and needs should be addressed.
- Support should be provided to them throughout the child's illness and death, given that their suffering is often underestimated.

### 3.3 ETHICAL NEEDS

**Standards**

- Each decision should be taken according to the four basic ethical principles: best interest principle, risk–benefit proportionality principle, distributive justice, autonomy.
- Each decision of care should be based on the principle of the "child's best interest", as shared between the patient, family and clinician.

### 3.4 ADVANCED CARE PLANNING

**Standards**

- Advance care planning discussions should continue throughout the disease trajectory as much as possible, and may include, but are not limited to: the wishes about the care of the child, the definition of the goals of care and reconsideration of goals when the child's health worsens, plans about "what to do" in case of emergencies, and end-of-life care. All options should be kept open and revised regularly.
- Specific guidelines for advance care planning should be established in each institution.
- Healthcare professionals should receive proper training in advance care planning.

## 4. END-OF-LIFE CARE

### Standards

- During the entire disease course, the possible evolution of the disease should be discussed.
- The end-of-life stage and its setting should be prepared and defined according to the wishes of the child, the family, and available resources.
- Distressing physical and psychological symptoms should be addressed and treated.
- The child's dignity must be respected by ensuring an appropriate environment and the presence of loved ones.
- Spiritual and religious services, appropriate to the family's beliefs and practices, should be offered before and after death.
- Children at the end-of-life should be cared for by trained healthcare providers and, when possible, by an interdisciplinary team.
- The family should be prepared for physical changes associated with the dying process.
- The family should have time to properly say goodbye to the child according to their spiritual and family culture/religious practices.
- Siblings must be granted adequate time with the dying child.
- The body should be treated with due respect and with extreme attention and care according to the family's culture and religious practices.
- Healthcare providers must respect all different strategies of coping with loss.
- Bereavement support should be offered to the family for as long as needed, within the resources available

## 5. CARE MODELS AND SETTINGS OF CARE

### Standards

- Paediatric palliative care offered by trained healthcare providers should be ensured to all eligible children and their families, regardless of their financial or health insurance status.
- Each child and family must have a defined point of contact for paediatric palliative care, who should co-ordinate the care plan.
- The support of a specialised paediatric palliative care team should be available continuously, when possible, all days of the year, 24/7.
- Paediatric palliative care should be offered in all settings of the child's life (home, hospice, hospital, school), by ensuring continuity of care.
- The paediatric palliative care team should be supported to ensure self-care and prevent them burning out.
- The gold standard for the place of care is where the child and family want to be and feel the most supported.
- The paediatric palliative care team will ensure that children's symptoms are assessed and managed appropriately.

- If necessary, respite care should be made available for families or other caregivers.
- Telemedicine should be integrated into current care models according to local resources.
- Perinatal palliative care should be considered in routine obstetrics and neonatal care.
- Hospitals providing neonatal and maternal care need to develop perinatal palliative care pathways.
- Perinatal palliative care may be provided in the delivery room, post-partum ward, in the neonatal intensive care unit, at home, or wherever is thought to be most appropriate and provided this approach is consistent with family goals of care.
- For critically ill children with an unknown diagnosis, goals of care, and potential incurability, professionals in the emergency department should evaluate the clinical situation and contact paediatric palliative care teams.

## 6. PPC IN HUMANITARIAN EMERGENCIES

### Standards

- Paediatric palliative care (PPC) should be made available during all humanitarian emergencies.
- Paediatric palliative care in humanitarian crises should be integrated into each country's healthcare system.
- Paediatric palliative care activities must be included in the planning and implementation of the social and healthcare response.
- Guidelines' education and mentorship should be provided to healthcare providers.
- Essential paediatric palliative care medications should be available in humanitarian crises.
- The child/family relationships should be ensured as much as possible during an emergency, using all appropriate tools.
- Paediatric palliative care staff working in humanitarian settings should be properly supported and protected.

## 7. CARE TOOLS

### Standards

- Standardised tools, when possible, validated for the specific language and culture of the child and the family, should be used in order to assess and measure the needs of children and families; the paediatric palliative care plan must be reconsidered accordingly.
- The development of tools to objectively measure the paediatric palliative care programme's effectiveness should become a priority.

- The tools to assess the needs of the child and family should preferably be based on a multidimensional approach that is culturally adapted.
- The assessment tools and the outcomes of the evaluation should be available to all professionals of the interdisciplinary team.

## 8. EDUCATION AND TRAINING FOR HEALTHCARE PROVIDERS

## Standards

- Paediatric palliative care education must be a core part of all paediatric healthcare professionals.
- Interdisciplinary education should be promoted, with members of different disciplines learning interactively to improve interprofessional collaboration and the well-being of patients.
- Curricula (goals and competence) should be adapted to the three levels of paediatric palliative care provision: the palliative approach by all healthcare providers (1st level); the generalised paediatric palliative care education (2nd level); and the specialised paediatric palliative care education (3rd level).
- Education should provide knowledge, skills and development of attitudes appropriate to the paediatric palliative care principles, as well as the implementation of interprofessional practice and abilities for self-awareness and proactive practice.
- Specialist paediatric palliative care competencies should further include paediatric palliative care advocacy, leading and developing services, policymaking, service evaluation, conduction of paediatric palliative care research and engagement in training and education.
- Every country must develop specific education curricula for all professionals in paediatric palliative care.
- Referral centres and academic institutions for specialist paediatric palliative care education must be identified.

*Source*: Benini, F., Pappadatou, D., Bernada, M., Craig, F., De Zen, L., Downing, J., Drake, R., Friedrichsdorf, S., Garros, D., Giacomelli, L., Lacerda, A., Lazzarin, P., Marceglia, S., Marston, J., Mukaden, M. A., Papa, S., Parravicini, E., Pellegatta, F., Wolfe, J. (2021). International Standards for Pediatric Palliative Care: From IMPaCCT to GO-PPaCS. *Journal of Pain and Symptom Management.* https://doi.org/10.1016/j.jpainsymman.2021.12.031

# Index

Page references in **bold** indicate boxes; page references in *italic* indicate tables or figures, alphabetised by letter.